Equine Lameness

Equine Lameness

Geraint Wyn-Jones
BVSc, DVR, MRCVS
86 Meadowbank
Holyway
Holywell
Clwyd CH8 7EF

BLACKWELL SCIENTIFIC PUBLICATIONS

OXFORD LONDON EDINBURGH

BOSTON PALO ALTO MELBOURNE

© 1988 by
Blackwell Scientific Publications
Editorial offices:
Osney Mead, Oxford 0X2 0EL
  (*Orders*: Tel. 0865-240201)
8 John Street, London WC1N 2ES
23 Ainslie Place, Edinburgh EH3 6AJ
Three Cambridge Center, Suite 208
  Cambridge, Massachusetts 02142
  USA
667 Lytton Avenue, Palo Alto
  California 94301, USA
107 Barry Street, Carlton
  Victoria 3053, Australia

First published 1988

Set by Setrite Typesetters Ltd
Hong Kong

Printed in Great Britain by
Butler & Tanner Ltd, Frome and London

DISTRIBUTORS

USA
  Year Book Medical Publishers
  200 North LaSalle Street
  Chicago, Illinois 60601
  (*Orders:* Tel. 312-726-9733)

Canada
  The C.V. Mosby Company
  5240 Finch Avenue East
  Scarborough, Ontario
  (*Orders:* Tel. 416-298-1588)

Australia
  Blackwell Scientific Publications
  (Australia) Pty Ltd
  107 Barry Street
  Carlton, Victoria 3053
  (*Orders:* Tel. (03) 347-0300)

British Library
Cataloguing in Publication Data

Wyn-Jones, G.
  Equine lameness.
  1. Lameness in horses
  I. Title
  636.1'08967   SF959.L25

  ISBN 0-632-01543-8

Contents

Preface   vii

1   The Diagnosis of the Causes of Lameness   1

2   Radiography   23

3   The Hoof   28

4   Conditions of the Foot and Lower Limb   42

5   Conditions of the Upper Forelimb   104

6   Conditions of the Upper Hind Limb   138

7   Deformities of the Appendicular Skeleton   194

8   Tendon Injuries   224

9   Fracture Fixation Techniques   237

10   Degenerative Joint Disease (Osteoarthritis, Arthritis)   273

References   292

Index   295

Preface

The lame horse has been a perennial veterinary problem since time immemorial, and as we, his masters, manipulate his genetics, distort his evolution, accelerate his development and find stranger and stranger ways of testing his endurance and ability it is likely that it is a problem which will be with us for a long time to come.

New causes of lameness are being discovered constantly but, because of the problems of researchers, lack of funds and the difficulties of using horses as experimental animals, there are too few answers to both the new and the old problems. However, in fairness, there have been enormous advances in the science of equine orthopaedics over the last two decades and therefore time brings with it, as in most medical and veterinary disciplines, an increasing complexity, rather than simplification.

A less tangible obstacle to progress in diagnosis, treatment and prevention of equine lameness lies in the fact that the roots of equine orthopaedics are buried in a morass of magic and mythology and that the potent mix of fact and fantasy still holds a great fascination for many of those who have dealings with 'the noble animal'. To these, the arcane powers of the green salve, or the red blister are infinitely preferable to a logical work-up, a concrete diagnosis and advice on rest and controlled exercise, and the 'character' who can diagnose the cause of a lameness whilst leaning casually over a stable door is far more attractive than those of us who need the help of nerve blocks, flexion tests and X-rays.

The newcomer, whether he be undergraduate or graduate dealing only occasionally with horses, is often daunted at the formidable prospect of entering this world so full of supposedly knowledegable and confident people and sometimes coming into direct confrontation with them.

One of the purposes of this book is to try and counteract this obstacle by encouraging a logical and methodical approach to lameness diagnosis and treatment and by emphasizing that such an approach will provide answers and the right ones: whilst one cannot be a competent diagnostician, etc., without a reasonable knowledge of anatomy, pathology, radiology and surgery, one does not have to have 30 years' experience and ride to hounds in order to 'get it right'.

The book is not intended for the experienced orthopaedic specialist; rather it caters for the undergraduate and those who require a broad base of general knowledge on the subject. It should enable a non-specialist to cope with most situations competently and to know what can be done, and, as importantly, what cannot, in the present state of knowledge. Techniques which are the province of the specialist clinician are attended to though they are not fully described. However, enough information and detail have been provided in the text to enable the clinician to explain and discuss these cases with owners and to present them with those facts necessary to make decisions on the animal's future.

References have been kept to a minimum, however, anyone interested in an individual topic should find an easy entry into the literature through the 'suggested further reading' lists at the end of each section. This is, however, a time of rapid advancement in the subject, new information appears all the time, and there is no substitute for regular reading and generally 'keeping up with the literature'.

It is the author's intention that this book be a compilation of the latest thinking on the various aspects of limb lameness in horses, coupled with a fairly personal view of the subject developed over many years of referral practice in equine orthopaedics. It seeks to encourage a methodical pragmatic approach based on the scientific principles of observation, deduction, factual knowledge and common sense! It is to be hoped that it will go some way to dispel the aura of mysticism which has far too long shrouded the professions dealing with 'the lame horse'.

Geraint Wyn-Jones

1: The Diagnosis of the Causes of Lameness

Introduction

Lameness is a *symptom*; it is *not* a disease in its own right. It is an alteration in the animal's normal stance and/or mode of progression caused by pain or mechanical dysfunction.

These facts must be understood before a clinician can begin the process of diagnosis. Terms and diagnoses such as 'shoulder lameness' or 'back lameness' should be avoided as being nonsensical and every effort made to realize that every lame horse has, as the cause of the gait abnormality, a pathological process, either mild, severe, acute or chronic.

Although in a proportion of cases the onset of lameness is coincidental with obvious trauma, the gait abnormality is frequently the first, and often the only, outward indication of a pathological process within the limb. It is, therefore, a reliable indicator of pathology; horses and ponies do not pretend to be lame nor do they adopt abnormal gaits of their own volition; the animal which is 'unlevel' but not lame is a myth. Another fact which should be realized at the outset is that the gait or stance abnormality is present because, (a) to adopt it eases the pain and, therefore, facilitates progression; or (b) the animal is forced to adopt it because of some mechanical constraints imposed, usually, by chronic (long term) changes within the limb. We have only to look at ourselves when we limp to realize that these are the purposes of the gait change which we call lameness.

The examination

Record everything in writing — this may seem overly careful, but the first experience of trying to recall in a court of law *exactly* what happened 2 years previously is a salutory one, and, on a less dramatic note, a case record of some detail is invaluable at the end of examination to 'bring it all together', and when a case is re-examined months or years later.

A shorthand, to simplify the task, is useful but only abbreviations which are well understood should be used as other clinicians may need access to the information contained in the notes.

Objectives of an examination

The objectives of an examination are:
1 To decide whether the animal is lame.

2 To determine which leg or legs are affected.

3 To determine which portion(s) of the leg are affected.

4 To determine whether a pathological process can be identified.

5 To assess the significance of that pathological process in terms of therapy and prognosis.

The case history or anamnesis

It is a gross, but convenient, simplification that the origins of lameness can be traced to three basic causes: trauma, infection and degeneration; the latter being subdivided into the degeneration of abnormal structures which cannot withstand normal wear and tear, and that of normal structures which fail to stand up to the rigours of abnormal husbandry or a too strenuous lifestyle.

Each cause tends to have a certain pattern of evolution and it is these which one tries to find during the taking of a case history. As a rule of thumb, the lameness due to the pathology of trauma will have a sudden, severe onset, improving subsequently; pain and lameness due to infection will have an imperceptible or sudden, mild onset, increasing rapidly in severity over a few days; and degenerative conditions will show an insidious onset and slow progression in severity. Therefore, it is trends which are significant, and specific dates or occasions, while all important to the owners, are generally irrelevant; the only notable exception might be the relationship of the onset of lameness to shoeing.

Other factors which must be borne in mind are the poor powers of observation of the general public, legendary in police forces worldwide; poor recollection and the desire of clients to tell the clinician what they think he wants to hear. In combination these factors can often produce frankly misleading scenarios. Their effect can be compounded by poor questioning technique; a query such as 'did the lameness start suddenly?' often eliciting a positive reply since most lamenesses are 'suddenly' noticed by the owners or handlers.

A more profitable part of history taking is often that which concentrates on aspects such as performance in the past, aspects which the owners often consider irrelevant. For example, a lameness noticed only some 6 weeks ago may have been undetected for a long period and be responsible for disappointing performance extending back months or even years.

The taking of a good history has long been a concept dear to the heart of the classical clinical teacher. However, the author suggests that, at best, such a history is of limited use in lameness *diagnosis* and at worst can be franky misleading. Its value lies in establishing a trend for the pathological process, which subsequently is of use in establishing an overall picture of the condition, its aetiology and probable pathogenesis.

Case histories should, therefore, be taken but then promptly ignored and the animal examined with a completely open mind.

Detection of lameness

Depending on the nature and severity of the disability, the animal may well show indications even when at rest. Observation of the animal should therefore concentrate, amongst other things, on whether there is any constant inequality or abnormality of stance. A 'normal' horse or pony will not rest or remove weight from either forelimb other than during locomotion. However, it will ease its weight off one or other hind limb by part flexing of the leg and adopting the characteristic pelvic tilt, though neither will be rested preferentially. In general terms, easing of weight from a forelimb either by advancing and extending the limb or by partial flexion indicates some discomfort. As in all matters relating to random movements, constancy is all important; such movements should not be considered significant unless they are repeated constantly.

If the animal is severely lame then observation while it is at rest, coupled with the owner's story, may be all that is needed to indicate which leg is to be examined. Indeed, forcing the animal into a trot under such circumstances may be contraindicated, for example in the case of a fracture, and it could also be regarded as inhumane!

In more nebulous cases an assessment of whether the animal really is lame may be a necessary first step. Many amateur owners, and occasionally even the professionals, will be wrong and convinced of the presence of a lameness which is non-existent. More important however, are those cases which are presented as, say, suspected cardiac or respiratory problems, usually because of a fall-off in performance or a disappointing standard of attainment, which when properly 'worked-up' are found not to suffer from any of these problems, but in fact to be lame. Also the diagnosis of whether a horse is lame is an integral part of 'suitability for purchases' examinations.

The trot is the only gait at which symmetry of stride can be assessed; all other gaits are asymmetric and their interpretation is difficult and confusing. It is the author's preference to examine the animal without tack and trotted in hand. A rider can inadvertently, and occasionally deliberately, mask the gait inequality, and even leading on a bridle can limit the all important head movements. The ideal surface under foot is smooth and non-slip, such as concrete or asphalt and, if at all possible, the animal should not be assessed if it has had its shoes removed within the last week. If this is unavoidable then allowances will have to be made for the possible concussive effects. Animals with flat soles especially can become extremely lame if exercised for any length of time and, of course, this can obscure a pre-existing problem and confuse the interpretation of nerve block results.

The animal is first trotted in a straight line; the trot should be slow and the head movements should not be restricted in any way. The prime objective is to assess, in cases of forelimb lameness, the symmetry of the head carriage, and in cases of hind limb lameness, the symmetry of pelvic movement. These are the easiest parameters to evaluate and the clinician should concentrate on them initially.

Where there is pain in one foreleg the animal will attempt to limit it by reducing the force of impact of that leg on the ground. It does this by keeping its head and neck up during the time that the painful leg is weight bearing, and bringing them down when the pain-free limb is in contact with the ground. This results in a rhythmic up and down movement with the animal 'nodding on the good leg'. The amplitude of the motion is, in crude terms, directly proportional to the degree of lameness. When a hind limb problem is present it would seem that, in most cases, the animal attempts to restrict leg flexion during the forward phase and weight bearing during the backward phase of the stride. This causes the pelvis on the affected side to move in an up-and-down motion, pivoting at the hip of the sound limb. The net effect is that the hip of the painful leg rises and falls when viewed from behind, whilst the hip and pelvis on the sound side appear to remain at the same level. (Video tape evidence indicates that even the sound hip may be somewhat elevated generally to lift the pelvis and increase ground clearance during the forward phase of the painful leg stride.) Contrary to popular opinion this characteristic pattern of movement is seen whatever the cause and site of the pain, so that different causes of lameness cannot be identified simply by watching a horse's gait (May and Wyn-Jones 1987). In mild cases the oscillation of the pelvis may be difficult to see, but it can be made much more obvious by taping white markers to the greater trochanter area on both sides. This renders even a mild asymmetry visible and is a technique which is to be recommended to teachers, novices, clients and even to experienced clinicians in equivocal cases. Another consequence of the disinclination to flex a hind limb is toe dragging or 'trailing'. This can be seen, and usually heard, during the forward phase of the stride and it will also leave its mark as a 'scuffing' on the top of the foot or shoe.

It has long been a feature of classical lameness teaching that observation of head movements is important to hind leg lameness too. This undoubtedly occurs in some instances and is noticeable especially in the more severe cases. The head is dipped as the lame leg and its diagonal come to the weight bearing part of the stride, i.e. the animal nods on the *opposite* side to the lame hind leg. Abolition of the painful focus by local analgesia will in these cases result in an abolition of the head movement. However, a head nod can also indicate a concurrent forelimb problem and the author has experience of many animals, lame in the hind leg, whose head nod has been entirely due to a forelimb problem demonstrable with forelimb nerve blocks.

Having grasped the principle that asymmetry of gait is linked to asymmetry of pain or mechanical dysfunction it then becomes clear that an animal which is bilaterally and symmetrically lame will not show an asymmetry of gait. When forelegs are involved the head carriage remains level, and a similar situation in the hind legs results in no detectable, abnormal pelvic motion. However, where there is a bilateral but unequal lameness then the asymmetry will again be manifest as if the animal were lame on one leg, that is, the one worst affected.

Score systems

In order to have some means of describing the severity of lameness, several score systems have been devised. A commonly used system involves the gradation of the severity of lameness on a scale of 1—10. On this scale 0/10th is not lame and 10/10th is non-weight bearing. Others use a very similar percentage scale. Although open to criticism for its obvious subjectivity it is a simple system essential for recording and communication.

It has to be emphasized that this is only a scale of visible lameness. An animal may be 4/10th lame on its left leg and 6/10th lame on its right, but initially, at the straight trot, it will be seen as only 2/10th lame on its right, i.e. the difference between the two legs. However, should the pain in the right be abolished by nerve block then the 4/10th left lameness will become apparent.

Ancillary aids to the detection of lameness

In the literature much emphasis is laid on the recognition of alteration in the arc of flight of the lame leg. These changes, for example a reduction in the length of the anterior phase of the stride, are said to be characteristic of certain conditions, and there is the implication that failure to recognize them can lead to inaccurate diagnosis of the cause of the lameness. Experience indicates that these alterations, which undoubtedly occur, can be difficult to recognize even when the animal is moving at a slow trot. It is often possible to say that there is something wrong with the movement of the leg or legs but it is far more difficult to say exactly what! Overdiagnosis here is a mistake, but it is a diagnostic sin often committed, usually as a means of impressing clients or colleagues.

Most painful stimuli and mechanical dysfunctions lead to a reduced freedom of movement of the limbs and this stilted action is recognizable as an entity and given such names as a 'proppy', 'footy' or 'pottery' gait. What must be realized is that these gait abnormalities, frequently and unfortunately elevated into conditions in their own right, are simply general manifestations of lameness and are symptoms of underlying pathology. Their recognition is important, especially in cases where superficially there may only be indications of a problem in one leg but where a bilateral 'stiffness of gait' betrays the involvement of more than one limb. Also important are the highly individual but comparatively rare gait alterations produced by such conditions as 'fibrous myopathy' of the semimembranosus and semitendinosus muscles, or stringhalt.

Lunging

Lunging is an invaluable aid in the detection of lameness. In most horses a lameness on the inside leg will be made more noticeable simply because the animal is forced to lean inwards and therefore, (a) puts more weight on the inside leg, and (b) the trunk/ground distance is shortened on that side, necessitating increased flexion of the limbs to clear the ground in the forward phase of the stride. In a small percentage of animals lame in the forelegs, lunging will exacerbate the lameness in the outer leg. Why this occurs is not clear, though it is a plausible theory that it is due to weight bearing stress in the distal limb articulations whilst they are held in the partially flexed state necessary to achieve the extra length required of that 'outside' leg.

Animals should be lunged without tack on *hard*, even ground. Although this causes many raised eyebrows amongst the horsey fraternity it is by far the best means of exacerbating and establishing the levels of lameness. If an area free from metal grids or pot holes is chosen, the risk of slipping is very small, and of injury even less. The concussion-reducing properties of soft ground and especially tan-chip arenas will often cancel out the exacerbating effects of lunging, although there is a suggestion that lameness due to soft-tissue injuries will be rendered more noticeable on soft ground or sand pits. Ideally one should use both! If it can be avoided then a bridle should not be used; rather a lunging cavesson should be substituted for a head collar where an unruly horse is to be examined. If an animal proves difficult to lunge in the conventional manner then 'leading it out' is often the solution. This entails a second person running outside the lunging circle leading the horse or pony on a lead rope. The clinician should, if possible, be on the outside of the circle, since it is difficult to evaluate the gait while actually doing the lunging. Decreasing the radius of the circle will increase the stress on the legs and lunging on a tight circle should be part of every suitability of purchase examination. It is also important to remember that, when evaluating an animal's response to nerve blocks, it should be lunged on the same diameter circle each time.

Flexion and extension tests

Flexion and extension tests are procedures in which joints or joint complexes are stressed and the animal then evaluated for the appearance, or an exacerbation, of lameness in that leg. When using these tests it is important to realize that there are very definite limits to their specificity. It is virtually impossible to stress a single articulation without also stressing other structures through attached ligaments and tendons. In the hind leg the problem is even greater because of the unavoidable action of the 'reciprocal' apparatus which does not allow flexion of, say, the hock, without concurrent flexion of every other hind limb articulation. Other difficulties arise over the amount of stress to be applied; the animal's response varying greatly depending on the vigour and duration of the flexion and extension. As a general rule the same person should carry out all the tests on a patient and for the same time period to ensure a reasonable degree of constancy. Other problems arise over interpretation of the results: firstly, the degree of lameness produced will vary enormously. In my view, only the production of a readily discernible gait abnormality, persisting well after the animal has settled into a steady trot, is of significance. A four-stage grading of response from negative to +++ is the most accurate that can be hoped for and, although again extremely subjective, is valuable for recording and communicating results. Secondly, the significance of a positive result is open to argument. Having seen, in many instances, flexion tests give very misleading information, I believe that they should only be used to produce or exacerbate lameness. Their prime use is, therefore, to convince the clinician and, no less, the owner that a horse has problems in a particular leg, and to elevate the severity of a mild lameness to the point where it can be evaluated with regional or intra-articular anaesthesia.

Although the principles outlined above can be applied to most articulations, only four variations are used commonly.

Distal interphalangeal (DIP) joint extension. DIP joint extension is traditionally used exclusively in the evaluation of suspect navicular disease. A piece of wood, about 2–3 cm thick, (traditionally a hammer handle), is placed beneath the toe of the hoof under examination and the animal made to bear weight on the leg; after 30 seconds to a minute the animal is trotted off. There is no doubt that animals suffering from navicular disease will be rendered more lame by this technique, but it would be naive to think that this was the only disease entity which would be rendered more painful — laminitis, diseases of the extensor process of the 3rd phalanx, even solar sepsis are some of the conditions which could react positively.

Fetlock flexion. Fetlock flexion is used in both fore and hind legs. A consideration of the anatomy shows that this is likely to elicit a more specific response from the fore fetlocks and a positive result should be an indication of problems in or around that joint. The situation in the hind leg is more complex. Firstly, the mechanics of performing a simple fetlock flexion, without exerting stress on the hock, are difficult and it is a frequent observation that very positive fetlock flexion tests can be elicited in cases subsequently proven to be tarsal osteoarthritis or 'spavin'. Positive hind leg fetlock flexion tests should not, therefore, be taken to indicate fetlock problems until the fetlock has been anaesthetized and the positive response abolished.

Hock flexion. Hock flexion *cannot* be achieved without flexion of all the other joints of the limb. In an attempt to reduce the stress on the fetlock the leg should be grasped at mid-cannon. However, it is difficult to support the weight of a limb (and occasionally the horse too) with such a grip. Inevitably the leg must be grasped just above the fetlock joint and inevitably some stress will be imparted to it via this pressure and by passive flexion. In addition, forced hock flexion results in forced flexion of both stifle and hip, reducing the specificity even further.

Full hind limb flexion. There is no doubt that full limb flexion will often elicit a lameness when separate hock and fetlock flexion tests do not. It is therefore the most efficient way of showing up an incipient or subclinical problem, or of exacerbating a mild one to the level where it can be seen and worked-up with nerve blocks. In fact, such is the non-specificity of the other flexion tests that there is a strong case for saying that they are superfluous and that only full flexion is necessary followed by diagnostic regional anaesthesia.

Physical examination

When the affected legs have been identified by the previous examination the next step is to use hands, eyes, ears and even nose to detect the presence of pathology. Alterations in shape, swellings, pain on pressure or manipulation, restriction in movement, crepitus and heat are all factors which may identify a problem site. However, in any discussion on the identification of the abnormal, one is forced as a prelude to resort to such cliches as 'a knowledge of normal is a prerequisite to the recognition of the abnormal'; and 'normal', of course, applies to such diverse factors as basic anatomy, range of movement in a joint, temperature of feet, etc.

Fortunately, in the equine limb we are dealing with a bilaterally symmetrical structure and a check on the normal can usually be quickly and conveniently carried out on the opposite leg. Beware, though, of the possible presence of bilaterally symmetrical pathology and, if in doubt, one should have no qualms about making comparisons with other animals.

A physical examination of a leg should be carried out slowly and methodically whilst trying to appreciate what structures are being palpated. One should not palpate a 'fetlock joint', rather one should feel the sesamoid bones individually, appreciate the degree of distension of the palmar pouch and sesamoidean sheath, palpate the insertion of the suspensory or interosseus ligament, etc. Only by resorting to a conscious effort each time can one be sure that major abnormalities will not be missed and that minor ones stand a good chance of being discovered. Also, constant, conscientious repetition builds up a store of personal knowledge of what is or is not normal and what is or is not significant, i.e. that oft-maligned attribute — *experience*!

In general terms it is in the acute or recent onset lameness that clinical examination is likely to reveal findings of significance; here pain, heat and swelling will be at their most detectable stage. In chronic, long term problems, acute pathology, it if were ever present, has subsided and the source of pain is usually detectable only by regional anaesthesia.

In any clinical assessment, but in particular a lameness examination, the clinician is often reliant upon subjective impressions. These impressions may be coloured by many factors: inexperience, complacency, owner pressure, ambient temperature, bigotry, etc. These factors must be borne in mind at all levels of clinical expertise and care taken to neutralize their effects. Reliance on a constancy of reaction, little or no weight given to equivocal findings, a methodical approach, logical thought and a healthy scepticism towards that which cannot be proven are excellent qualities in an orthopaedic clinician.

Hoof testers

As with many other aids to diagnosis, the results of an examination with hoof testers or pincers must be treated with caution and over-interpretation avoided. Animals vary greatly in their response to pressure applied to the hoof and it is therefore important to check the reaction on at least one normal foot, and to keep the pressure level constant. Excessive compression of hoof structures, such as that exerted by large, long-handled pincers applied enthusiastically, will make even the most stoic and normal of horses flinch. Only moderate pressure should be applied and only *repeatable* vigorous reactions considered significant; equivocal reactions should be ignored as being difficult to interpret and often misleading.

These factors therefore render this device of little value in the assessment of chronic, poorly localized pain and limit its value to the detection and/or localization of more substantially painful foci such as in the case of solar sepsis or pedal bone wing fractures. Hammers, the handle of a hoof knife, even hands, can make an effective substitute for purpose built hoof testers since it is the principle which is important, not the instrument.

Diagnostic nerve blocks

The clinical examination described thus far may well have identified the lame limb or limbs, and may even have suggested the region of interest within the limb; rarely, though, will it have positively identified the pain source. In many instances, too, there will be no indication whatsoever as to which part of this metre-and-a-half long appendage is causing the problem. The success of nerve blocks lies in the fact that the horse does not malinger; if its leg hurts; it is lame; if it does not, it is not lame. It is a quality which is to be appreciated as it is a considerable compensation for the animal not being able to tell one where it hurts. Nerve blocks themselves do not seem to affect the animal's gait in any way and, done correctly, carry little or no risk. Intra-articular anaesthesia obviously must be undertaken only when routine aseptic precautions have been taken. Provided these are practised, the frequently met paranoia about intra-articular infection is unjustified.

As good technique, and for medico-legal reasons should the unlikely happen, always clip the site of injection and wash with antiseptic soap and spirit. Always use a *new* syringe and needle for each injection, and always a *new* bottle or vial of local anaesthetic for each examination. For intra-articular injections extend the precautions by preparing a larger site and, ideally, wearing sterile, surgical gloves.

For routine nerve blocking, the needle should be small enough to minimize discomfort to the horse yet of sufficient bore to allow rapid injection: 25 × 0.7 mm (22 g × 1″) is ideal. Also, the minimum size of syringe for the volume to be injected allows a faster injection and is less clumsy to handle.

Always have adequate restraint of the animal and in this regard the owner's wishes must be secondary. It is often a good plan to allay fears by explaining carefully beforehand why nerve blocks are necessary and why restraint is essential to prevent damage to horse, handler, or veterinary surgeon (though not necessarily in that order). A twitch and a leg-up are all that is usually necessary.

In the UK it is common practice to hold up the leg which is not being injected but in America and European countries the clinician will usually raise the leg which is being blocked. This latter course is only feasible where the preponderance of horses are well trained and well-behaved, i.e. most certainly not the UK. Sedation of an intractable animal is not feasible since the level required to allow blocking will most certainly affect the gait also.

Injection technique is important; the needle puncture should be quickly executed without the syringe being attached and with probing or stabbing at the site to be avoided at all costs. This is helped by assessing the point of insertion carefully and gauging the direction of insertion to allow for the fact that the site of deposition of the local may be up to one inch from the site of skin penetration. Redirection is occasionally necessary, if for example, the needle enters a vessel, but the redirection should be done not by bending the needle, but by partial withdrawal and swift repenetration.

Bleeding from the puncture site is common as most major nerves run in company with large vessels, but should be minimized with pressure; and it is also good practice and public relations to wash off the bulk of the skin soiling. It is similarly good practice to apply a firm pressure bandage for 24 hours following multiple blocks, as quite substantial subcutaneous reaction and swelling can occur, even with the cleanest technique.

Following injection, the extent of the denervation must be checked prior to evaluation of lameness. Whilst only an approximate guide, skin desensitization is the only means available. Blocks which are supposed to be highly selective, such as the palmar digital nerve block should be checked early (5 minutes) since spread of local anaesthetic solution to influence other nerve branches will confuse, and render inaccurate, any inferences drawn from the consequences of that block. A sharp-blunt instrument, such as a ball-point pen tip or a straightened paper clip, makes an ideal tester, producing adequate stimulation and yet no blood!

Local anaesthetic agent

Local anaesthetic agents act at the nodes of Ranvier, increasing the permeability of the cell membrane to Na^+ and preventing depolarization of the nerve. Two drugs are commonly used

1 Lignocaine hydrochloride BP (lidocaine hydrochloride INN) used as a 2% or preferably 3% solution. It should be used with added adrenaline (epinephrine) to ensure persistence at the site. Effective anaesthesia without adrenaline is approximately 30 minutes; with adrenaline it is approximately 60 minutes.

2 Mepivacaine (Carbocaine — Winthrope Laboratories). Produces minimal reaction. Effective anaesthesia is 1½–2 hours.

When only a single diagnostic block is to be done, the duration of anaesthesia is immaterial. However, when multiple sequential blocks are necessary the duration of desensitization becomes critical and only those agents which have a long action should be used.

Regional blocks of the forelimb

Palmar digital nerve block (PDNB)

A PDNB anaesthetizes the navicular bone, navicular bursa, lateral cartilage and variable amounts of palmar or plantar hoof, depending on the level of injection. To obtain maximum specificity, inject as distally as possible. The ideal site is at the level of, and medial to, the lateral cartilages. The needle should be directed distally, dorsally (forwards) about 40° to the vertical, and slightly towards the mid-line (Figs. 1.1, 1.2 and 1.3). Two millilitres is the maximum amount to be injected

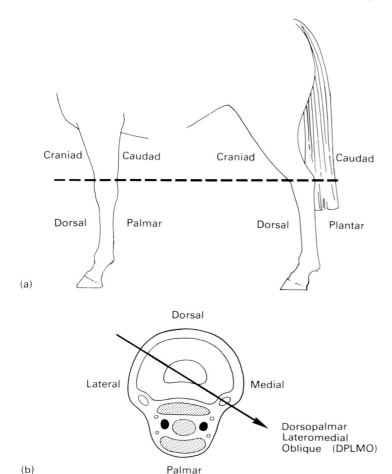

Fig. 1.1 Diagrams illustrating the directional nomenclature used in this book.

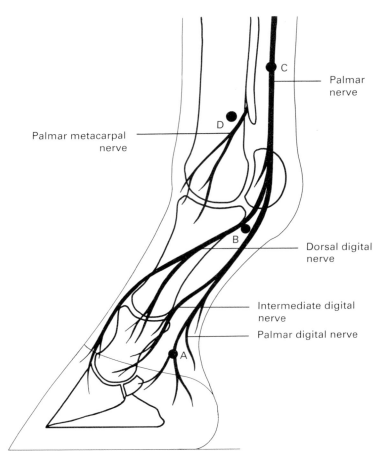

Fig. 1.2 Schematic representation of the distribution of nerves in the distal forelimb. A, B, C and D mark the sites for palmar digital, abaxial sesamoid, palmar and palmar metacarpal nerve blocks respectively.

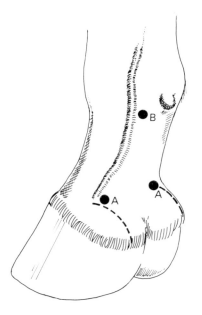

Fig. 1.3 A marks the site of injection for a PDNB and B for an ASNB. The dotted line represents the palpable proximal border of the lateral cartilage.

and the block should be tested by skin pricking within 5 minutes. At this time only the skin between the lateral cartilages should have been desensitized: left longer, the level of cutaneous anaesthesia will 'creep' forwards and, although there is no absolute relationship between the area of skin affected and the anaesthesia of the deeper regions, there is inevitably a loss of confidence in the specificity of the technique.

Abaxial sesamoid nerve block (ASNB)

The bifurcation of palmar nerve into dorsal and palmar digital branches is at a variable level, though mostly at about mid-sesamoid. It is tempting to inject at that level since the branches are travelling together. However, retrograde, proximal flow of the local up the fascial planes surrounding the nerve trunks can result in much of the lateral and medial fetlock being anaesthetized too. For maximum specificity inject at point B (Figs. 1.2 and 1.3) below the base of sesamoid bone. Insert the needle palmar to the large vessels which are palpable in this region and direct it subcutaneously forwards and slightly downwards at about 20° to the horizontal.

Inject 2−3 ml of local as the inch long needle is withdrawn. In this way the effects of the anaesthesia will be limited to the desired area.

Palmar block

The medial and lateral palmar nerves are distal continuations of the median and ulnar nerves respectively. They are joined in mid-cannon region by a communicating branch which crosses the palmar surface of the superficial flexor tendon (SFT) subcutaneously, where it can be palpated. *NB* the lateral palmar nerve runs in the groove between the suspensory ligament and deep flexor tendon (DFT) but the medial palmar nerve runs in the groove between the DFT and the SFT. The nerves should be blocked some 6 cm (2½″) proximal to the sesamoid bones using about 3 ml of local anaesthetic each side (Fig. 1.2).

The palmar block will anaesthetize all the area covered by the ASNB, also the palmar 50% of the fetlock joint though excluding the proximal 25% of the sesamoids and the proximal palmar pouch of the fetlock joint capsule.

To anaesthetize the dorsal 50% of the metacarpal phalangeal articulation it is necessary, in addition to the palmar block to block the palmar metacarpal nerves as they emerge from under the distal end of the splint bones, the so-called 'four-point block' (Fig. 1.4). The needle is inserted just proximal and dorsal to the 'button' at the end of the splint and directed distally to lie against the bone; 2 ml of local are injected as the needle is withdrawn. When this block is checked it must be remembered that the skin over the dorso-medial aspect of the fetlock is innervated by the terminal fibres of the medial cutaneous antebrachial nerve, and will probably still be sensitive.

For most conditions of the fetlock, the four-point block provides sufficient relief from pain to enable a diagnosis to be made. However, residual lameness may persist due to the innervation of the proximal sesamoids and palmar pouch by branches of the palmar metacarpal nerves not affected by local injected at the sites described above. These branches, and the palmar metacarpal nerves, run distally, protected by the splint bone abaxially and the suspensory ligaments, to which it sends branches, axially. These nerves may be blocked by a single infiltration where they originate in the sub-carpal area.

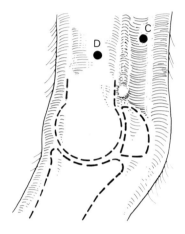

Fig. 1.4 C marks the site of injection for anaesthesia of the lateral palmar nerve. D marks the site of injection for a palmar metacarpal block. Anaesthesia of these nerves on both sides of the leg makes up the 'four-point block'.

Sub-carpal block

Both the lateral and medial palmar metacarpal nerves originate from the ulnar, or at this level, the lateral palmar nerve just distal to the distal border of the accessory carpal bone. Practically, it can be difficult to locate the palmar nerve in this area and best results are obtained by laying down a barrier of anaesthetic agent. The needle is inserted some 1 cm distal to the accessory carpal bone and approximately 6−8 ml of local is distributed into the area (Fig. 1.5). Desensitization of the skin on the lateral aspect of the metacarpus is a reasonable indication of a successful block.

The median and ulnar blocks

The entire carpal area and lower leg can be anaesthetized with these two blocks. However, they have little practical use in the diagnosis

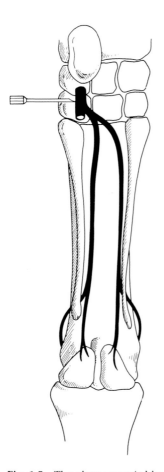

Fig. 1.5 The ulnar nerve is blocked just distal to the accessory carpal bone, thus ensuring that both palmar metacarpal nerves are fully anaesthetized.

of lameness. From the carpus proximally, intra-bursal or intra-articular anaesthesia is of far greater value.

The median nerve is blocked on the caudal aspect of the radius and cranial to the muscular portion of the flexor carpi radialis muscle. The 3.75 cm (1½″) needle is inserted through skin and fascia about 5 cm (2″) distal to the elbow joint. Ten to twenty millilitres of local should be injected to cover a wide area as the nerve, though large, has a slightly variable course.

The ulnar nerve is most accessible about 10 cm (4″) proximal to the accessory carpal bone. The needle is inserted in the groove between the flexor carpi ulnaris and ulnaris lateralis muscles and 10−20 ml of anaesthetic solution are deposited at depths varying from 1−2.5 cm (½−1″).

Regional blocks of the hind limb

The plantar digital and the abaxial sesamoid blocks are performed as in the forefoot. However, the dorsal fetlock receives a significant innervation from the lateral and medial *dorsal* metatarsal nerves. Therefore, to achieve full anaesthesia of the dorsal 50% of the fetlock it is necessary to carry out a virtual 'ring' block some 10 cm (4″) proximal to the joint, in addition to the four-point block as described for the forefeet. For most routine examinations however, a four-point block is usually adequate. For suspected lesions on the dorsum of the foot, the additional ring block may be necessary.

Tibial and peroneal blocks

As in the forelimb, the higher blocks have limited practical application, though they have been advocated in the diagnosis of hock conditions following the elimination of distal digit problems by preliminary four-point blocks.

The tibial nerve is often palpable as a flat, pencil-sized structure just cranial to the Achilles tendon. This is best done with the weight off the leg and by pinching over the tendon with thumb and fore-finger. With a fine needle, place a skin 'bleb' of local anaesthetic about 10 cm (4″) proximal to the point of the hock and over the nerve. Then, infiltrate about 20 ml of local around the nerve through a longer, wider bore needle.

The superficial and deep peroneal nerves are usually blocked in conjuction with the tibial nerve. Locate the groove between the lateral and long digital extensors on the lateral aspect of the leg. Place a skin bleb over the groove some 10 cm (4″) proximal to the level of the point of the hock. A 5 cm (2″), wide bore (18 g) needle is inserted to the hilt at this point and 15−20 ml of local anaesthetic solution is infiltrated into a large volume of tissue by frequent redirection of the needle. This is necessary as there are no further landmarks to aid location of this deeply situated and variably positioned deep peroneal nerve. The superficial peroneal is also variable in position and as the needle is retracted, a further 10−15 ml of local is injected at depths of 0.7−2.5 cm (¼−½″) to ensure anaesthesia of this branch.

If the nerves are completely anaesthetized, the occasional animal will show extensor weakness which may confuse a lameness evaluation, especially in relation to 'toe dragging'.

As a general rule the hock and joints proximal to it are best investigated with intra-articular anaesthesia.

Intrabursal and intra-articular anaesthesia

Intrabursal and intra-articular anaesthesia are much more specific means of detecting painful foci than the regional blocks. They may be used in two ways: firstly, as a supplement to regional anaesthesia, when the latter has indicated an area of interest, and secondly, as a first diagnostic line where clinical findings indicate strongly that a synovial structure is involved.

In the past, clinicians have been reluctant to inject into joints and bursae, principally because of the risk of infection. However, if adequate sterile precautions are taken, with careful preparation of the site and a 'no touch' technique, where the skin at the point of entry is not touched after its preparation, and only new needles, etc. are used, the risks are very small. As with regional blocks, a new bottle or vial of local anaesthetic solution should be used for each case. Mepivacaine is the ideal solution because of its low irritability; however, 2 or 3% lignocaine hydrochloride is used routinely by many workers without causing problems. It is good technique initially to insert a skin bleb at the site of injection. This allows painless redirection of the needle and enables a larger bore to be used. Insertion of the second needle should be done without the syringe attached and then redirected until synovial fluid flows. Only then can one be sure that the local will be within the synovial compartment and the results of the block valid. Adding contrast medium to the local anaesthetic solution, followed by radiography, will achieve the same ends but more tediously.

Whilst the creation of the initial skin bleb is easier when the leg is weight bearing and the contralateral leg raised, the insertion of the wide bore needle is often helped by raising the affected leg, this having the effect of relaxing the joint or bursal walls. However, this will also reduce intra-articular pressure and occasionally synovial fluid will not emerge from the needle. Gentle manipulation sometimes helps but a return to weight bearing to increase intra-articular pressure must be done only when it is certain that joint surfaces, etc. will not trap the needle or be damaged by it.

Over-distension of joints should be avoided, and ideally an equivalent amount of synovial fluid should be removed prior to injection of a volume of local. An alternative technique which works well is to inject the local and allow intra-articular pressure, helped by aspiration, to remove an equal amount of synovial fluid/local mixture. The plunger is depressed several times to ensure thorough irrigation of the articulation with the local anaesthetic solution. This latter technique is useful in the smaller 'tight' synovial structures such as the navicular bursa.

The interpretation of the results of intrasynovial blocks is not difficult, provided it is certain that the local has entered the joint and it is recognized that only intra-articular structures will be anaesthetized. Problems of interpretation can also arise in cases of joint trauma, for example, where fibrous joint capsule or collateral ligaments are damaged and painful; in these animals improvement in lameness may be minimal despite intra-articular damage.

Techniques

Navicular bursal block

The navicular bursal block can be done in the standing, unsedated animal. The site of injection is immediately proximal to the coronary band in the mid-line of the heels, and this area should be thoroughly prepared. Inject 1−2 ml of local as a skin bleb with the affected leg down and weight bearing. Continuing to apply restraint, lift the affected leg and insert a needle, minimum length 6 cm (2½″), immediately proximal to the skin horn junction. The direction of insertion should be exactly sagittal and, in the vertical plane, on a line half way between the horizontal and the line of the coronary band. The bevel of the needle should be uppermost. Insert the needle until bone is struck. Synovial fluid may or may not emerge. Weight bearing should not be allowed, as the needle tip may damage important structures as the anatomical relationships change. Any difficulty depressing the syringe plunger indicates that the needle tip is not in the bursa. If synovial fluid has not emerged then overdistension of the bursa *must* be avoided by using the irrigation technique.

Where bursal pathology exists, the effects of the block are dramatic, improvement being detectable literally within 1−2 minutes after injection. It is also an extremely specific block, useful in cases of dispute.

Distal interphalangeal (DIP) ('coffin') joint block (Fig. 1.6a)

First, insert a skin bleb in the dorsal mid-line some 1.5 cm (½″) proximal to the coronary band with the leg weight bearing. Insert a 6 cm × 1 mm (2½″ × 18 g) needle 1 cm (½″) proximal to the coronary band, advance it through the thick extensor tendon and, keeping the needle shaft almost vertical, on until bone is struck. Usually synovial fluid flows immediately; if not, redirect the needle by 'walking it' along the dorsal surface of the 2nd phalanx until it falls into the dorsal synovial pouch. If the bevel of the needle is uppermost (caudal), it is less likely to damage articular cartilage at the dorsodistal edge of the 2nd phalanx. This technique may also be performed with the leg raised, advanced, and with the foot placed on the operator's knee.

Proximal interphalangeal (PIP) (pastern) joint block (Fig. 1.6b)

The skin and subcutis is anaesthetized with a skin bleb placed exactly in the dorsal mid-line some 2 cm (¾″) proximal to the line of the joint. The minimum of anaesthetic solution is used to avoid anaesthesia of larger branches of the dorsal digital nerves, which would, of course,

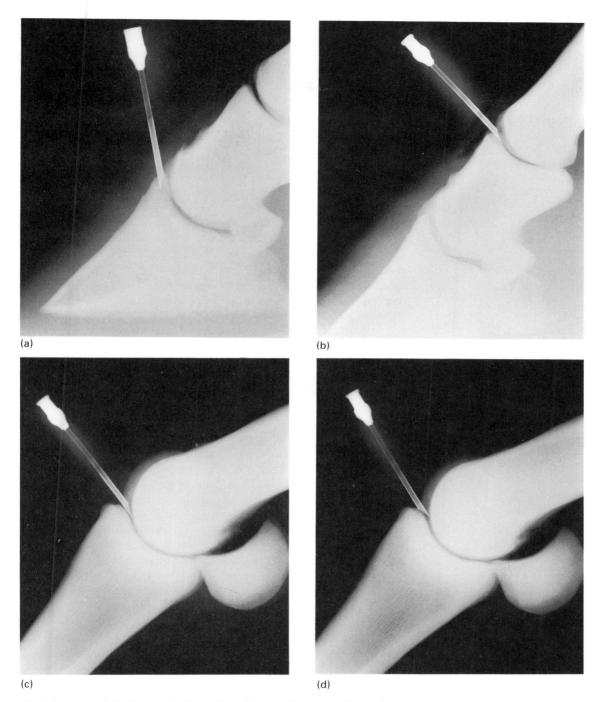

Fig. 1.6 a, b, c, d. Radiographic illustration of the position of needles in the DIP, PIP and MCP articulations. Fig. 1.6d shows how inserting the needle bevel downwards can result in damage to cartilage. (Cadaver specimens and large bore needles were used for clarity.)

17

ruin the specificity of the block. The longer needle is then advanced through the skin 1 cm (½″) proximal to the joint, (that is, slightly distal to the bleb) in the mid-line, through the extensor tendon and onto bone. With the shaft of the needle held about 45° to the vertical, its point is walked distally until it falls into the dorsal joint space when synovial fluid will emerge and may be collected for analysis.

The metacarpophalangeal (MCP) (fetlock) joint block
(Figs. 1.6c and d)

Two techniques are routinely used for fetlock joint blocks and the choice is really one of personal preference. The more conventional one aims to inject into the dorsal palmar or plantar pouch. Following the placement of a superficial skin bleb, a 4 cm × 1 mm (1½ × 18 g) needle is directed axially from a point just proximal and dorsal to the proximal tip of the sesamoid bone, so that its point comes to lie in the mid-line just palmar to distal cannon and in the dorsal palmar pouch. Occasionally, much haemorrhage is encountered using this technique and villonodular synovitis lesions in the pouch may preclude a free flow of synovial fluid.

The author finds a more satisfactory technique to be injection into the dorsal pouch. This can be done with the leg weight bearing or raised, extended and placed on the operator's knee. Because of the central articular eminence of the distal cannon bone, the needle must be inserted to one side of the mid-line and especially so if the semi-flexed position is chosen. A skin bleb is inserted whilst the leg is weight bearing and a 4 cm × 1 mm (1½″ × 18 g) needle is introduced with the shaft held at about 30° to the vertical, so that as it is advanced its tip strikes the intra-articular portion of the dorsoproximal margin of the 1st phalanx. The bevel of the needle should be inner-most so that the point does not damage the articular cartilage of the cannon. Ten to 12 ml of local anaesthetic solution can be injected into this comparatively spacious joint without causing problems. Sometimes synovial fluid will not flow when the needle enters the joint. If it is reasonably certain that the joint has been entered a test injection can be made when there will be virtually no resistance to the flow of local anaesthetic.

Carpal blocks

The carpus has three main articulations though only the proximal two contribute to the flexion of the joint complex; the carpometacarpal joint is immobile. The proximal radiocarpal joint has, in the majority of animals, its own intact synovial sac, whilst the intercarpal and carpometacarpal sacs communicate between the 3rd and 4th carpal bones. These synovial sacs penetrate in between the individual carpal bones and/or between the interosseous ligaments. All three sacs share a common fibrous capsule, over the dorsal surface of which course the three main ancillary synovial structures, the tendon sheaths of extensor carpi radialis, common digital extensor and abductor digiti I longus (extensor carpi obliquus).

Injection of both sacs is best done from the dorsal aspect and slightly medial to the mid-line to avoid the tendon sheaths. The line of the articulations and tendon sheaths are usually easily palpated in the absence of swelling, and individual joint distension makes identification even simpler. However, periarticular swelling can mask anatomical detail and if periarticular infection is suspected the technique should be abandoned for fear of introducing infection into the joint. Five to 10 ml of local anaesthetic solution, depending on the size of the animal, can be introduced into both the proximal and distal joint complexes without causing problems of overdistension.

Humeroradial (elbow) joint block

This is an extremely difficut joint to penetrate consistently, unless it is significantly distended. The joint should be flexed several times so that the position of the articular line can be determined. Following adequate aseptic preparation and the creation of a skin bleb a needle is inserted at a shallow angle to the skin so that its shaft is a tangent to the joint line. When it strikes bone, 10−15 ml of local anaesthetic solution can be injected. Alternatively a long needle can be used in an attempt to enter the caudal pouch of the flexed joint proximal to the anconeal process.

Scapulohumeral (shoulder) joint block

This is a block which can be done with relative ease in the standing animal. Following adequate aseptic preparation and the creation of a skin bleb, a long (6 cm × 1.2 mm) needle is inserted into the notch between the processes of the lateral tuberosity of the humerus. The caudal process can easily be clearly palpated so that the needle is passed cranial to this and then directed slightly upwards and caudally on to the articular surface.

Ten to 15 ml of local anaesthetic solution can be injected into this articulation.

The hock articulation

Tarso-crural (tibiotarsal) joint block

This joint capsule is voluminous, making penetration a relatively simple matter. Where the capsule is not distended, the best site is on the dorsal surface of the joint, medial to the medial condyle of the talus and extensor tendons, and lateral to the prominent saphenous vein. Here a depression can be palpated and it is at the centre of this that, after suitable skin preparation, the 5 cm × 1.2 mm needle should be inserted horizontally and in a dorsoplantar direction. Distension of the tibiotarsal joint capsule simplifies matters even further, the site of injection bulging dorsally as it is relatively unsupported by periarticular structures. Fifteen to 20 ml of local anaesthetic solution may be injected to anaesthetize this articulation, and the proximal intertarsal joint with which it is in communication dorsally and distally.

Distal intertarsal (DIT) and tarsometatarsal (TMT) joint blocks

Local anaesthesia of these joints is advocated as part of the diagnostic work up of a suspected tarsal osteoarthritis (bone or occult spavin). Injection at the conventional sites, i.e. on the dorsomedial and medial aspects of the joints is doomed to a high failure rate, because of the close fit of the margins of the joints, the tightness of the fibrous joint capsule and the absence of accurate external landmarks. Moreover the combined thickness of the articular cartilage is usually less than that of a 25 g needle. Sack and Orsini (1981) suggest that the TMT joint be injected from the lateroplantar surface between metatarsus 4 and the 4th tarsal bone by advancing a 2.5 cm (1″) needle in nearly a sagittal plane and directing it dorsodistally (Fig. 1.7). Four or 5 ml of local anaesthetic solution may then be injected.

In a proportion of horses (approximately 8%) there is communication between the TMT and DIT joints negating the block's specificity to a certain extent. The DIT is usually anaesthetized in concert with the DMT joint but it is a difficult block to achieve consistently. The method suggested by Sack and Orsini (1981) again seems to be the most reliable: they advise injecting the DIT joint through the gap between tarsal bones 1 and 2, the 3rd tarsal and the central tarsal bones on the medial side (Fig. 1.7) by placing a 2.5 cm (1″) needle as far proximally in the gap as possible and advancing it not quite to the hub so that its tip remains within the joint. If the gap is not palpable they suggest laying a straight edge between the palpable distal tubercle of the talus to the palpable space between metatarsus 2 and 3. In the extended hock the needle is then inserted where this line is intersected by the palpable distal border of the cunean tendon, and directed caudolaterally.

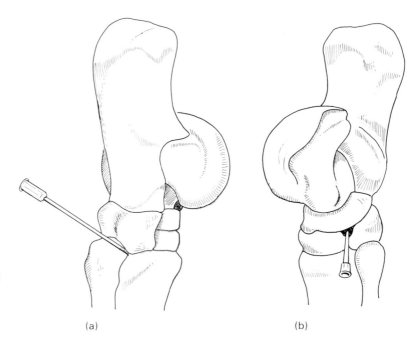

Fig. 1.7 A lateral (a) and medial (b) view of an equine hock showing the position of needles for anaesthetizing the tarsometatarsal and distal intertarsal joints respectively.

(a)   (b)

When DIT and TMT joints were injected with latex (Sack and Orsini 1981), the compound was invariably found at dissection to have permeated dorsally to involve the tendons of peroneus tertius, tibialis cranialis and the long digital extensor muscle, and to come close to the medial and lateral dorsal metatarsal nerves which innervate dorsal fetlock and digit upto and including the coronary band. Local anaesthetic solution is likely to do likewise and, therefore, the effects of injection into these joints cannot be regarded as being purely intra-articular.

Cunean bursal lesions are also implicated in the pathogenesis of tarsal osteoarthritis (spavin). Anaesthesia of this structure is achieved by sliding a 2.5 cm (1″) needle proximally under the palpable cunean tendon on the medial aspect of the hock and injecting 5–10 ml of local anaesthetic solution.

Summary of DIT and TMT joint blocks

Diagnostic regional local anaesthesia of the hock region is of somewhat limited value. The techniques are often difficult and even when they are performed successfully, they lack the specificity to allow precise clinical judgements to be made. Intra-articular anaesthesia, however, is a much more precise tool and is the technique of choice for most suspect hock conditions. Fortunately, the two most frequently needed blocks, the tarsocrural and the TMT are relatively simple to do and give clear, unequivocal results.

The stifle

The equine stifle in reality consists of two joints, the femoropatellar and the femorotibial articulations. Its joint capsule is capacious and has three basic compartments, the femoropatellar and the medial and lateral femorotibial sacs. The femoropatellar and medial femorotibial sacs almost always communicate through a slit-like aperture which is usually covered by a synovial membrane flap, occasionally occluding it: about 20% of horses have a similar connection between the femoropatellar and lateral femorotibial sacs. Therefore, unless distension of the sacs allows the presence or absence of these intercommunications to be detected, when local anaesthetic solution is injected into one compartment it cannot be assumed that it has not permeated the whole stifle. Statistically, however, to anaesthetize the entire complex, one must inject the femoropatellar and lateral femorotibial sacs.

Despite their large size and voluminous synovial sacs, the compartments of the stifle are not easy to inject. The classical texts describe penetration between the straight patellar ligaments as being the approach of choice to the individual femorotibial articulations but the author has, as yet, found no consistently reliable technique and considerable probing and redirection is often needed. Injection into the femoropatellar, and hence the medial femorotibial sac is often easiest through a cranial approach, the needle being angled caudally and proximally into the patella/trochlea space which can be widened by having the leg in extension and by grasping the patellar firmly and elevating it off the femur. If the medial femorotibial pouch is to be anaesthetized with this technique one must allow permeation from one compartment to another; this can be encouraged with light exercise. Injection of the lateral femorotibial compartment is much more difficult but fortunately is very rarely required.

Coxofemoral (hip) joint

Injection into the coxofemoral joint is feasible; it requires a 15 cm (6") needle which should be directed axially and ventrally from the only landmark available, the greater trochanter. The needle should ideally be walked up the neck of the femur until the joint is entered; much redirection and luck is needed.

Suggested further reading

Derksen FJ (1980) Diagnostic local anaesthesia of the equine front limb. *Equine Practice* **2**(1), 41–7.

Dyson S (1986) Problems with the interpretation of the results of regional and intra-articular anaesthesia in the horse. *Vet Rec* **118**, 419–22.

Nyrop KA, Coffman JR, DeBowes RM, Booth LC, (1983) The role of diagnostic nerve blocks in the equine lameness examination. *Compendium cont Ed* **5**(12), 5669–76.

Sack WO (1975) Nerve distribution in the metacarpus and front digit of the horse. *JAVMA* **167**(4), 298–305.

Sack WO and Orsini BS (1981) Distal intertarsal and tarsometatarsal joints in the horse: communication and injection sites. *JAVMA* **179**(4), 355–9.

2: Radiography

It is a myth, which needs to be dispelled, that high quality radiographs cannot be taken under practice conditions. Adherence to some basic rules should result in consistently good and useful films. On the other hand, even high quality radiographs will not provide all the answers on their own and radiography and radiology must be recognized as being only part of a complete work-up.

Equipment

The generator

The generator is usually a practice fixture and therefore immutable: given the choice, it should be based on compromise between a high power output, enabling short exposure times to be used, and mobility and portability. With the advent of ultrasensitive, rare earth screens and an increasing use of radiography in equine practice, high output has become less critical and ease of use and ruggedness have assumed greater importance. As important in some ways is the acquisition of a good light beam diaphragm (LBD): careful alignment of beam direction is a feature of successful diagnostic radiography and this, along with limitation of beam size for safety and economy, is only achievable with an LBD.

Ancillary equipment

Although much attention is paid to the choice of generator, principally because of the capital outlay involved, it is rare to find a similar degree of care displayed in the choice of the other equipment used in radiography. These items are often relegated to the level of accessories, yet they are as important, if not more so, than the generator. It is reassuring to know that if your generator will produce X-ray photons, good ancillary equipment and techniques will enable you to take good radiographs!

Grids

Grids are *not* necessary for most radiogrpahic examinations of the equine limb, where bone provides good inherent contrast and tissue thicknesses are such as to produce little 'scatter'. Where grids are used they cause little or no improvement in film contrast and counter any benefits by (a) requiring a much greater exposure intensity, reflected usually in a longer exposure time, (b) obscuring fine detail by virtue of their linear construction, and (c) requiring accurate alignment with the main beam especially if they are of the 'focused' variety. This is usually difficult to achieve in the hurly-burly of practical equine radiography.

The only exceptions would be the dorso-palmar views of the navicular bone, grossly swollen carpi or hocks and the largest draught breeds, in all of which tissue thickness will produce noticeable scatter necessitating the use of a grid.

The choice of a grid, which is an expensive item, requires some thought. There are many factors to be considered and a compromise to be struck between the grid's efficiency in removing scattered radiation and the inevitable increase in exposure factors, degree of alignment needed, and, not least cost, associated with such improved efficiency.

Some terms used in description of grids are

1 Grid ratio. The ratio of the height of the lead strips to the width of the gaps between them. It is a measure of the grid's efficiency in absorbing scattered radiation. The higher the ratio number, the more efficient the grid.

2 Lines per inch or cm. The greater the number of lines per inch or cm, and the closer together they are, the more efficient the grid becomes.

3 Grid factor. This is the factor by which, if the grid is used, the exposure (mAS) will have to be increased to produce the same density (blackness) of film as when the grid was not used. It rises with grid ratio and with the number of 'lines per inch, or cm'.

4 Parallel and focused grids. In parallel grids all the lead strips are vertical. Focused grids have their lead slats symmetrically inclined towards a point of a specified distance from the grid centre, i.e. they are focused at a specific distance and *must* be used at that distance from the tube *anode* or target (not the front of the tube or LBD). They *must* always be accurately centred on the main beam centres and their plane of symmetry *must* be at right angles to the central part of the main beam. It is virtually impossible to use a focused grid properly without a LBD. Parallel grids are more forgiving in their needs, but are correspondingly less efficient.

The choice of a grid is, therefore, a complex matter and individual requiremens should be discussed with an experienced radiologist.

Cassettes

Cassettes have a tough life in large animal practice; accordingly they should be checked often for damage which could lead to light leaks or the poor screen/film contact. They should be handled gently and never placed under a horse's foot without the protection of a wooden bridge. The newer, synthetic plastic types are more resistant to wear and tear but should still be handled carefully to prolong their life.

Screens

Traditionally the veterinary radiographer has opted for fast screen/film combinations to minimize the all important exposure time. However, speed is always 'traded off' against sharpness, since faster speeds are associated with larger grain size and hence graininess of image. The use of fine-grain screens with their increased inherent contrast characteristics and absence of discernible granularity improves definition enormously and the increased exposure they require is offset completely by the abolition of the grid as a factor. If rare earth, fine-grain screens are used, substantially lower exposure factors can be used than with the conventional variety and, of course, the rare earth screen's affinity with higher photon energies (higher 'KVs'), without losing contrast, can also be used to reduce mAS and therefore exposure time.

In summary, fine-grain screens used with conventional film will give the best possible definition in equine distal limb radiography; rare earth, fine-grain screen/film combinations give almost as good a result but with a much reduced exposure. These combinations can be used for all techniques to above carpus and hock and for the thinner portions of the upper limbs such as olecranon or patella.

Screens should be kept clean by *regular* gentle washing with mild detergents and warm water, wiping clean and being allowed to dry open in a dust-free environment.

Films

Non-screen films have been superceded by fine-grain screen/film combinations and have no real place in routine examination of the limb. One technique has been described where simultaneous images of navicular bone and pedal bone can be obtained by placing a non-screen film envelope above the grid and cassette when carrying out the dorsopalmar navicular projection. They can be useful for intra-oral examination of the horse and other species. Non-screen films are developed for the same times as conventional films but require double the 'fixing' time.

Rare earth screens emit green light as opposed to the blue of conventional ones, and special film is required to absorb this emission. Rare earth type films and conventional ones should be kept separately and it must be remembered that if rare earth films are introduced, new appropriate safe lights must be obtained too.

A recent development in film emulsion technology is a restructuring of the halide grains giving them a much greater light catching capacity. These films are faster than their conventional counterparts with no diminution in definition.

Processing

Surveys consistently show that most film faults are caused during processing. An X-ray film is a piece of high technology: treated well by being stored, handled and processed properly it will give consistently good results. Its requirements are few and simple. Film boxes should be stored upright, not piled one on top of another, and in a cool, dry climate; films should be handled gently with dry hands and they should be processed in *fresh* chemicals, at the *correct* temperatures for the *correct* time under the *correct* safelight.

Dish developing is undoubtedly best in practice conditions were throughput is low. Large, hospital type tanks require a lot of chemicals, take a long time to reach the required temperatures, or, if left on permanently without proper replenishment, result in rapid oxidization of developer and other chemical changes which greatly impair film quality.

Where the economics justify, then small automatic processors are the most satisfactory solutions to processing problems, though even these devices require careful maintenance.

Viewing

After processing, viewing is the most neglected aspect of radiography. Use a proper viewing box with tubes of the correct intensity and colour values. View in near-darkness and mask the area of viewing base not covered by the film: this is not a counsel of perfection; it makes a dramatic difference! Use a bright light viewer, or simply a small desk lamp to illuminate the darker areas, and reveal detail obscured by relative over-exposure. Where detail is rendered unclear by poor inherent contrast, e.g. navicular bone invaginations, the situation can sometimes be improved by rotating the film to an angle of 45° to the viewing box; this increases the film emulsion thickness as seen by the observer resulting in enhanced contrast.

Techniques

Examination of individual areas will be mentioned in association with specific conditions. There are, however, general principles which apply to all examinations.

1 Standardize as much as possible — there are enough unpredictable variables as it is! Keep the tube/film distance constant; use the same screen/film combinations; record all exposures, a legal necessity now anyway; select the exposure values giving the best results and use them consistently.

2 Be versatile, do not be hidebound by what the textbook says. 'Shoot for the lesion'.

3 Use the LBD to 'cone down to the area of interest', do not unnecessarily expose large areas of tissue: this improves quality of films; improves radiation safety and is economical in that with appropriate 'coning' at least four views of a fetlock, etc. can be had on one 20 × 34 cm piece of film.

4 Be critical! do not accept poor quality; there is always a reason for it and usually a simple remedy. If in doubt ask someone who *knows*.

Suggested further reading

Clayton-Jones DC and Webbon PM (1979) Observations on the technical quality of radiographs submitted to a veterinary college. *Vet Rec* **104**, 576–8.

Equine Veterinary Journal, Commissioned Articles *Interpreting Radiographs* 1983 **15**(4) and 1984, **16**(1, 2, 3 and 5).

Jeffcott LB and Kold SE (1982) Radiographic examination of the equine stifle. *Eq Vet J* **14**(1), 25–30.

May SA, Wyn-Jones G and Peremans KY (1986) Importance of oblique views in radiography of the equine limb. *Eq Vet J* **18**(1), 7–13.

Shively MJ and Smallwood JE (1980) Radiographic and xeroradiographic anatomy of the equine tarsus. *Equine Pract* **2**(4), 19–34.

Smallwood JE and Shively MJ (1979) Radiographic and xeroradiographic anatomy of the equine carpus. *Equine Pract* **1**(1), 22–8.

3: The Hoof

Hoof horn

Horn is produced by the stratum germinativum of a much modified epidermis. The underlying dermis or corium is formed into multiple papillae at the coronary band and on the solar surface of the digit so that the epidermis, which closely follows its contours, produces rods of horn; these quickly lose their centres to become cylinders or tubules of highly keratinized cells pointing downwards and forwards. They are bound together by unstructured horn produced by the inter-papillary epidermis to form the wall and sole of the hoof. Damage to the coronary band, or any other part of the horn-producing structures, can result in temporary or permanent discontinuity in the horny integument.

The coronary band has a second, more superficial, component called the perioplic layer. The perioplic horn produced by it is softer and more flexible; it extends down over the wall horn for a variable distance in the adult and in the caudal aspect of the foot it forms almost the entire thickness of the soft expandable heel bulbs. Its function is said to be prevention of water loss from the wall and to increase the flexibility of the heel region.

The sloping walls of the pedal bone are covered by a corium which is thrown up into approximately 600 primary lamellae running radially from the coronary band. These are bound to the pedal bone by a much modified, highly vascular periosteum. The lamellar corium produces horn which blends and bonds with the tubular horn growing down from the coronary band. This lamellar horn is unstructured, unpigmented and together with horn tubules formed from papillae at the distal end of the laminae, forms the 'white line'. The interdigitations of the lamellae, each of which has about 100 secondary components, allows for an enormous area of bonding between the horny hoof and the tissues deep to it.

At the skin—horn junction, a too abrupt transition between the soft tissue of skin, etc. and the relatively unyielding hoof is prevented by an encircling, fibroelastic transitional layer called the coronary cushion.

The sole is also formed of horn tubules produced by a papillar solar corium. Its ground surface is concave, mirroring the concavity of the solar surface of the pedal bone, and its curvature is greater in the hind feet. It maintains its thickness by exfoliating in flakes. Caudally it blends with the complex frog structures which are also formed of horn tubules though these are sinuous, not straight, less keratinized and have a greater water content, all of which confers a much greater elasticity. The function of the frog has long been the subject of debate. It is the author's belief that its complex, bellows-like structure is simply a device for permitting expansion and contraction of the heels; if the sole were to be flat all over, such movement would not be possible.

Growth of wall horn is uniform at about 7 mm (¼") per month all round the coronary band; making the youngest horn at the bearing surface that of the heel. A hoof therefore takes 9–12 months to grow out. The rate of growth is slowed down by cold weather and accelerated by warmth. The wall is substantially thicker at the toe, diminishing gradually towards the heel; its average inclination to the ground at the dorsum of the forefoot should be 50° with the hind being slightly more vertical at 55°.

The ergot is commonly regarded as the vestige of the hooves of the 2nd and 4th digits while the chestnut is a remnant of the 1st: the latter is absent in the hind legs of donkeys.

Conditions of the hoof

Abonormalities of growth and wear

Overgrowth

In the natural state growth and wear are finely balanced. Overgrowth occurs when wear is reduced; in unshod animals this happens when conditions underfoot are soft and/or exercise is limited. Shoes also prevent wear over most of the bearing surface except at the heels where differential movement occurs between shoe and horn. The shod hoof has, therefore, a tendency to grow long in the toe.

Resistance of horn to wear and its hardness are governed by several factors, principally the degree of hydration; dry horn is harder than moist horn (the only rational use for a bran poultice is as a means of hydrating a rock-hard hoof to allow easier paring).

An overgrown foot should be pared in the following sequence. Firstly, the sole is cut back to the correct shape and thickness; the shape should be slightly concave and the thickness can be judged with thumb pressure; if any discernible depression can be caused by firm downward pressure then the remaining sole is some 7–8 mm (¼") thick or less. When the sole is at its correct thickness, the second step is to trim the wall to shape using pincers, keeping the plane of cut parallel with the ground and bearing in mind that all weight should be borne on the walls and on no more than 7–8 mm (¼") of the solar margin. During shaping of the wall, frequent sighting along the dorsopalmar direction is needed to ensure symmetry. If the toe is 'turned up' great care should be exercised in removing the surplus: the two steps of the above sequence should be followed and the remaining excess can be carefully trimmed away or rasped. If the distortion is great the correction must be done gradually over several months and may never be completely achieved.

The frog is the last to be trimmed. Contrary to popular opinion there are no drastic consequences to cutting the 'sacred' frog: being rubbery in texture it is difficult to cut and a sharp knife is essential. Its shape should be restored and sufficient depth should be left so that it just comes into contact with the ground. On a shod horse this depth can be correspondingly greater.

Overwear

This rarely occurs over a whole hoof unless unshod animals are used excessively on hard ground. It can occur over part of a hoof if a painful condition or conformational abnormality causes the animal to bear a greater proportion of weight on one side of the foot. Identification of the cause of the foot misplacement is obviously the important initial stage in correction. Removal of a painful focus will allow the animal to place the foot normally though it must be remembered that if a significant inequality of wear has taken place then self-correction is not possible, and corrective trimming will have to be undertaken.

Horn quality varies greatly in response to such factors as climatic conditions, diet, disease and environment. Although much research has been carried out in pigs and cattle, little has been done in the horse and this area of veterinary medicine abounds with myth and folklore. Many 'experts' and owners have their own special remedies, and fashions in treatment come and go: all that can be said for most is that they do little harm, even if they do little good! Most of the superficially more rational treatments are based on supplementation of diet with amino acids. Powdered milk has been advocated (60−120 g/day) for its lysine content; methionine at 10 g/day for its action in forming the basic disulphide bond of horn and, more recently, the vitamin biotin.

Methionine has a theoretical role to play in horn formation and is advocated in the treatment of laminitis to promote new horn growth. Biotin has an established pedigree, especially in pigs, as a factor in producing good quality horn, and evidence has been produced to show that it exerts a beneficial effect on weak flaking equine horn (Comben *et al* 1984). According to the authors its effect is not confined to new horn, even existing horn somehow showing an improvement.

Hoof oils

Many commercial brands are available, with endless varieties of 'home brews'. Most have a turpentine base with the addition of various oils (fish, neatsfoot, etc.) tars and waxes. Popular opinion is that these oils moisten the hoof and keep it supple, however, the true action is somewhat different; the oils, in fact, provide a waterproof coating retaining moisture within the hoof, and, of course, excluding it too. Oils are therefore contraindicated in hard, dry brittle hooves unless they are adequately soaked in water prior to being oiled. Hosing or standing in water is a much more rational treatment for this condition, along with regular routine hoof trimming to remove flaking horn, and dietary supplementation with amino acids, etc. Recently, new synthetic coating materials have appeared on the market, some claiming to strengthen the hoof wall and act as a replacement for the periopic layer. If used rationally, these products could have a place in foot care procedures. However, they should not be regarded as a panacea for all the ills that befall the equine hoof.

Hoof cracks (sand cracks, grass cracks)

Whatever names are given to them, cracks fall into two categories (a) the crack which starts at the coronary band and eventually grows down to extend along the whole length of the wall (Fig. 3.1a) and (b) the crack which begins lower down in the wall and extends distally to the bearing surface of the hoof (Fig. 3.1b). The first category is due to a fault, either congenital or acquired, in the coronary band epidermis which leads to a failure in the production of horn tubules or their bonding. The second category is probably due to imperfect bonding which fails at a certain level of imposed strain causing the crack to remain at the same level despite the fact that the horn is growing down around it.

Many horses have cracks which give no trouble since they do not penetrate the deeper layers of the wall. Occasionally some factor, e.g. increased stress or keratophilic organisms extend the breach to the sensitive structures below; infection then becomes established leading to pain and lameness. The area is very sensitive to pressure and tapping with a hoof knife elicits a constant response. Later, coronary band swelling, separation of horn from the coronary band and exudation occur. Initial treatment is with antibiotics, with radical local treatment indicated if, as is likely, antibiotic therapy alone fails to effect a complete cure. Removal of wall horn is indicated in most cases of sepsis of the sensitive laminae and is the *only* consistently effective treatment for hoof cracks. *It is wise to explain the rationale of drainage and debridement to the owner before embarking on surgery; also to warn of the long convalescent period.*

Technique

Removal of wall horn can be done under local nerve block but general anaesthesia is preferable in anything other than the most tractable animal.

Centering on the crack, or a probe placed into the infected track, cut away a 1 cm wide strip of horn. An oscillating plaster saw is ideal but a hoof knife will suffice, especially if the hoof has been hydrated and softened by the application of a bran poultice for 24 hours.

In the case of laminar sepsis the full thickness of wall should be removed to expose the whole length of the infected track; it is likely that separation will have occurred at the coronary band but care must be taken here to avoid damage to the horn-forming tissues. In long standing cases underrunning of horn can be extensive and septic pedal osteitis may be present. All underrun horn and necrotic tissue, including pedal bone, *must* be removed. Stabilize the free edges of the horn wall by drilling a hole through the wall thickness and fashioning a wire loop (Fig. 3.2) (thick coat-hanger wire is ideal). Apply a firm

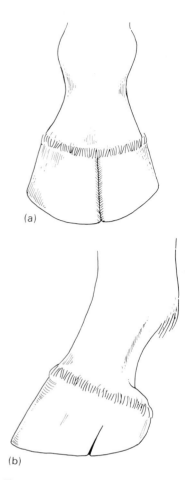

(a)

(b)

Fig. 3.1 Horn cracks. (a) A full length horn crack extending from the coronary band down to the bearing surface. (b) A quarter crack. These probably occur at this site because it is the region where the flexible, expansile heel gives way to the thicker more rigid toe horn. Also, it is the approximate site of the most caudal shoe nail. Dorsal to the hoof will be rendered more rigid by being nailed to the shoe.

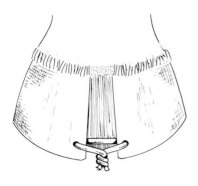

Fig. 3.2 A full thickness horn defect can be given a degree of temporary stability by being wired together like this. The wire should not be tightened excessively!

pressure bandage and start appropriate antibiotic therapy. As healing occurs, the wound will dry and become relatively pain-free: persistence of moisture and pain indicate residual infection which *must* be treated by further removal of tissue.

At about 2 weeks post-surgery the first new horn is detectable and this increases in thickness with time. Not until there is a solid layer of dry, pain-free horn in the base of the wound should filling of the defect be considered.

In the case of a hoof crack, the whole wall thickness need not be removed, only sufficient to ablate the fissure line. If the crack extends to the coronary band then the horn strip around it must be similarly removed up to the coronary band. Since no sensitive soft tissue has been exposed the horn defect created can be filled immediately. If, inadvertently, blood is drawn, then filling *must* wait until the wound has a thick horn covering.

Filling technique

All the fillers used are epoxy or polyester resin-based. All have good gap filling properties but relatively poor adhesion to horn. Technovit (Kulzer) is probably the best and it has a very rapid setting time. The margins of the cleft should first be underrun to create a reverse wedge effect, the two edges must be bound together using either staples or wire lacing, see Figs.3.3a and b. Staples can be mae from discarded Steinman pins and obviously have shallow points. Degrease the horn using acetone then apply the filler and rasp to shape.

The filler plug eventually grows down and is removed during hoof trimming. A shoe with quarter-clips each side of the defect will provide additional stability and should allow the animal to work normally.

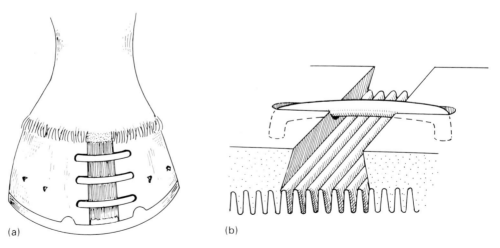

(a)   (b)

Fig. 3.3 (a) Staples bridging the two sides of a horn defect preparatory to filling it with a filler paste. Additional stability is given by the shoe which has clips at each side of the breach. (b) A close up view of how the horn is shaped, providing a reverse wedge shape to hold in the filler paste. The staple can also be seen recessed into the horn so as not to stand proud of the filler.

Thrush

Thrush is an infection of horn and horn-forming tissues. It results in separation of the horn of the frog and adjacent sole from the underlying corium which can become thickened and produce abnormal soft, cheesy horn. An abundant foul smelling exudate is also present.

Causes

Thrush invariably occurs in animals in dirty, wet underfoot conditions. Poor hoof care and maintenance predispose to the development of the infection. Fungi and anaerobes have been implicated as the main instigating organisms, but virtually any bacterium can be isolated from an established case.

Diagnosis

Diagnosis is often initially by smell or the discovery of horn flaps or exudate in the frog clefts. There is usually a history of poor husbandry or wet conditions underfoot.

Treatment

Treatment may not always be successful in advanced cases. Antibiotics alone will *not* effect a cure; most broad spectrum antibiotics have been used, but anecdotal evidence suggests that the antibacterial metranidazole can be more effective than most. Radical local treatment is necessary and should be directed towards removing *all* underrun horn and cutting back diseased and abnormal horn to expose the corium. Following initial bandaging to control haemorrhage the author has used several treatments ranging from astringents such as $CuSO_4$, 5% formalin foot baths and, most effectively, applying a shoe which has two bars welded to the bearing surface so as to raise the foot some 2–3 cm clear of the ground. Provided the animal is not on soft, wet bedding, this allows aeration of the frog and sole and frequent cleaning with a hosepipe jet. Regular re-examination is necessary with any suspect tissue being removed. *Treating a case of thrush can be a long and expensive job* with some cases being totally refractory.

Solar penetrations

Penetrations of the sole and frog by sharp objects are relatively common occurrences. The outcome of such trauma can vary from the trivial to the very serious and can culminate in the destruction of the animal. An appreciation of the likely sequelae to penetration of each part of the foot is vital both for decisions about therapy and the all-important prognosis. Four factors are crucial — *site, direction, depth* and *duration* of penetration. If the penetrating foreign body is metallic then ideally it should be radiographed *in situ*. Two projections at 90° to each other are essential to position the object within the hoof. Failing this, the depth and direction of penetration should be assessed

(a)   (b)

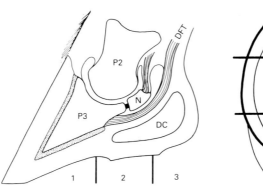
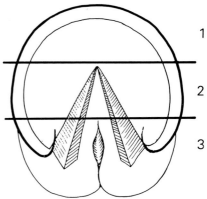

Fig. 3.4 (a) Mid-sagittal section of an equine hoof showing the three zones of penetration. P2 = second phalanx; P3 = third phalanx or pedal bone; N = navicular bone; DFT = deep flexor tendon; DC = digital cushion. (b) Solar view of hoof showing the three zones.

and some idea gained of where the tip of the penetrating object 'ended up' within the foot.

The foot can be roughly divided into three zones (Figs. 3.4a and b). Penetrations in the dorsal or anterior zone come up against corium and pedal bone; infection is trapped between corium and horn and a build-up of pus pressure causes separation of these two structures

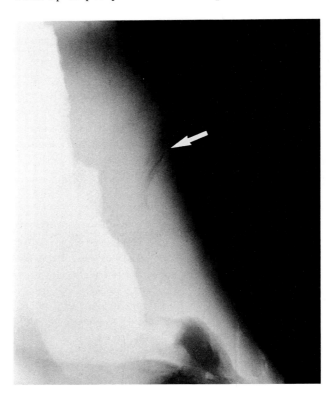

Fig. 3.5 Radiograph of a lateral hoof showing the thin air lucency (arrowed) which marks the separation of horn from underlying coronary band. Note too the solar lucency caused by paring the sole at the site of penetration.

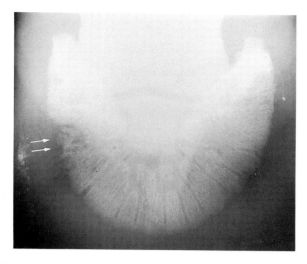

Fig. 3.6a Early osteopenia (lysis) of the bone in septic pedal osteitis (arrowed). An overlying lucency is caused by superficial horn paring. Some mineralized material (dirt) is seen abaxial to the lesion.

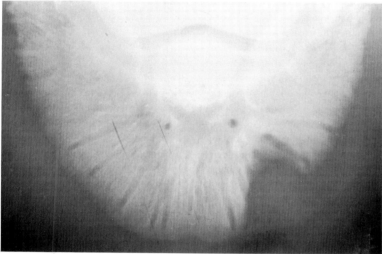

Fig. 3.6b A more well established case with much focal osteopenia.

and, as time goes on, increasingly large areas of underrunning. Occasionally infection 'turns the corner' and runs up the laminae to the coronary band (Fig. 3.5), and in some cases a septic pedal osteitis develops with osteopenia and sequestration of bone fragments (Figs. 3.6a and b). Long-standing cases should be radiographed and care taken not to confuse the 'crena' with an area of osteopenia (see pedal bone section, p. 42).

Treatment should consist of following the penetration track down to the horn–corium separation and the removal of *all* underrun horn. Most recurrences of infection are due to inadequate initial treatment; even a small amount of underrunning can act as the focus for further extension of the infective process and horn should be pared away until the horn and corium are contiguous. The removal of horn should extend up the wall if necessary. If a portion of the pedal bone is infected, it too must be removed; this is a simple task and can be done with a hoof knife or currette. Healthy pedal bone cannot be cut with either and the technique is simply to pare away necrotic tissue until solid, 'grating' bone is felt under the knife blade.

This type of work is far better done under a general anaesthetic if at all possible and following the application of a tourniquet.

Penetrations in zone 2 are potentially lethal. Whilst implantation of infection at the corium–horn junction will have the same consequences as elsewhere, deeper penetration is not blocked by the pedal bone but will probably affect the deep flexor tendon and, maybe the navicular bursa. Forcible penetration can even fracture the navicular bone or lead to direct contamination of the coffin joint (Fig. 3.7).

Prognosis in these cases is vital and ideally radiography should be used before the nail, etc. is removed. Alternatively a probe can be directed up the track, should this be patent. In the absence of radiography the likely position of the nail or probe point should be gauged by measurement of the depth and angle of penetration.

Early cases of deep zone 2 punctures may respond to intensive broad spectrum antibiotic therapy, but often the response is temporary — foreign material is usually implanted with the nail, etc. and acts as a nidus for infection. However, such treatment is worthwhile even if the chances of recovery are slim. Flushing of the track has been recommended though it is likely to achieve little apart from pushing contamination deeper into the tissues. Irrigation of the navicular bursa is feasible using the same technique as for bursal anaesthesia; it may help in early cases of confirmed intrabursal contamination but is unlikely to achieve anything in established infection.

The development of a severe 8–10/10th lameness over a period of a few days, following a puncture of this nature is a very poor prognostic sign. If the initial vigorous antibiotic therapy has failed then chances of subsequent successful treatment is virtually nil and early euthanasia must be considered. It is wise to warn owners at the outset of the likely consequences of this type of injury: most have

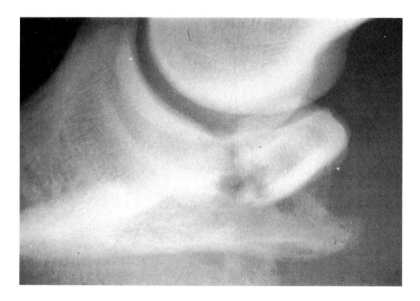

Fig. 3.7 Lateromedial projection of a foot showing a fracture of the distal horizontal border of the navicular bone. This horse had stepped on a nail seven days prior to the radiographic examination. There is also evidence of focal osteopenia (lysis) in the region of the fracture suggesting that infection has become established. The animal was 10/10th lame and was euthanased.

understandable difficulty in appreciating how a small nail prick can lead to the death of their horse or pony or how impotent the clinician is in this situation. A little time spent on explanations at the outset is time well spent!

Deep penetration of zone 3 can have widely differing sequelae depending on depth and site of puncture. Shallow penetration will have the same relatively trivial consequences as in zone 1 or 2. Deeply implanted infection in the central region often gives rise to abscessation of the digital fibroelastic cushion. Pain and swelling of the heel bulbs are the usual consequences and the animal will be reluctant to bear weight on the heel. This can lead to confusion between heel abscessation and an infectious navicular bursitis. The former usually has less severe symptoms and usually responds to antibiotic therapy, in that the degree of lameness improves as the infection is 'walled off' and persists at a lower level subsequently.

If the abscess is large it may discharge externally in the region of the heel, if not then its location can often be found by probing under local anaesthesia with a wide bore needle. If constant suction is applied to the needle through an attached syringe then pus will flow as soon as the needle penetrates the capsule. Aspiration on its own is rarely sufficient; a more consistently successful way is to establish drainage by cutting along the aspiration needle left *in situ*, entering the abscess cavity, preferably in two places and passing a seton through the drain hole. (A seton is a loop of bandage which maintains the patency of drainage tracks and promotes the formation of granulation tissue.) Daily irrigation of the abscess cavity along with systemic antibiotic therapy should result in rapid healing.

Deep penetration of zone 3 abaxially can result in trauma and infection of the lateral cartilages, the so-called 'quittor'.

Quittor

Quittor is infection and necrosis of the lateral cartilage of the pedal bone (see pedal bone section, p. 42). Classically this condition occurred in draught horses and it was said to be caused when the outer foot stepped on the heel of the inner as the animal was turned sharply at the end of a furrow. The protruding cartilage was traumatized and possibly skin damage occurred leading to the access of infection. Cartilage is avascular and when traumatized or infected is not protected by the normal body defences. It therefore provides a centre for a chronic, grumbling infection which leads to initial swelling, fibrous reaction and later discharging sinuses in the abaxial heel region above the coronary band.

The classical aetiology for quittor is supported by the high percentage of draught horses or large crossbreds amongst the sufferers. However, it does occur in the more nimble thoroughbreds and ponies suggesting a different route for entry of infection. This concept is reinforced by the large number of cases which are found on surgical exploration to have tracks extending down to the abaxial frog, sole and wall region of zone 3.

The condition is characterized by a very chronic and low grade

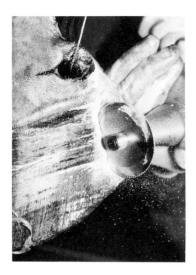

Fig. 3.8 An oscillating saw is being used to cut away a section of hoof wall to obtain access to infected tissues in this case of quittor. A probe is seen within the original sinus track above the coronary band.

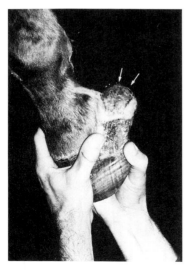

Fig. 3.9 An old wire cut has caused damage to the coronary band and heel region in this pony. A granuloma (arrowed) has forced the wound edges apart causing significant distortion.

course and as such it may be that the initial penetration is regarded as a trivial solar penetration and no association made between it and the development of a discharging sinus above the coronary band months later. Indeed the initial trauma is almost never recognized or recalled by the owners.

It presents initially as a firm, variably painful swelling in the region of the lateral cartilage or adjacent coronary band associated with an unpredictable degree of lameness. The formation of a sinus track is usually only a matter of time, it coincides with a reduction in the lameness level and leads to a modification of the diagnosis of quittor from provisional to firm.

Quittor is refractory to conservative antibiotic therapy. Prolonged courses may sometimes lead to a remission with a drying of the discharge and healing of the sinus. However, a recurrence is inevitable and unless anticipated can be extremely disappointing and discouraging. The reason for the recurrrence is that infected and necrotic cartilage forms a nucleus for infection and a centre of foreign body reaction which must be physically removed before healing can occur.

The surgical technique advocated in the literature involves incising over the lateral cartilage and literally 'scraping out' the infected tissue with a special 'quittor knife'. However, the lack of precision and dependant drainage dooms it to a high failure rate.

In contrast, surgical extirpation of all the infected and necrotic material through a lateral approach following removal of a section of hoof wall (Fig. 3.8) has a high success rate even in advanced and extensive cases. General anaesthesia and the application of an Esmarch's bandage are essential as is a radical attitude. Infected tissue and cartilage, recognizable by its colour, varying from purple through dull red to muddy yellow, and its glistening pulpy texture, must be cut or curretted away no matter how extensive it might be. It is often necessary to cut or even remove sections of coronary band to expose the tissue and similarly sections of normal cartilage may have to be removed to get at tracks which lie deep to it. Healing is by second intention and is slow: re-operation is often necessary to excise secondary tracks or slits in the granulation tissue and cut back the latter if it becomes exuberant. Eventually horn grows from reformed corium, though it is somewhat amorphous and requires constant attention to prevent fissuring. Differential movement between the two sides of the horn breach can delay healing indefinitely. This is best prevented by severely cutting back the wall caudal to the breach so that it bears no weight. A full shoe, nailed well back will maintain the stability of the foot in the meantime.

Occasionally complete healing seems to occur only to be followed some weeks later by the development of another sinus track. It is as well to warn owners of this possibility in advance, it avoids acute disappointment on their part and not a little embarrassment to the clinician.

Traumatic heel wounds

Wire and sheet metal cuts to the heels are common injuries: they often look apalling but most respond to relatively simple management. Suturing is, in general, contraindicated because of the inevitable initial contamination and the extreme difficulties in keeping such wounds clean subsequently; also the degree of post-trauma swelling is such that most of the sutures will probably tear out. Partial suturing of the extreme proximal commissure of the wound can be indicated if the laceration extends up the pastern, but drainage is all-important and the surgeon should resist the temptation to close the last few distal inches. Instead the wound should be debrided, cleansed thoroughly and tightly pressure bandaged.

If these wounds are left untreated or not adequately bandaged, granulation tissue forces the cut edges apart and distorts the heel (Fig. 3.9). At this stage pressure bandages alone are not sufficient and the wedge of granulation tissue must be excised so that the two sides of the wound can be reasonably apposed. This procedure may have to be repeated once or twice and skin grafting should be considered to hasten healing. Using this technique, severe, long-standing wounds with significant distortion of the heel can be made to heal with only minimal distortion. Cartilage damage is likely with this type of wound and delayed healing or the development of sinus tracks should be viewed with concern as they may indicate the development of a quittor-like lesion.

'Corns'

The downwards and forwards growth of the wall horn inexorably moves the shoe in a similar direction in relation to a fixed point on the foot. This causes the incurving heels of the shoe to be pulled forward off the wall and to make contact with the sole in the angle of the heel (Figs. 3.10a and b). Infrequent shoeing and poorly fitting shoes contribute greatly to the problem. The trauma to the solar corium results in haemorrhage and the production of poor quality horn, or no horn at all over the affected area. The condition is painful and causes lameness.

The alteration in horn quality leads to an increased susceptibility to trauma, fissuring, cracking and bacterial assault. If infection then penetrates, the corium separates from the overlying horn and pus is produced.

Diagnosis

The animal will present with a lameness of variable severity, possibly involving more than one foot. Badly fitting shoes or shoes seated far forward should arouse suspicion and, of course, the lameness will block out with a palmar digital nerve block (PDNB). Shoe removal may reveal no obvious lesion, the discoloured horn only coming to light with exploratory paring. In other animals discoloured horn, fissured and appearing moist, may be evident.

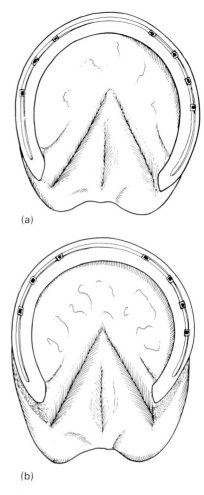

(a)

(b)

Fig. 3.10 (a) The shoe is fitted correctly. (b) Because of the forward and downward growth of the wall, this shoe, left on too long, has been pulled dorsally relative to the heel. The heels of the shoe now rest partially on the sole.

39

Treatment

Treatment consists initially of removing the offending shoe. If no infection has penetrated, this should be sufficient; the damaged corium heals and horn growth begins anew. With time the discoloured haemorrhagic horn grows out. However, if infection is present then the lesion must be treated like any other solar abscess, with removal of all underrun horn and necrotic tissue followed by pressure bandaging, antitetanus therapy and 3—4 days of systemic antibiotics.

Preventive measures are directed towards proper and prompt shoeing, with regular examination of the affected area.

Keratoma

Keratomas are aberrant masses of horn produced by focal areas of abnormal corium. They can arise either at the coronary band or from the lamellar region and grow distally, sandwiched between the wall and the pedal bone. They are rare. They seem to cause little discomfort until they have grown down to the bearing surface of the hoof where their lack of continuity with the surrounding horn allows infection to track upwards. This is despite their presence causing local resorption of pedal bone. When infection penetrates, a lameness is noticed and initial paring will usually reveal a circumscribed round or ovoid island of horn some 1—2 cm in diameter at the white line. Further paring shows the core to extend proximally as a distinct entity. X-ray examination will usually show a discrete lytic depression in the adjacent pedal bone (Fig. 3.11).

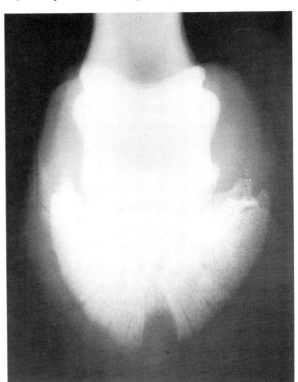

Fig. 3.11 The discrete lytic depression in this pedal bone caused by the presence of a keratoma can be difficult to differentiate from the consequence of pedal sepsis. The bone defect produced by a keratoma *tends* to be more clearly marginated.

Treatment by superficial paring and antibiotics will have no effect. The tumour must be removed in its entirety along with its covering of wall horn. An important point is to identify its origin and excise the offending section of germinative epithelium and corium. If this is not done the tumour will regrow. The epithelial defect will heal and begin producing horn again. The breach is dealt with subsequently in the usual way (see section on hoof cracks and pedal sepsis, p. 31).

Suggested further reading

Camben N, Clark RJ and Sutherland DJB (1984) Clinical observations on the response of equine hoof defects to biotin supplementation. *Vet Rec* **115**, 642−5.

4: Conditions of the Foot and Lower Limb

The 3rd phalanx (pedal or coffin bone)

The 3rd phalanx, or pedal bone, is entirely enclosed by the hoof to whose shape it conforms in a general way. Its ossification is peculiar in that while the proximal articular part is still cartilaginous, a perichondral cap of bone forms against the hoof and later extends to the upper or proximal part. This may account for the high incidence of adult horses in whom the extensor process appears to be a separate centre of ossification, often leading to radiographic misdiagnosis of fracture of the process. The general radiographic anatomy is pictured in Fig. 4.1a and b. Figures 4.2a and b show the distribution of vessels within the pedal bone and hoof.

From the proximal angle or wings of the pedal bone arise the rhomboid-shaped lateral cartilages which extend above the hoof walls on either side. They have the radiodensity of soft tissue and are therefore *not* visible unless ossified.

Radiography

Good preparation of the foot is essential, not just desirable; irregularities on the sole and frog can mimic convincingly areas of lysis, or fractures. The solar surface and the frog should be cleaned, not by brushing or scraping but by paring, especial care being taken with the depths of the frog clefts where underrun margins of the central eminence can trap air. These air pockets can lead to linear lucences being projected on to the pedal bone in the 60° dorsopalmar (DP) view. The solar irregularities and the various sulci of the frog should then be packed with thick soft soap or Playdoh. Shoe removal is not necessary unless part of the shoe is likely to cover the area of interest. However, the packing should not completely fill the hollow made by the shoe since this would simply add an overall soft tissue density and reduce contrast. Finally the foot is bandaged to retain the packing and prevent mess.

A 60° dorsopalmar (DP) and a straight lateromedial (LM) are usually adequate for initial screening. Other useful views are the horizontal, weight bearing DP and the 60° dorsopalmar lateromedial (DPLM) and dorsopalmar mediolateral (DPML) obliques. The flexor view can provide useful information on the wings of the pedal bone or ossified lateral cartilages. Fine-grain screen/film combinations give excellent detail and grids are *not* necessary. The tapering thickness of the pedal bone makes it difficult to visualize all its parts with one exposure;

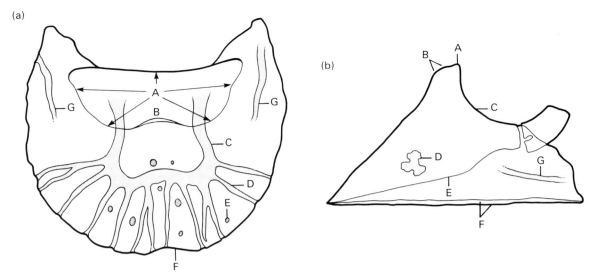

Fig. 4.1 (a) A diagrammatic representation of a 60° dorsopalmar oblique radiograph of a pedal bone. A = margins of the DIP articulation; B = the extensor process; C = the semilunar vascular canal; D = one of its radiating branches; E = a vascular canal seen 'end on'; F = the 'crena' or notch — a normal feature which should not be confused with a lytic depression; G = the dorsal vascular groove. (b) Diagrammatic representation of a lateromedial projection of a pedal bone. A = the joint margin; B = the extensor process; C = the glenoid or articular surface; D = the semilunar canal seen 'end on'; E = the cortex at the point of the greatest concavity of the sole surface; F = the two solar extremities, often separated by beam angulation; G = the dorsal vascular groove. NB the lateral cartilages are *not* visible unless they have undergone calcification.

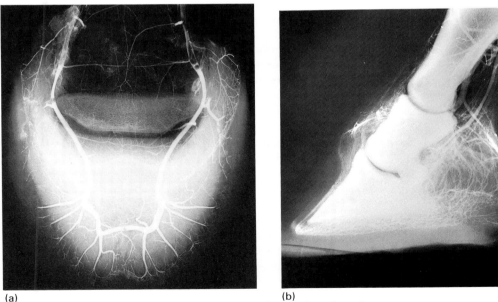

(a)   **(b)**

Fig. 4.2 (a) A post mortem angiograph showing the distribution of arteries within the pedal and navicular bones. The 2nd phalanx has been removed. (b) The rich plexus of blood vessels which supply the coronary, laminar and solar corium.

two are needed, or more economically, one exposure for the thicker portions with the film being viewed by bright light illumination to show its periphery.

Laminitis

Aetiology and pathogenesis

Rations high in carbohydrates (including lush grass and clover), retained placenta, mastitis, intake of excessive amounts of cold water, over-exercise on hard ground and excessive weight bearing on one leg following injury or surgery to the contralateral limb have all been implicated in causing laminitis. Apart from the latter two, where simple, mechanical stress overloading of the laminar and solar corium would seem to be the cause, the others probably exert their effects through bacterial endotoxin release.

A high carbohydrate intake, either at a constant absolute high level, or a sudden increase to a relatively high level, markedly alters the balance of the intestinal (large bowel) bacteria. The lactic acid-producing bacteria find conditions to their liking and multiply rapidly at the expense of others. The pH of luminal contents drops rapidly causing lysis of the gram negative bacteria and releasing vasoactive lipopolysaccharide compounds (endotoxins). These are absorbed by the gut mucosa which has been rendered more permeable by the highly acidic conditions, and, along with lactic acid, pass into the blood stream.

The endotoxin causes arteriovenous shunting and ischaemia of target organs. Amongst these are the sensitive laminae of the feet and here ischaemia causes laminar degeneration and clinical laminitis. The liver is also affected, preventing adequate detoxification of the toxic compounds.

Other changes include increases in plasma renin, aldosterone and catecholamines resulting in hypertension; also platelet aggregation and increases in plasma cortisol, probably as a result of stress. It is likely that direct endotoxin absorption occurs in metritis and endometritis. *These changes can occur very quickly, in a matter of only a few hours.*

Laminar degeneration follows very rapidly with haemorrhage and thrombosis of laminar vessels. Separation occurs at the horn−corium junction and the pedal bone loses its dorsal support. However, it is supported caudally by the navicular ligaments, and its attachments to the 2nd phalanx and the digital cushion via the lateral cartilages, etc., so that the downward thrust of weight bearing causes it to rotate around a pivotal point situated in the caudal hoof. The normally concave sole becomes flattened or convex and the 2nd phalanx sinks into the hoof creating a noticeable depression at the coronary band. In general, the degree of rotation is related to the severity of the laminitis and again *it can take place in a matter of hours*. The pedal bone tip can penetrate the solar horn within a few days resulting in severe infection of the degenerate corium. Also, separation of horn and the underlying soft tissues of the coronary band can occur, becoming evident initially as an exudation along the proximal margin of the hoof. Both of these are extremely poor prognostic signs.

In less severe cases the corium repairs itself and starts producing horn again. The changes at the coronary corium produce characteristic horn ridges lying parallel to the coronary band and the laminar corium produces amorphous horn which fills the gap between the dorsal pedal bone and the hoof wall. This eventually grows out to produce a crescentic area of crumbly, poor quality horn at the dorsal white line which is given the colloquial name of 'seedy toe'.

Repeated attacks of laminitis result in a progressive aggravation of signs.

Diagnosis

Symptoms can develop very rapidly in a few hours. The animals are distressed, with elevated pulse and respiration rates and the more severe cases will tremble and sweat. A reluctance to move is almost always evident with the more severely affected animals, not responding to even the severest provocation. Some are recumbent and characteristically lie on their sides with their legs stretched out. When they stand they usually adopt a classical stance with both fore and both hind legs advanced, they then appear as if they are leaning backwards.

Local signs

Any or all four feet may be affected. There is pain on pressure on both walls and sole; heat is definitely a feature and steam may rise from damp hooves. There is often a *bounding* arterial pulse in the digital arteries (moderate pulsation of these vessels can be palpated in normal animals). In severe and well established cases venous distension can sometimes be seen in the lower limb. After a few days the nature of the solar horn can change to become friable with visible haemorrhage; the solar contour will become concave as the pedal bone rotates, and the development of a crack just in front of the frog apex heralds the penetration of the pedal bone tip.

Radiography will show the degree of rotation; a *straight* lateral view using relatively low exposure intensities is used and the divergence of the dorsal wall of the pedal bone and the dorsal hoof wall outline is assessed (Fig. 4.3). The solar surface should not be used for comparison as it can be altered by paring or wear.

The lameness has been classified by Obel (1984) into four degrees of severity:

1 Grade I. Incessant paddling of affected feet. Not apparently lame at the walk, but the trot is slow and stilted.

2 Grade II. The walk is stilted, but a forefoot may be lifted without difficulty.

3 Grade III. The animal moves most reluctantly and will not allow a forefoot to be lifted.

4 Grade IV. The horse will not move without being forced.

45

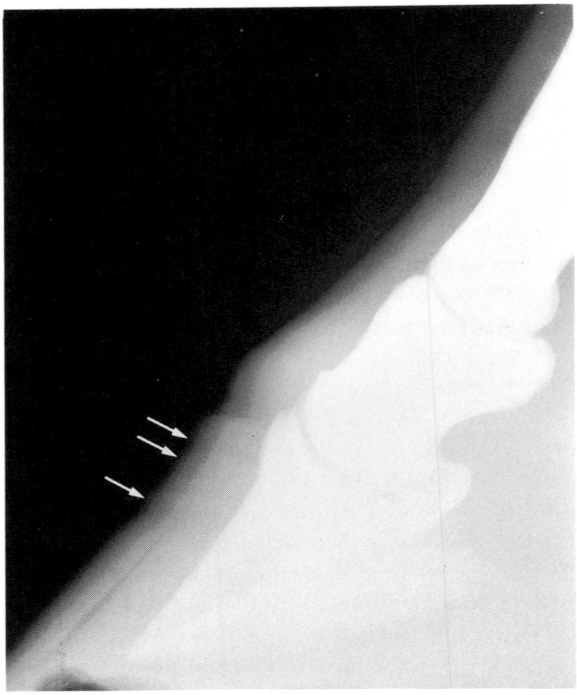

Fig. 4.3 A lateromedial projection of a pedal bone showing a mild degree of rotation. The typical linear radiolucency is visible between the horn and the dorsal pedal bone. It represents air between the separated planes of horn. Some 'ridging' of the horn (arrowed) is apparent, suggesting that this might be a chronic laminitic animal.

Epidemiology

Males and females are at equal risk with the highest risk times being 7–10 years and 4–7 years respectively.

More ponies suffer from laminitis than horses, but the latter in general show severer symptoms because of the increased ratio of body mass to weight bearing area.

The lush growing seasons are the times of greatest risk for ponies and infrequently used horses; the showing season with its attendant stress and high concentrate feeding regimes is another.

Treatment

Acute laminitis is an *emergency* — irreversible changes occur within hours of the development of lameness. *The animal is probably worse than either owner or veterinary surgeon realize.*

Initial treatment

Give a *mineral* oil purge — mineral oil is used because its laxative action is combined with an endotoxin blockade effect. (Salt purges are not indicated as they only compound dehydration already present.)

Restore blood flow to the feet and inhibit platelet aggregation by moderate exercise — this *must* be achieved even if all four feet have to be nerve blocked — intravenous phenylbutazone is effective in less severe cases, and to maintain the analgesia of nerve blocks. The nerve blocks may need to be repeated daily for 2–3 days if the animal will not walk without them.

Sodium is, in general terms, vasoconstrictive and hypertensive. Therefore remove any source of sodium and give approximately 30 g potassium, which is vasodilatory, orally every day.

Both isoxsuprine and phenoxybenzamine have been advocated in the treatment of laminitis; the former because of its vasodilating effect and the latter because it inhibits the effects of those vasoactive compounds causing the vascular changes.

Because laminar degeneration is likely to have taken place, broad spectrum antibiotic therapy is necessary.

The animal experiences much relief, and the pedal bone is prevented from rotating, by supporting the sole. The easy way is to put the animal on deep litter; the most effective way is using plaster shoes. Plaster of Paris bandage is layered concertina fashion in the sole concavity and passed over the front of the hoof to construct a 'slipper' of plaster of Paris. The sole must not be permanently hidden by Technovit or a metal shoe with pads.

Corticosteroids are contraindicated — they can cause and exacerbate laminitis by potentiating the effects of the vasoactive substances! (Eyre *et al* 1979). Cold hosing is theoretically contraindicated too; yet it may offer some symptomatic relief.

Long term therapy

Provide a disulphide-based substrate by the oral administration of 10 g methionine daily for one week with 5 g/day for three subsequent weeks.

Eliminate grain from the diet and substitute roughage which provides a volatile fatty acid source and no substrate for lactic acid-producing bacteria.

Hoof trimming

If the pedal bone has rotated then trimming is directed at restoring the pedal bone/ground relationship. The results, unfortunately, are often disappointing. The technique involves cutting back the heels and removing horn and therefore weight off the toe (Figs. 4.4a and b). Remove the horn slowly with a rasp as it will be of unknown thickness. A shoe should be fitted which supports the heel and exposes the toe. An egg bar shoe or more simply a normal shoe fitted back to front, will have the correct effect. Temporary packing can be fitted to apply pressure to the sole. Over the months the hoof can be 'rotated' around the pedal bone by repetition of this trimming procedure. The use of 'heart-bar' shoes which have a forward pointing tongue to support the sole has been much advocated recently and would seem to have much to recommend it.

If there is infection in the foot then the horn preventing drainage must be removed and the foot bandaged. Constant attention is required with repeated removal of underrun horn and infected tissue. The prognosis is very poor.

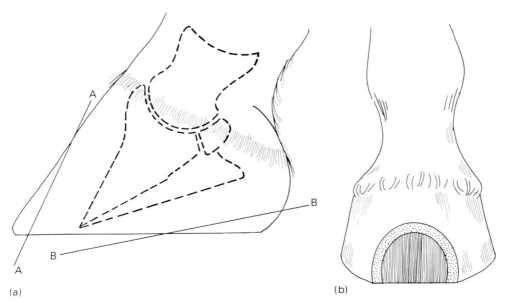

(a)   (b)

Fig. 4.4 (a) AA and BB show the line along which the laminitic hoof is trimmed. The process of correction is slow and since it relies on horn growth, as well as trimming, it cannot be hurried. (b) Illustration showing that trimming the toe will expose initially the horny laminae, and, if taken deeper, the sensitive laminar corium.

There are reports of animals being nursed through months of recumbency following complete sloughing of one or more hooves; the ethics of this are open to debate, though there is no doubt that with care and total commitment some do make remarkable recoveries — again full and frank discussion with the owners is advisable!

Prevention

Feed a diet with a high roughage to grain ratio. Avoid sudden increases in the concentrate ration or unrestricted access to lush grazing. Prevent unrestricted cold water intake after vigorous exercise.

Remove retained placenta as early as possible or use vigorous antibiotic therapy if this is not possible. Avoid heavy or long term corticosteroid therapy.

Suggested further reading

Eyre P, Elmes PJ and Strickland S (1979) Corticosteroid-potentiated vascular responses of the equine digit: a possible pharmacologic basis for laminitis. *Am J Vet Res* **40**(1), 135–8.

Garner HE (1980) Update on equine laminitis. In *Veterinary Clinics of North America — Large Animal Practice*. Symposium on Equine Lameness, Vol 2, Part 1, pp. 25–32. Ed. W Moyer, WB Saunders, Philadelphia.

Hood DM (1979) Current concepts of the physiopathology of laminitis. *Proc Am Assoc Equine Prac* **25**, 13–20.

Moore JN, Garner HE and Coffman JR (1981) Haematological changes during development of acute laminitis hypertension. *Eq Vet J* **13**(4), 240–2.

Pedal osteitis

The term 'pedal bone osteitis' has a very specific meaning, defining an inflammatory condition of the bone of the 3rd phalanx. As a description of a type of pathological reaction which is a sequel to most insults to bone it has a legitimate use. However, the term 'pedal osteitis' has over the years been increasingly misused so that it is now used extensively to signify a condition in its own right. It has also been dignified by inclusion in some reputable texts. The existence of this 'condition' is based on the presence of a uni or bilateral low grade chronic lameness of indefinable origin accompanied by radiographic changes which have been variously described as a demineralization, new bone formation or an increase in numbers and diameter of the vascular channels of the pedal bone.

Even more unfortunate is the tendency to lump together under the broad heading of pedal osteitis any chronic lameness for which, on casual examination, no obvious cause can be found.

There is no doubt that, even after a careful work-up, no specific pathology can be demonstrated in a small percentage of chronic foot problems. With the advent of more critical nerve blocks, intra-articular anaesthesia and better quality radiography, fewer such cases remain unsolved. There is, however, little or no justification for classifying these insoluble few under the arbitrary heading of pedal osteitis.

Rendano and Grant (1978) carried out a radiographic survey of pedal bones from normal horses and discovered an immense individual variation in contour, degree of roughening of solar margin and in the number and diameter of vascular channels. This, and the author's personal observations, would indicate there is enough variety in the physical characteristics of the pedal bones to preclude a radiographic diagnosis of pedal osteitis based on these factors.

In occasional animals, pain can be located to the dorsal solar region and radiography demonstrates marginal fractures of the pedal bone. These fracture lines follow the external contours of the solar margin leaving a halo of fragments some 1–2 mm wide (Fig 4.5). The cause is not known though it is probably trauma. With rest, healing occurs and the animals become sound. With little justification the phenomenon has been included under the umbrella term of pedal osteitis; although the term 'marginal fracture' would seem much more appropriate.

Outgrowths of periosteal new bone on the marginal solar border, usually towards the wings, have been similarly called pedal osteitis. These are often found incidentally on otherwise normal horses and great care must be taken not to overinterpret their presence.

Horses and ponies with flat or minimally concave soles will often exhibit great discomfort when exercised on hard or stony ground. They are often said to be suffering from pedal osteitis. There is no doubt they can suffer considerable pain if the exercise is prolonged, but it is likely that the cause is trauma to the sensitive solar corium and its subsequent inflammatory response. Prolonged trauma may also instigate a periosteal response resulting in the production of new bone. Again the term pedal osteitis would be incorrect.

49

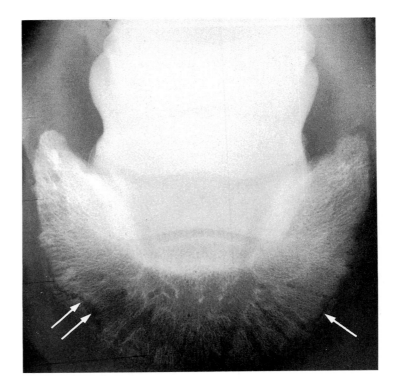

Fig. 4.5 Marginal fractures (arrowed) of the pedal bone.

'Pyramidal disease', 'buttress foot'

'Pyramidal disease' is new bone formation and associated soft tissue reaction at the extensor process of the 3rd phalanx or pedal bone.

Aetiology and pathogenesis

Excessive strain on the common digital extensor tendon at its insertion on the extensor process of the 3rd phalanx can cause tearing of the insertion and possibly avulsion of small flakes of bone. The subsequent periosteal reaction produces new bone, or 'enthesiophytes' as they are more properly termed; this, and the accompanying soft tissue reaction and tendon inflammation and fibrosis produce a swelling of varying degree at the dorsal coronary band, and, of course, pain.

Clinical signs

Clinical signs include, initially, a sudden onset of moderately severe lameness with a tendency to hold the foot in the 'neutral' non-weight bearing position with the toe just touching the ground. There may be swelling or pain on pressure in the dorsal coronary band region. In the more chronic stages there is a lameness of variable severity with no particularly definitive characteristics. A firm swelling is often palpable at the dorsal coronary band and it may or may not be painful on pressure. The lameness will block out with an abaxial sesamoid nerve block (ASNB), though not with a palmar digital nerve block (PDNB).

Radiography

The DP view is not usually helpful, only the straight lateral projection is of use. Films taken early will show no change unless a fracture has occurred. Later, moderately aggressive, irregular new bone develops on the extensor process. *NB* the normal shape of the extensor process is very variable, and it is frequently separated by a slight groove from the dorsal articular margin. The latter, along with the dorsodistal joint margin of the 2nd phalanx should also be evaluated for osteophytes which would indicate associated degenerative disease of the coffin joint.

Treatment

If there is no fracture then rest alone is indicated. In the very early stages pressure bandaging of the area will serve to disperse some of the inflammatory exudate and minimize the area of subsequent fibrosis. It will also result in some immobilization of the area. Analgesics are not indicated as a reduction in pain could lead to greater use of the foot. Box rest for a minimum of 2 weeks should be followed by controlled exercise for 3 months. In the chronic case, there is no treatment of any practical value other than permanent non-steroidal anti-inflammatory drugs such as phenylbutazone, or a dorsal digital neurectomy.

Fracture of the extensor process

Occasionally the extensor process will fracture in such a way as to produce a large proximal fragment. The cause is probably external trauma or an excessive extensor pull, although this is not certain.

Clinical signs

With the fracture there will be a sudden onset of severe, non-weight bearing lameness with swelling and pain in the dorsal coronary band region. After a few weeks, if untreated, the lameness will diminish slightly, but, because the fracture is always intra-articular and subject to the movement of the joint and distraction by the extensor tendon, it persists at a relatively high level. Later degenerative joint disease (DJD) of the distal interphalangeal (DIP) articulation will maintain the disablement.

Radiography

A straight lateromedial projection is the most useful single view with maybe some slightly oblique views centred on the extensor process to clarify the position of a fragment. In more long standing cases the DIP joint should be evaluated for signs of DJD (Fig. 4.6).

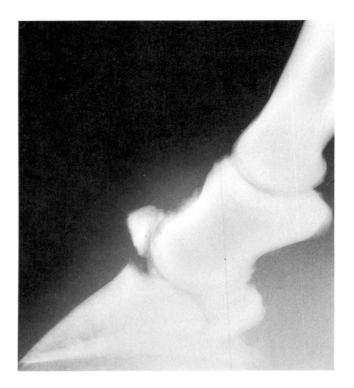

Fig. 4.6 A fracture of the extensor process of the pedal bone. The pull of the extensor tendon has distracted the fragment proximally. There is much new bone production on the dorsal aspect of the 2nd phalanx and osteophytes on the palmar articular margins of the DIP joint indicate the presence of degenerative joint disease.

Treatment

Small fragments can be removed through a window cut in the hoof just below the coronary band. They are difficult to identify and remove, as they are invariably buried within extensor tendon and camouflaged by inflammatory or fibrous change. Larger fragments may be amenable to internal fixation. The piece of bone must be large enough to accept a screw without splitting and the fracture must be recent. Figure 4.6 illustrates how distraction of the fragment occurs and if this is consolidated by fibrous reaction, then reduction may be impossible. The approach is through an incision immediately above the coronary band with the screw being directed distally and with a slightly palmar angulation. Wound healing can be a problem in this area and in the long term coronary band damage and DIP joint DJD can affect the prognosis. Nevertheless, failure to treat a fracture of this kind will result in the situation in Fig. 4.6 and a permanently lame animal.

In selected cases, a dorsal digital neurectomy would considerably alleviate pain. However, if DJD is extensive it is unlikely to be other than a palliative procedure.

Suggested further reading

Rendano VT (1979) Radiographic interpretation — pedal osteitis. *California Vet* **33**(10), 27−9.
Rendano VT and Grant B (1978) The equine third pahlanx: its radiographic appearance. *J Am Vet Rad Soc* **19**, 125−35.

The navicular bone

Anatomy

The navicular bone is a small shuttle-shaped bone lying between the
deep flexor tendon (DFT) and the palmar aspect of the distal interphalangeal (DIP) joint, contributing about 30% to the distal articular
surface. It is a sesamoid bone lying in the palmar inter-osseous
ligament. Proximally this acts as the suspensory ligament of the
navicular bone. Distally, where it is given the name of the 'distal

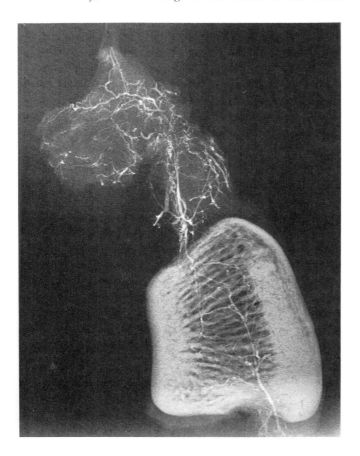

Fig. 4.7 An angiographic study of
a slab of navicular bone showing
arteries entering the bone through
the proximal and distal navicular
ligaments.

navicular ligament', it is less substantial and holds the navicular bone
tightly against the palmar aspect of the pedal bone. Nutrient arteries
run into the sesamoid through both the proximal and distal ligaments
(Fig. 4.7). In the normal adult, the proximal supply is greatly reduced.
The articular surface is covered by articular-type hyaline cartilage,
while the palmar surface, over which the DFT runs, is covered by
fibrocartilage. Between the DFT and the navicular bone lies the
navicular bursa which in life is virtually a potential space bounded at
its extremities by a flimsy synovium and containing a minimal
amount of synovial fluid. The main function of the navicular bone is
probably to provide a smooth change in course for the DFT and to
ensure a constant angle of insertion into the pedal bone.

Navicular syndrome (Navicular disease, podotrochleosis chronica aseptica)

Navicular syndrome was first described as a clinical problem in the mid nineteenth century. Since then, opinions as to its aetiology, pathogenesis, symptomatology, diagnosis and therapy have been the subject of continual debate, dispute, fashion and change. Poulos (1983) quotes John Godfrey Saxe (1936):

*And so these men of Indostan
Disputed loud and long,
Each in his own opinion
Exceeding stiff and strong
Though each was partly in the right
And all were in the wrong.*

*So oft in theologic wars
The disputants, I wean,
Rail on in utter ignorance
Of what each other mean
And prate about an elephant
Not one of them has seen.*

Whilst apt in the context of many veterinary debates, this criticism applies particularly to the field of navicular research. It is likely that the occasional widely differing results of research into this condition are not contradictory, but complementary, building up a picture of a complete syndrome with multifactorial aetiology, pathogenesis and diverse clinical and pathological manifestations.

Aetiology and pathogenesis

Three main schools of thought exist. One incrimates concussion, vibration and third order acceleration as a cause of trauma to, and subsequent degeneration of, the fibrocartilaginous surface of the navicular bone and the DFT (Rooney 1977); the second, that arterial occlusion within the foot, though principally in the distal navicular arteries, leads to bone ischemia which is painful (Colles 1979). The third cites the changes in the navicular bursa synovium and in the vasculature of the navicular bone itself, in addition to alterations in subchondral bone pressure-drop curves as being strong evidence that navicular disease is basically an osteoarthrosis (Svalastoga 1983; Svalastoga and Nielson 1983; Svalastoga and Smith 1983). The fact that navicular disease is often found in association with degenerative disease of the metacarpophalangeal (MCP) and interphalangeal joints adds weight to the latter theory.

Since good cases can be made for all three scenarios, it is probable that all have a part to play, interacting with additional factors such as hoof pastern angles, general conformation and maybe level of work during early, immature years and subsequently.

One explanation for the lack of progress in understanding the disease is that no one has yet produced it experimentally; clinical cases are the only source of research material.

Clinical signs

The classical image of navicular disease is that of a gradual onset, low grade lameness affecting one or both forefeet. The stride length is reduced, the animal may stumble at the trot, and at rest it may 'point' or ease its forefeet. The lameness is variable in severity with periods of complete remission in the early stages. In established cases there is reduced wear and contraction of the heel region and the foot assumes the characteristic 'boxy' appearance with a small 'atrophic' frog.

It is, however, rare that an animal will be initially presented with these signs. It is likely that at first examination the history will be of a suddenly noticed lameness or gait asymmetry; maybe on a turn, on one diagonal or, commonly, going downhill. Often, on close questioning, the owners will comment on a reduction in performance, a disinclination to work or some other change in the animal's behaviour pattern in the previous weeks or even months. In these cases the animal has probably been lame for some time either at such a low grade that it is passed unnoticed by inexpert eyes or equally, that it was suffering from uniform bilateral lameness which only became obvious when one leg became worse than the other. This affords another explanation for the apparent periodic remission which is so characteristic of the disease. If an animal is, say, 2/10th lame on its right fore, it is noticeable; if the left fore then worsens to a 2/10th level the animal would then appear not to be lame unless examined very critically. This view is supported by the number of horses and ponies which have a history of poor performance, are not overtly lame, even on the lunge, but when a PDNB is performed on one leg become obviously lame on the other.

Occasionally, bizarre manifestations of forelimb problems are encountered such as a refusal to jump, or even lying or falling down when mounted.

The clinician must be wary of prejudging such cases, especially as they often present with lay, or sometimes professionally applied labels of 'shoulder lameness' or 'back problems'.

Diagnosis

1 A history of an insidious onset, usually low grade lameness affecting one or both forelimbs and possibly a fall off in performance over weeks, months or longer. (Beware the 'sudden onset' lameness meaning that the lameness has been 'suddenly noticed'.)

2 A clinical examination which reveals a stilted, 'proppy' or 'pottery' gait, with possibly an overt lameness on the straight trot or lunge in one or both forelegs; also an inequality in hoof size or shape and a tendency to rest one or other forelegs during the examination. The clinician should exclude other possible causes such as corns or pedal sepsis.

3 A positive response to a flexion or extension test of the lower limb.

4 An abolition, or a substantial reduction, in lameness following a PDNB or, more sensitively, a navicular bursal block. This will probably lead to the demonstration of a bilateral lameness in which case a

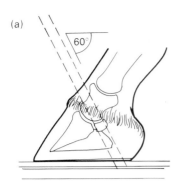

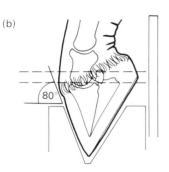

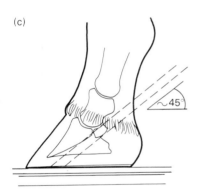

Fig. 4.8 (a) The 'high coronary' or dorsopalmar projection with the beam centre at 60° to the horizontal. (b) The 'upright pedal' projection. With the dorsal hoof at an angle of 80° to the horizontal the image of the navicular bone is thrown clear of the DIP joint. (c) The 'flexor' projection of the navicular bone. The beam angulation shown is only an approximate guide. It may have to be altered if the animal is small, with little height under its thorax, to avoid superimposition of the palmar fetlock; also in those animals which will not lean forward as shown in the diagram and in those animals with very low heels.

PDNB should also be performed on the second leg.
5 Radiographic examination.

Radiography of the navicular bone

Good preparation of the foot is essential if radiographs of diagnostic quality are to be taken. In the most commonly used 60° dorsopalmar (DP) or 'high coronary' projection, the frog is superimposed on to the image of the navicular bone; material within the sulci can obscure detail, while air-filled depressions or clefts can convincingly mimic areas of navicular bone osteopenia, synovial fossae or even fractures.

To prepare the foot the surface horn must be pared, not scraped, clean; frog clefts should be opened out and ragged horn, especially around the central sulcus, cut off to leave a smooth, unpockmarked surface. The clefts can be packed with soft soap or Playdoh. The former, though messier, fills better and is squeezed into cracks by the animal's weight. Finally, a protective *cotton* bandage is applied.

Projections (Figs. 4.8a, b and c)

Three projections are needed to evaluate the navicular bone completely. The first two produce almost identical views, though the horizontal beam technique with the 'Hickman block' should produce more consistent angulation of the navicular bone to the beam centre. This is because the relationship of foot to beam is not affected by heel length or foot shape as in the 60° dorsopalmar (DP) view.

The lateral and flexor views are often omitted. However, they are useful for confirming the presence of changes such as osteophyte production on the dorsal navicular border, alteration in lateral profile, flexor erosions, DFT calcification and eliminating artefacts. Artefacts caused by superimposition can also be spotted if two DP projections are made, angled 10° apart and the position of the suspect lesion relative to the navicular bone compared. Frog artefacts will move, whilst genuine lesions maintain their relationship with the bone outline.

Often the scope of the examination is limited by the type and versatility of the X-ray machine.

The DP projections should be well exposed to penetrate adequately the combined thickness of the 2nd phalanx and navicular bone.

Radiographic interpretation

Note there is large grey area between normality, as defined by the absence of *detectable* pathological change, and patent abnormality. The significance of any radiographic interpretation is in relation to clinical findings and nerve block evidence; some horses with clinical navicular disease have radiographically 'normal' navicular bones, others have severe radiographic changes but apparently may not appear lame unless critically examined.

Many criteria may be used to establish a radiographic diagnosis; controversy rages over the significance of some but a measure of agreement exists over others. It will be useful to consider these radio-graphic changes in relation to the histological appearance of the lesions they represent.

The synovial fossae (vascular channels — nutrient foraminae)

Increase in numbers and change in shape of these triangular or cone-shaped radiolucent areas on the distal border of the navicular bone have long been held to be a significant indicator of disease. Until recently they were said to be nutrient foraminae; in fact the visible lucencies represent fossae dorsal to the nutrient arterial channels and have been reported to be lined with synovial membrane (Poulos 1983). Proximal enlargement of these fossae producing the inverted flask or 'lollipop' shape (Fig. 4.9) is not due to vascular proliferation but probably to synovial proliferation into the navicular marrow cavity in the acute phase of the disease (Poulos 1983). Guidelines as to numbers and shapes which are 'normal' have been given by Colles (1982). In general terms, any fossa which is dilated proximally can be regarded as abnormal; all others are normal. In addition, more than seven normal shaped fossae, fossae on the sloping distal borders and prominent 'vascular channels' on the proximal horizontal border are all said to be abnormal and indicative of the presence of navicular disease.

Focal osteopenia, 'lucencies' within the navicular bone, 'cysts'

These changes are easily reproduced by frog artefacts, so beware! Seen as well-demarcated, focal areas of osteopenia, (Figs. 4.10a and b), they are, in fact, areas of cortical and medullary erosion arising on the flexor surface of the navicular bone. Fibrocartilage is first lost with erosion of the adjacent flexor tendon; synovial tissue then establishes itself in the defect and erosion progresses to involve the cortex and medulla. Adhesions between the area of the defect and the deep flexor tendon are always present but they cannot be detected radio-graphically. Occasionally cortical defects can be seen on the flexor view when they are not deep enough to be visible on the DPs. Their presence indicates moderate to advanced disease.

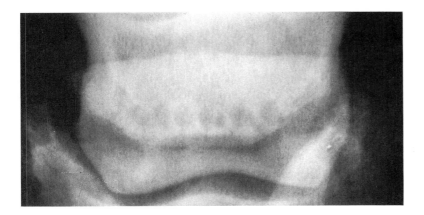

Fig. 4.9 A 60° dorsopalmar projection of a navicular bone showing numerous proximally dilated synovial fossae ('lollipops' or 'flasks').

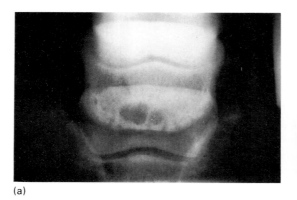 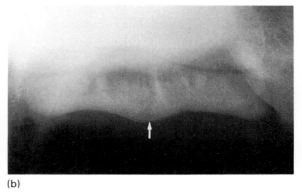

(a)   (b)

Fig. 4.10 (a) A 60° dorsopalmar projection of the navicular bone showing well demarcated areas of osteopenia (lysis). (b) A 'flexor' view of the same navicular bone confirming the presence of osteopenia and, in addition, showing lysis (arrowed).

Osteophytes ('spurs')

Much controversy exists over the significance of these signs. Osteophytes are found on the extreme 'wings' of the navicular bone, on the dorsal surface at the attachment of the suspensory ligament and at the origin of the distal navicular ligament. Here they should more properly be called enthesiophytes. All are indicative of secondary joint disease and in the case of the navicular bone are probably caused by chronic trauma, DJD or, as Rooney (1977) suggests, third order acceleration.

Although no definite correlation has yet been made, it is likely that they form part of the complex navicular disease syndrome and their presence should be viewed with some suspicion especially if clinical evidence suggests the presence of navicular pain.

Medullary sclerosis or 'apparent loss of medullary cavity'

This is probably an artefactual appearance caused by cortical or trabecular thickening compounded by poor radiographic technique. It has not been shown to exist histologically.

Mineralization of the DFT

Mineralization of the DFT occurs in cases of severe tendon damage. It may be simple calcification or ectopic ossification or a combination of both. It is regarded as a poor prognostic sign and may precede rupture of the DFT.

Chip fractures of the distal navicular border

These 'fractures' (Fig. 4.11) are usually found at the junction of the distal, palmar, horizontal and sloping borders. There may be two

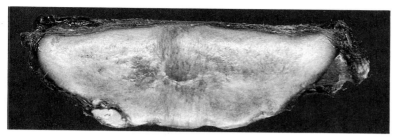

Fig. 4.11 A so-called chip fracture of the distal horizontal border of a navicular bone.

fractures in a single bone and they are often bilateral. They are not found in the hind feet nor in the absence of clinical navicular disease. Excellent radiographic technique is required to visualize them, and it is certain that they are far more common than is realized. Some controversy exists as to whether they are true fractures, or ossicles within the distal navicular ligament. If they are true fractures it is likely that their presence indicates a poor prognosis for any treatment other than simple pain alleviation.

Treatment of navicular disease

There are three main categories of treatment
1 Reduction or abolition of pain.
2 Drugs which affect the blood supply to the navicular bone.
3 Hoof trimming and corrective shoeing.

Pain alleviation

Analgesics

Two non-steroidal anti-inflammatory drugs (NSAIDs), phenylbutazone (PBZ) and meclafenamic acid, have provided the mainstay of analgesic treatment in navicular disease. Of these, PBZ is most frequently used. Oral preparations are available and the dose rate is kept to the minimum compatible with alleviation of clinical signs. In most cases of the disease, some improvement is seen following its administration, and some horses may be 'worked' satisfactorily on PBZ. However, the drug must be used on a permanent basis, it does not effect any cure and the disease process will usually worsen despite its use, necessitating periodic increases in dosage. Fortunately PBZ has few side effects in *adult* horses. However, at some stage, which can vary from months to years after the onset of treatment, the increased level of lameness will not be masked and drug therapy alone will be ineffective.

The additional expense of the other NSAIDs is not usually justified by any increased potency of effect against navicular pain.

Intrabursal injection of cortisone preparations is practiced by some workers. The relief offered is said to be good but temporary and the risk of adverse reactions such as metastatic calcification of the DFT or introduction of infection makes the technique unattractive. There is too the risk that it will adversely affect the ability of the flexor fibrocartilage to withstand wear and tear, thus exacerbating the condition.

Neurectomy

Probably the earliest form of treatment for navicular disease. Initially the lateral and medial palmar nerves were sectioned but the complications of loss of proprioception and occasional sloughing of the hoof wall led to the adoption of the technique of lateral and medial palmar *digital* nerve section.

Incomplete desensitization because of aberrant subcutaneous branches running to the heel region, painful neuroma formation and only partial relief because of concurrent DIP joint arthritis, are the main drawbacks to this operation. Surveys report success rates (i.e. returning the animal to useful work) of between 67−80% but with a diminishing success rate in years subsequent to the first 12 months after surgery (year 1, 80%; year 2, 67%; year 3, 48%; year 4, 40.5%). Painful neuroma formation is a significant post-operative complication to this surgery. Many techniques have been devised to prevent the problem arising, including epineural capping, cautery of nerve ends, diverting the stump into a hole drilled in the 1st phalanx and others. It would seem, however, that careful atraumatic and rapid surgery involving the minimum of interference to the nerve stump will produce just as good a result. Despite the advent of new modes of therapy, neurectomy should still be considered in cases where other treatments have failed.

Alcohol injection and cryoneurectomy have been practiced with varying success rates. Alcohol block desensitizes for between 1−6 months whilst cryocautery carries a high risk of post-operative infection.

Drugs which affect the blood supply

Warfarin

Colles and Hickman (1977) and Colles (1979) demonstrated thrombosis of the distal navicular nutrient arteries in horses affected with navicular disease. Colles (1979) suggested that warfarin might have a beneficial effect by allowing the development of a secondary blood supply. Its action is not fully understood although it appears to reduce blood viscosity and affect red blood cell morphology. Initially therapy is aimed at increasing the one-stage prothrombin time by 2−4 seconds from its 'normal' range of some 11−17 seconds; this is done by starting at an initial dose rate of 0.018 mg/kg (10 mg for an average horse) and increasing the dose by 20% increments until the desired effect is achieved. Final dose rates are variable; from 0.012−0.75 mg/kg in the initial work, with a mean treatment time of 7 weeks for the horses to respond. In the experience of the author and others, an increase of 2−4 seconds is difficult to monitor. The one-stage prothrombin test is very subjective and variations of 2−4 seconds in the same sample are possible. Also, in many animals no clinical response is seen until the one-stage prothrombin time is doubled!

Principal and often overwhelming disadvantages are (a) the necessity for continuous and expensive monitoring of one-stage prothrombin times; (b) the samples must, ideally, be taken at the same time of day and with the same relationship to feeding and exercise; (c) the practical difficulty of getting accurate and reproducible laboratory results; (d) the difficulties experienced in stabilizing the dose, and (e) interactions with other drugs. Warfarin interacts with many drugs, therefore warfarin and these drugs must not be used simultaneously. Protein-binding compounds such as phenylbutazone release active warfarin into the circulation with the risk of fatal haemorrhage or haemarthroses.

Long term results are variable. Some horses remain sound for long periods, others regress within months. Changes in diet, workload or even monitoring laboratory staff may have an effect too. In a follow-up study of 100 horses, 77% became sound while being treated. In the event of haemorrhage, 1 mg/kg of vitamin Kl should be given intravenously.

Isoxsuprine hydrochloride

This is a peripheral vasodilatory drug initially used in man. It has a direct effect on vascular and non-vascular smooth muscle; it also causes a reduction in blood viscosity in man and the horse.

Rose *et al* (1983) conducted a double-blind trial in which isoxsuprine hydrochloride in paste form and a placebo were administered to horses with clinical navicular disease. The results showed a highly significant effect of the drug with seven out of eight horses in the isoxsuprine group becoming sound.

Studies have shown that the minimally effective dose rate is 0.6 mg/kg. This is the dose level recommended for the first 3 weeks of treatment. If there is no response then a higher dose rate of 0.9 mg/kg and even 1.2 mg/kg may be used without side effects for a further 3 weeks.

Animals becoming lame again following a course of treatment should ideally be re-evaluated with nerve blocks and if appropriate, a second course of isoxsuprine hydrocloride administered over 6—8 weeks. The time for which horses remain sound is very variable and usually unpredictable, except that in general terms, horses which have been lame before treatment for less than 12 months show a good response to the drug and the duration of drug action is longer.

The only published contraindications are that the drug should not be administered to pregnant mares, within 14 days post partum or after recent arterial haemorrhage.

Hoof trimming and corrective shoeing

Broken hoof/pastern axis, upright pasterns and contracted heels have all been implicated in the development of navicular disease. The former is a result of the fashion or fad for long toes and short heels which has been prevalent for many years, and also a result of the natural wear pattern of shod hooves (see section on hoof wear, p. 29); the latter two may be results rather than causes.

Corrective trimming should be aimed at achieving an unbroken hoof/pastern axis with neither heels nor toes being too long. This can be a slow process, and in the interim similar results can be achieved

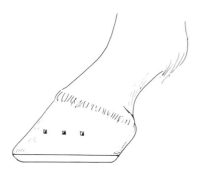

Fig. 4.12 A shoe with a 'rolled' toe exerts less leverage on the foot at the 'break over' point of the stride, i.e. when the heel is lifted at the beginning of the forward phase of the stride.

by shoeing with wedges placed between hoof and shoe. Bar shoes are generally held to be beneficial though little factual evidence exists to support this. Chamfering the bars of the shoe on their solar aspect is also said to exert a widening effect on the heels. However, the initial narrowing of the heels is due to reduced weight bearing on the heel region, and widening of itself has no intrinsic merit. On the other hand, nailing shoes too far back along the bars may restrict normal heel expansion with a possible reduction in concussion absorption. A rolled toe (Fig. 4.12) is also said to be beneficial since it reduces the leverage on the toe at the break-over part of the stride.

Few detailed assessments of corrective trimming and shoeing have been undertaken, though from an Australian study it appears that short term improvement can be expected in 50% of horses treated solely by these techniques. The eggbar shoe is specifically recomended by Ostblom *et al* (1982). It is egg-shaped in outline, the caudal part of the oval forming a 'bar'. It has a 'rolled toe' and has only three nail holes a side, presumably to facilitate heel expansion.

'Grooving' the heels with vertical and horizontal cuts has achieved some popularity. No concrete evidence exists as to its efficacy.

Section of the navicular suspensory ligament

Section of the medial and lateral suspensory navicular ligaments has been recently advocated as a 'cure' for navicular disease. The ligaments are cut at their origin on the distal lateral and medial aspects of the 1st phalanx. At the present time, there is insufficient evidence as to the efficacy of this treatment. Some horses do seem to benefit in the short term, but the percentage improves, and the long term results still await evaluation. Wright (1986) reports the technique and good results in 13 of 16 horses 6 months after surgery.

Summary

Navicular disease is a complex syndrome with a host of variable presenting signs, a number of suggested aetiologies and numerous forms of treatment. Even the all-important diagnostic criteria are the subject of intense argument and debate. Adding to the difficulty of both diagnosis and treatment is the fact that, with the use of more precise and full nerve block work-ups it has become clear that a high proportion of cases responding positively to PDNBs show a residual lameness, indicating pain higher up the limb. Investigation of this phenomenon with further regional and intra-articular blocks has shown *repeatedly* that this pain is located in some combination of the three distal limb articulations. Radiography of these joints often shows the characteristic changes of DJD. The author also sees many animals presented with what would be regarded traditionally as classical navicular disease which are, on further evaluation, also lame in one or both hind limbs; DJD in one of its manifestations being the culprit here too. A disturbing feature is that these animals are often young; 4 and 5 years olds being commonly affected; few are over 8 years of age. The inescapable conclusion is that navicular disease, at least in cases seen at the author's clinic, seems not to occur in isolation but frequently in association with a polyarthritis syndrome.

If this is the case nationwide, then it could account for the disturbing poor success rate in the treatment of the condition known as navicular disease.

The plethora of treatments which have been advocated over the years as fads and fashions have come and gone is a good indication that no single one has provided the answer, and it is likely that unless any individual treatment takes into account the presence of concurrent disease, none ever will.

When nerve block evidence shows that only navicular pain is present, and whilst on this point, residual lameness after bilateral PDNBs should not be simply dismissed as the block not having worked properly, then the choice of treatment must depend on several factors. One of these is that the rules of many equestrian sports do not allow the use in competition of animals treated with certain prescribed substances; among these are NSAIDs such as phenyl-butazane (PBZ), or compounds such as warfarin. Other factors are: the value of the animal; its level of potential use; the ability and inclination of the owner to monitor medication, so necessary with warfarin for example, and last, but not least, the current fashion in treatment and the clinician's individual beliefs and preferences.

It is therefore not possible, with one exception, to give unequivocal advice as to the choice of treatment but rather to counsel that clinicians should tailor their therapy to the individual needs and constraints of their patient and its owner, bearing in mind what is, and what is not, known about each mode of treatment. The exception is the one form of therapy which has a broad consensus of approval, and that is foot care. Through all the changing fashions, the correction of incorrect hoof/pastern angles, long toes and poor shoeing techniques has emerged as an effective, continuous therapeutic thread.

In the present state of the science, the treatment of navicular disease syndrome is at best palliative, and with only temporary improvement to be expected whatever the choice of therapy.

As with many other conditions mentioned in this book, clinicians are well advised to discuss these points fully and frankly with owners before embarking on treatment.

When navicular disease is found in association with DJD of other joints, therapy aimed at the navicular problem alone may improve the situation, but never remove the lameness entirely. In animals intended for light work then simply tackling the navicular disease may remove a considerable burden of pain from them and allow their uncritical use. Similarly, a broad attack with a general systemic, analgesic, anti-inflammatory drug such as phenylbutazone may have an ameliorating effect. The most effective will be a combination of both. Unfortunately, those horses that need it most, i.e. the athletic competition horses, are prevented by the rules of the sport from benefiting from this blanket therapy. If this is the case then it is likely that their competitive working life is over and they will move down from the first team to the third or fourth or even out of the game entirely.

Suggested further reading

Colles CM (1979) Ischaemic necrosis of the navicular bone and its treatment. *Vet Rec* **104**, 133.

Colles CM (1982) Navicular disease and its treatment. *In Practice* March, 29–36.

Colles CM and Hickman J (1977) The arterial supply of the navicular bone and its variations in navicular disease. *Eq Vet J* **9**(3), 150–4.

Fricker CH, Riek W and Hugelshofer J (1982) Occlusion of the digital arteries — a model for pathogenesis of navicular disease. *Eq Vet J* **14**(3), 203–7.

O'Brien TR, Millman TM, Pool RR and Suter PF (1975) Navicular disease in the thoroughbred horse. A morphological investigation relative to a new radiographic projection. *J Am Vet Rad Soc* **16**, 39–50.

Ostblom L, Lund C and Melsen F (1982) Histological study of navicular bone disease. *Eq Vet J* **14**(93), 199–202.

Poulos PW (1983) Correlation of radiographic signs and histological changes in navicular disease. *Proc 29th Ann Conv Amer Ass Eq Prac* **29**, 244–55.

Rose RJ, Allen JR, Hodgson DR and Kohnke JR (1983) Studies on isoxsuprine hydrochloride for the treatment of navicular disease. *Eq Vet J* **15**(3), 238–43.

Saxe JG (1936) *The blind man and the elephant: The best loved poems of the American people.* Selected by Hazel Fellemen, Garden City Books, Garden City, New York.

Svalastoga E (1983) Navicular disease in the horse — a microangiographic investigation. *Nord Vet Med* **35**, 131–9.

Svalastoga E and Nielsen K (1983) Navicular disease in the horse — the synovial membrane of bursa podotrochlearis. *Nord Vet Med* **35**, 28–30.

Svalastoga E and Smith M (1983) Navicular disease in the horse — the sub-chondral bone pressure. *Nord Vet Med* **35**, 31–7.

Turner TA and Fessler JF (1982) The anatomic pathologic and radiographic aspects of navicular disease. *Comp Cont Ed* **4**(8), 5350–5.

Van de Watering CC and Morgan JP (1975) Chip fractures as a radiologic finding in navicular disease of the horse. *J Am Vet Radiol Soc* **16**, 206–10.

Wright IM (1986) Navicular suspensory desmotomy in the treatment of navicular disease: technique and preliminary results. *Eq Vet J* **18**(6), 443–6.

The phalanges and interphalangeal joints

The distal interphalangeal (DIP) joint (coffin joint)

The DIP joint is well protected from most external insults by the surrounding hoof. However, it will be involved in fractures of 2nd and 3rd phalanx and the navicular bone, in navicular disease, occasionally in traumatic penetrations of the sole or wall and by sub-chondral cysts of the pedal bone. The joint reacts to insult in the manner of all joints, degenerative disease being the sequel. This occurs only rarely in isolation from other conditions and it is usually masked by their presence. Degenerative disease of the DIP joint is often seen in association with navicular disease and degenerative joint disease (DJD) of the proximal interphalangeal (PIP) and meta-carpophalangeal (MCP) articulations as part of a 'polyarthritis syndrome' of the distal digit.

Clinical signs

Alone, arthritis would produce a non-specific lameness, and no external signs.

Diagnosis

A palmar digital nerve block (PDNB) might cause a partial improvement in the lameness which would be abolished by an abaxial sesamoid nerve block (ASNB). An intra-articular block would provide hard evidence.

Radiography

A straight lateromedial centred on the joint is the projection of choice. Variations in cartilage depth cannot be seen unless gross, but osteophytes on the dorsal and palmar articular borders may be visible (Fig. 4.13). Care should be taken to distinguish the articular margin of the 3rd phalanx from the adjacent extensor process. Lesions of the extensor process will also produce new bone but these are outside the joint and not on the articular margin. However, coffin joint degenerative disease and extensor process lesions can coexist and may have the same aetiology (see pyramidal disease pp. 50−52).

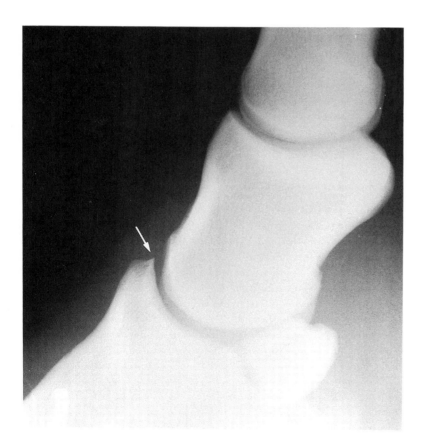

Fig. 4.13 A periarticular osteophyte is visible (arrowed) in this lateromedial projection of a pedal bone.

Treatment

1 Treatment of an initiating cause such as a fractured 3rd phalanx.
2 A NSAID such as phenylbutazone, to provide a general level of analgesia especially if there is extra-articular change or fracture of adjacent bones.
3 Digital neurectomy; both dorsal and palmar digital branches must be cut.
4 Hyaluronic acid in the rare cases of individual coffin joint DJD.
5 Surgical arthrodesis of the DIP joint is not feasible.

Phalangeal exostosis (ring-bone)

Definition

The term phalangeal exostosis describes a condition where new bone of periosteal origin forms usually on the dorsal, dorsolateral and dorsomedial aspects of the 1st and 2nd phalanx and the extensor process of the 3rd phalanx. When the new bone growth is on the distal 1st and/or proximal 2nd phalanx the lay term 'high ring-bone' is used, if on the distal 2nd and proximal 3rd phalanx it is 'low ring-bone'. It is further classified into 'periarticular' where the exostoses abutt the joint capsule, or 'articular' if periosteal, periarticular new bone growth is accompanied by the osteo and enthesiphytes of degenerative joint disease. Therefore a high articular ring-bone would involve the PIP joint and a low articular ring-bone the DIP articulation.

In many texts there is the inference that the periarticular reaction encroaches on the joint and eventually causes the articular pathology. This is doubtless true in some instances, but PIP and DIP arthritis can be a sequel to many insults, such as fractures or subchondral cysts, etc. To lump all cases of DJD of the PIP and DIP articulations under the common heading of 'articular ring-bone' is misleading.

Aetiology and pathogenesis

Trauma is the usual aetiology of phalangeal exostoses or 'ring-bone'. Direct blows, from fence rails, etc., excess strain on the collateral fibrous joint capsules and traction on the ligaments which bind the common extensor tendon to the phalanges can cause disturbances of the periosteum. This then reacts causing inflammation and new bone growth (Fig. 4.14). Instability of the PIP joint has also been blamed, as has poor conformation. 'Base wide' animals are said to be predisposed to changes on the medial side, with the converse occurring in 'base narrow' horses especially if they have a toe-in or toe-out deviation as well. One authority believes such conformational abnormalities, and therefore a predisposition to ring-bone, to be inheritable.

If the insertion of the common extensor tendon on to the 3rd phalanx is strained, then tearing of tendon fibres, periosteal attachments, or small avulsion fractures may occur, leading to extensive new bone growth on the extensor process. This is often included in

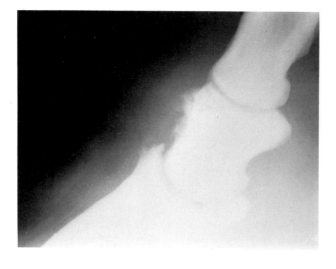

Fig. 4.14 This Shire stallion had suffered a blow to the dorsal coronary band region some years previously. Note the well established new bone on the dorsal 2nd phalanx, on the extensor process of the 3rd phalanx and on the articular margin of the DIP joint.

the 'low ring-bone' group, but, as a condition with a fairly specific aetiology, it is best regarded as a separate entity — commonly called pyramidal disease or 'buttress foot' (see section on pyramidal disease, pp. 50–52).

Periosteal exostoses on the palmar or plantar lateral or medial aspects of the 1st phalanx are sometimes seen as incidental findings. They may run the entire length of its shaft but since they do not occur at the insertion or origin of any structure and do not impinge on a joint they are of dubious significance.

Clinical signs and diagnosis of phalangeal exostoses

The condition occurs in both fore and hind limbs with or without PIP and DIP joint arthritis. The associated lameness is usually gradual in onset, and if the condition is bilateral, may be relatively advanced before it is noticed. It will be exacerbated by flexion tests and by lunging. It shows no particular characteristics to distinguish it from navicular disease, for example.

Physical examination may detect pain at the site and occasionally swelling, but the pain response must be consistent and the swelling marked before it is regarded as significant. (Coronary band swelling will make the hair in the region 'stand on end'.) To those unused to palpation, the region of the distal epiphysis of the 1st phalanx can feel abnormally large. Heat is always being felt by lay people in feet and again temperature differences must be marked before being taken into account.

In chronic cases there can be swelling at the dorsal coronary band and/or a 'thickening' of the pastern region, easiest to feel in thin skinned horses.

A PDNB will have little effect unless done high up the pastern, but an ASNB should abolish the lameness. Intra-articular blocks are *essential* where radiographic evidence is equivocal and surgical arthrodesis is being considered. Extensive periarticular new bone can make the technique difficult, though fortunately radiographic diagnosis is more certain in these cases.

Treatment

Early cases — before bone formation

Early cases are difficult to diagnose, but treatment must be rest for a minimum of 3 months. The ideal method is immobilization in a cast for 4 weeks; at the very least pressure bandaging to prevent accumulation of inflammatory products and reduce swelling and subsequent reaction.

Long-standing cases with new bone formation

If the new bone has, radiographically, an aggressive appearance but is away from the articulations, then adequate rest again is the answer, with immobilization if possible — pressure bandaging at the very least is indicated.

Chronic lesions not affecting the joints

If the lesion is long standing and of *proven* significance and the bony reaction is established, rest alone is unlikely to cause further improvement. In these cases NSAIDs such as phenylbutazone may produce some improvment, or a dorsal digital neurectomy will offer a more permanent solution. (First assess the effect of the proposed neurectomy with selective nerve blocks.) *NB* chronic lesions of this type, away from joints, are not common causes of lameness.

Lesions affecting the articulations

DIP joint.   Surgical arthrodesis of the DIP joint is not feasible so, if this is involved, the prognosis for a return to soundness is not good. NSAIDs or a dorsal digital neurectomy are the only possibilities for treatment. (Use selective nerve blocks to assess the effect of the proposed neurectomy.) *NB* once the dorsal aspect of the joint is involved, the whole articulation will become affected. Under these circumstances, a dorsal digital neurectomy will not be completely effective. Anti-arthritic drugs such as hyaluronic acid or the polysulphated glycosaminoglycans are also unlikely to be effective because of the periarticular changes.

PIP joint.   Surgical arthrodesis is the treatment of choice for DJD of the pastern from whatever cause when only this articulation is involved. If other joints are affected, then NSAIDs with maybe a reduction in work load is the only practical approach. Arthrodesis of the PIP joint carries a good prognosis, though better in the hind than the forelimbs. (Survey results are 80% return to working soundness for the hind limb, 60% for the fore.) Bilateral surgery is feasible.

Several techniques for surgical arthrodesis have been devised. The following technique has been used successfully by many people, including the author.

A C-shaped incision is made in the dorsal surface of the pastern. The PIP joint is exposed through a Z-plasty of the common extensor tendon. The joint is opened through section of its dorsal joint capsule and the articular cartilage completely curretted away. The subchondral bone surfaces are apposed and compressed by three or four cortical screws inserted 'lag' fashion from the 1st phalanx to the 2nd phalanx (Figs. 4.15a and b). The leg is immobilized in a cast for the anaesthetic recovery period. Although some surgeons will leave the cast on for 3 months the author has not found this to be necessary and removes the cast after 3–4 days, allowing proper wound care. Post-operative management is walking *in hand* for 3 months, increasing the amount of exercise slowly and then, if radiographic examination shows satisfactory progress, the animal is allowed to go to more strenuous work. The total lay-off period is 6–9 months.

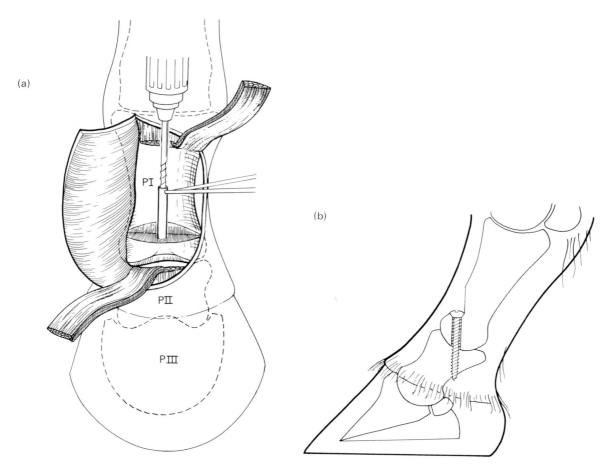

(a)

(b)

Fig. 4.15 (a) Illustration of the access obtained to the PIP joint and showing the drilling of the gliding hole in the 1st phalanx. (b) A lateral projection of the same area showing the relationship of the screws to the two phalanges.

Subchondral bone cysts

Subchondral bone cysts have been reported to occur in the stifle, and most articulations of the lower limb. The frequency with which they are seen at various sites seems to vary between, and even within, countries. This might be due to variations in the predominant type of animal, or maybe in management practices such as feeding or exercise and work patterns.

Aetiology and pathogenesis

Three possible causes have suggested for the cysts: infection, osteochondrosis and trauma. All implicate damage to the cartilage surface followed by penetration of synovial fluid under pressure into the subchondral bone. This aspect of the scenario is given credibility by the tendency for these cysts to enlarge over a period of months or years. However, it does not explain those cases where cysts are incidental findings and on further examination appear to have no contact with the joint at all.

When communication is present the pain associated with the cyst probably arises from two sources; firstly the release of irritant material into the joint cavity causing a synovitis and secondly the permeation of synovial fluid, under pressure, into the subchondral bone.

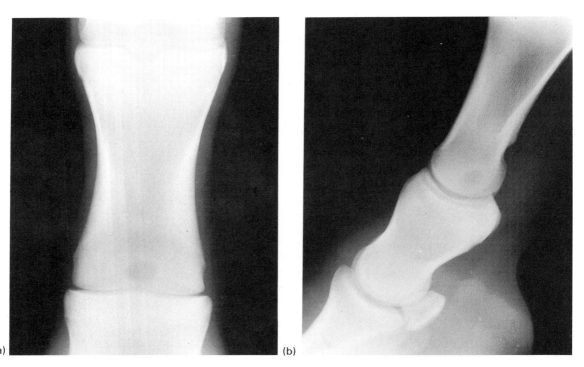

(a) (b)

Fig. 4.16 (a) A dorsopalmar projection of a 1st phalanx showing the subchondral bone cyst affecting the pastern joint. (b) A lateromedial projection of the same cyst.

Clinical signs

Whilst not exclusively so, the animal is likely to be young. The lameness onset is variable, though often sudden, and its severity too, varies considerably. Local signs are minimal, though usually there may be some local swelling and resentment to palpation of the pastern region.

Diagnosis

There is nothing particularly characteristic about the gait abnormality produced by subchondral bone cysts and they are usually discovered following a routine work-up and/or radiography of the area (Figs. 4.16a and b). Their significance can be checked by intra-articular anaesthesia of the PIP or DIP joints and this would be essential if arthrodesis were to be considered as a treatment. Also, contrast radiography, i.e. performing an arthrogram, would confirm the cyst's communication with the joint cavity. The technique is simple. Four or 5 ml of a water soluble contrast medium should be injected into the joint maintaining strict asepsis (see section on intra-articular anaesthesia, pp. 15–22, for details of the approach). The animal is then exercised lightly for 4 or 5 minutes and re-radiographed. The films are examined for evidence of penetration of contrast medium into the cyst cavity.

Treatment

Many animals respond well to a period of rest, 2–3 months, becoming sound over that period. Enclosing the distal limb in a cast has been suggested as a device to restrict movement and encourage healing. The long term prognosis is good enough to warrant this period of rest, though recurrence and the prospect of DJD must be considered and discussed with the owner. The ultimate treatment for cysts involving the pastern is, of course, arthrodesis. With its good success rate and minimum interference with the animal's function it is a very viable alternative and should be seriously considered in those cases which do not respond to simple conservative therapy.

Degenerative disease of the PIP joint

Degenerative disease of the PIP joint is often found as a clinical entity in association with DJD of the fetlock joint and clinical navicular disease. In these cases, which are often young animals of 5 years and upwards, bilateral involvement is demonstrable with both regional *and intra-articular* anaesthesia. In a proportion of cases there will be similarly demonstrable osteoarthritic changes in the hind limb articulations too, causing lameness which might initially be masked, but which will respond in the usual way to flexion tests. Radiographic examination shows variable degrees of periarticular osteophyte production (Figs. 4.17a and b). Where clinical navicular disease coexists, the presence of the concurrent multi-articular DJD will compromise the treatment of the navicular problem. In these cases treatment of

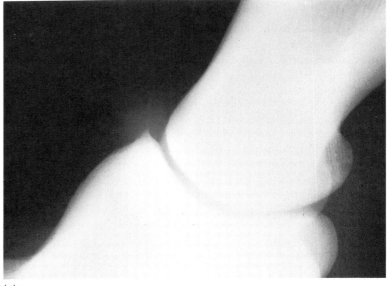

(a)

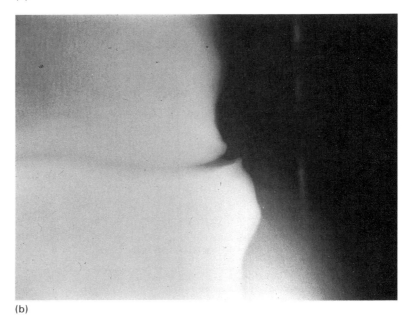

(b)

Fig. 4.17 (a) A pronounced periarticular osteophyte on the dorsoproximal 2nd phalanx. The fact that this change was associated with pain in the joint was demonstrated convincingly when intra-articular anaesthesia of this articulation produced a marked improvement in the animal's lameness. (b) A dorsopalmar projection of the same articulation showing that the osteophyte is not an isolated spur but extends as a 'collar' around the joint.

individual joints by, for example, intra-articular sodium hyaluronate or arthrodesis is not practical and the only feasible course of action is that the treatment of navicular disease must be supplemented by NSAIDs. The prognosis for complete return to soundness must be guarded.

Suggested further reading

Genetzky RM, Schneider EJ, Butler HC and Guffy MM (1981) Comparison of two surgical procedures for arthrodesis of the proximal interphalangeal joints in horses. *J Am Vet Med Ass* **179**(95), 464–8.

Hoffman KD, Pool RR and Pascoe JR (1984) Degenerative joint disease of the proximal interphalangeal joints of the forelimbs of two young horses. *Eq Vet J* **16**(2), 138–40.

Martin GS, McIlwraith CW, Turner AS, Nixon AJ and Stashak TS (1984) Long term results and complications of proximal interphalangeal arthrodesis in horses *J Am Vet Med Ass* **184**(9), 1136–40.

The metacarpo/phalangeal (MCP) (fetlock) joint

Diseases of the fetlock (MCP, MTP) articulation

The MCP or fetlock joint is susceptible to injury because its angular design renders it liable to extreme hyperextension as well as suffering the profound compressive, tensile and torque forces of hard athletic work. The hyperextension causes a marked tension on the palmar or plantar aspect of the joint and marked compressive effects dorsally. Heavy loads, tests of endurance or agility, lack of fitness, bad conformation, etc. all add to the stresses and strains imposed on this highly mobile and vulnerable articulation.

The anatomy of the fetlock joint is shown in Figs. 4.18a, b, c and d.

Fig. 4.18 (a) and (b) Diagrammatic representations of some important anatomical aspects of the fetlock articulation. (c) and (d) Diagrammatic illustrations of the relationship of the suspensory apparatus to the fetlock joints.

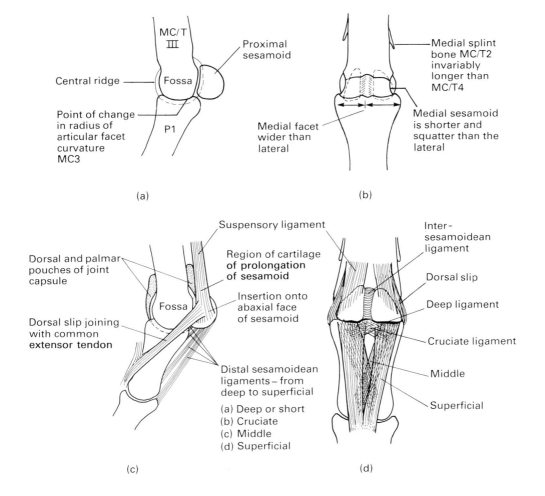

Type of lameness produced by fetlock disease

Fetlock pathology may occur in association with changes in other articulations especially the pastern, and is often not confined to one limb. It is frequently bilateral so that its effects on gait may be masked or merely a small part of the total lameness picture. It also occurs as a single joint problem as a result of trauma, infection, osteochondrosis, etc. It must be appreciated that all insults to joints have one common sequel, DJD; this may be the first thing that is recognized; the initiating injury to the joint may never be known.

Physical examination of the fetlock joint

Don't think about it as a 'fetlock', think of it as a metacarpophalangeal articulation with added sesamoids. A good analogy is to visualize the joint as a set of bones sitting in a springy armchair of suspensory ligaments and flexor tendons. An examination should aim at evaluating all the component parts of the articulation, paying especial attention to whether there is

1 Soft tissue swelling in subcutaneous tissue, collateral and suspensory ligaments and tendons.

2 Distension of the joint capsule, best appreciated as a variably tense, fluid-filled swelling *between* the cannon bone and the suspensory ligament (articular wind-gall or wind-puff).

3 Distension of the flexor or sesamoidean sheath; presenting as a tubular fluid-filled distension extending around the flexor tendons for some 5 cm proximal to the constricting volar annular ligament (tendinous wind-gall or wind-puff).

Local anaesthesia of the fetlock

Firstly, anaesthetize the limb distal to the fetlock with an ASNB. Then opt for either intra-articular anaesthesia or a four-point block (see section on nerve blocks, p. 12). *NB* four-point blocks do not *completely* desensitize the fetlock and intra-articular anaesthesia will not remove pain from extrasynovial structures affected by conditions such as osteoarthritis or some of the proximal sesamoid fractures. Therefore, no response to the local anaesthesia is no guarantee of non-involvement of the fetlock.

Where tendon sheath lesions are suspected, this structure too can be selectively anaesthetized by intrasheath local.

Radiography

The initial DP projection should be angled 30° downwards and centred on the joint itself. The cassette is held snugly against and parallel to the pastern. This projects the bone of the sesamoids clear of the MCP joint. To visualize the sesamoids clearly a well-exposed film is necessary.

The straight lateromedial projection is a good initial screening view. However, it will not demonstrate the distal borders of the sesamoids or the two slightly sloping dorsoproximal borders of the 1st phalanx.

Flexed laterals show the distal sesamoid outlines well and allow better evaluation of sesamoid and proximal 1st phalanx fractures.

Beyond these three basic screening views the radiographer has unlimited scope and should adopt a flexible approach, 'shooting for the lesion'. With a good light-beam diaphragm several projections of this compact area can economically be obtained on one film. Special views to demonstrate specific lesions will be mentioned in their context.

Contrast radiography can be useful to demonstrate space-occupying lesions such as villonodular changes, or to demonstrate the origin of sinus tracts. Contrast studies of the tendon sheath are also feasible (Fig. 4.19). Any water soluble contrast medium may be used: barium or oily iodine preparations must not be injected into synovial structures.

Sampling and examination of synovial fluid can provide some additional information (see section on synovial fluid analysis, p. 277) and synovial membrane biopsy, if feasible, is the best method of providing material for bacterial culture in septic arthritis.

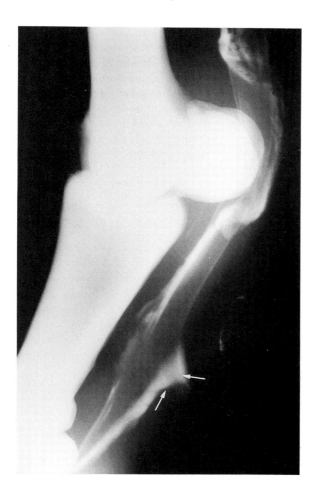

Fig. 4.19 Contrast medium injected into this flexor sheath has outlined a 'slip' of DFT (arrowed) which has become adherent to the deep face of a healed overreach wound on the palmar pastern. Following section of this slip of DFT, the animal's persistent lameness resolved.

Fetlock disease of the young animal

The first signs of fetlock disease can appear at a very early age. It is probably caused by stress, strain and concussion on the immature joints (see section on DJD, p. 273), aggravated by under-preparation and overwork of the young athlete, and exacerbated by conformational defects. *The pressures of the racing world make it inevitable that a high proportion of young stock will develop distal limb joint disease for these very reasons!*

The first signs are a serous arthritis with synovial effusion and the development of a joint capsule distension, the so-called articular wind-gall. (The same changes probably occur in the interphalangeal joints but are not obvious.) If the signs are not recognized and training continues then the degenerative process will progress with thickening of the joint capsule and eventually bony change.

In the early stages lameness is minimal and probably being bilateral will be very difficult to detect; however, the development of joint distension is the cardinal danger sign.

Treatment is rest or, at the very least, a substantial reduction in activity. Many 'cures' have been devised ranging from those with some pharmacological basis to frank witchcraft. All pander to the enormous economic pressures to keep a young horse working. Any treatment which maintains the animal in work is, however, simply creating and storing up problems for the animal's future. Following a period of rest the return to work should be gradual with close attention being paid to the state of the fetlocks.

Cases of capsular distension which do not respond to rest need more extensive investigation. In young adults osteochondritis dissecans of the sagittal ridge of the cannon bones has been described (Yovich *et al* 1985), and villonodular changes of the synovial membrane have been described (Nickels *et al* 1976) as a consequence of chronic irritation of the fetlock joint.

Osteochondritis dissecans (OCD) of the fetlock

Osteochondritis dissecans has been reported to occur primarily at two sites in the fetlock. One is the distal palmar aspect of the cannon and the other is the sagittal ridge. The condition is usually seen in young, well grown horses and often associated with the onset of hard training. There may be little lameness at first examination, though bilateral involvement, which is common, may mask a gait abnormality. Fetlock flexion tests will usually elicit pain and local examination of the joint will probably demonstrate a fluid distension of the palmar pouch of the joint capsule.

Diagnosis

The clinical signs therefore are not particularly specific for OCD and diagnosis is heavily dependant upon radiography. In the case of sagittal ridge lesions, good quality lateromedial (LM) projections exposed for peripheral bone detail will show flattening or erosion and irregularity of the sagittal ridge.

Lesions on the palmar articular surface are more difficult to demonstrate. They occur at, and palmar to, the transverse ridge which marks the point at which the radius of curvature of the articular facet changes. As such they will not be highlighted by a conventional dorsopalmar (DP) projection, nor will they be well visualized in an LM projection because of the thickness of superimposed bone. Hornof and O'Brien (1980) described a 125° DP metacarpal skyline projection (125° DPMS) which allows good visualization of this area and demonstrates the lesions as irregularly marginated lucencies of the subchondral bone. Whilst the projection is not the simplest to make, it offers the only means of evaluation of the site and should be attempted if the clinical signs warrant. It is also useful in determining if there is comminution of metacarpal condylar fractures (see section on cannon bone fracture, p. 254).

Treatment

Removal of fragments and debridement of the parent sites is the only effective treatment. Whilst this is feasible for the sagittal ridge lesions, either through an arthrotomy, or ideally, via arthroscopy, the same is not true of the palmar lesions. Their position makes them virtually inaccessible and the prognosis is extremely poor. Rest is a poor alternative, and the animals usually remain lame and progress rapidly to a chronic fetlock DJD.

A proportion of animals suffering from sagittal ridge lesions will, with early and thorough treatment, return to work. Unfortunately, a high proportion are not diagnosed until later when DJD has become well established.

Villonodular synovitis

Villonodular synovitis has been reported to occur in horses of all ages, except the very young. It is characterized by the development over a few months of a circumscribed mass within the joint cavity. The lesions bear a great resemblance to those seen in many joints in man. The similarity also extends to the fact that in neither horse nor man is the aetiology known for certain. It is an inflammatory lesion, not neoplastic, and chronic trauma is the most likely cause. The cortical erosion which it produces is the result of pressure of the mass on the bone.

Clinical signs

Initially the animals present with a non-characteristic lameness which is exacerbated by lunging and flexion tests. There may be few local signs at first but later fetlock joint distension becomes obvious and a firm soft tissue swelling becomes evident over the dorsal surface of the joint.

Diagnosis

Once the fetlock has been pinpointed as the source of the pain by clinical and nerve block examination, the diagnosis of villonodular synovitis is made on radiographic evidence. On lateromedial projections, smooth bordered depressions will be seen in the dorsal and/or palmar cortex of the cannon bone just proximal to their articular surface. The presence of a soft tissue mass at this site and elsewhere within the joint can be confirmed by positive contrast arthrography. This is a simple procedure and carries very little risk if aseptic precautions are adhered to. Five millilitres of a water soluble contrast agent is injected into the joint cavity and after a little exercise to disperse the contrast medium throughout the joint, the radiographic examination is repeated. The masses will show as obvious filling defects in the dorsal or palmar pouches.

Treatment

The only effective therapy is excision of the mass which must be carried out through an arthrotomy, or occasionally two parallel incisions if the lesion is very large. Following extirpation of the soft tissue mass, the exposed bone is curetted clean, the joint irrigated, and the incisions closed routinely. Post-operative management consists of early rest and pressure bandaging but with a slow introduction to exercise after 2–3 weeks of inactivity. Increasing amounts of hand walking will lead after 2–3 months to light trotting with a return to training delayed until 6 months post-surgery.

Examination of the masses show them to be composed mainly of dense collaginous connective tissue lined by a single layer of synovial epithelium. Occasionally there is some hyaline or osseous change within the stroma.

Suggested further reading

Hornof WJ and O'Brien TR (1980) Radiographic evaluation of the palmar aspect of the equine metacarpal condyles: A new projection. *Vet Radiology* **21**(4), 161–7.

Nickels FA, Grant BD and Lincoln SD (1976) Villonodular synovitis of the equine metacarpophalangeal joint. *J Am Vet Med Ass* **168**(11), 1043–6.

Yovich JV, McIllwraith CW and Stashak TS (1985) Osteochondritis dissecans of the sagittal ridge of the third metacarpal and metatarsal bones in horses. *J Am Vet Med Ass* **186**(11), 1186–91.

Chronic and advanced DJD (osteoarthritis)

The reaction to injury of any joint is limited and the end result of sustained insult is invariably chronic osteoarthritis of variable severity. Therefore in many cases, the degenerative changes will take over from the initiating cause, e.g. in the case of intra-articular chip fractures, as the prime cause of the pain and lameness.

Clinical signs

The main clinical sign is lameness of variable severity but with no particularly distinguishing characteristics which will be unaffected by an ASNB but wholly *or greatly* diminished by a four-point fetlock block or by intra-articular anaesthesia. Capsular distension is a variable feature as is periarticular thickening.

Radiographic appearance of osteoarthritis

Advanced cases of osteoarthritis will usually have radiographically identifiable and characteristic changes. Most are best seen on a flexed lateral and are

1 New bone formation (osteophytes) at the articular margins. Small osteophytes on the dorsoproximal border of the 1st phalanx often need bright light illumination to visualize them. Examples of these changes in profile are seen in Figs. 4.20 a and b.
2 Demineralization (irregularity) of the sagittal ridge (Fig. 4.21).
3 Concavities of the distal, dorsal and/or palmar cannon (Fig. 4.22) caused by pressure from villonodular lesions, fibrosis and inflammatory changes in the dorsal and volar capsular pouches.
4 Subchondral demineralization.

Controversy exists as to what level of change is 'normal' in older, hard working horses. In these, and younger animals, changes must, unless severe, be shown to be clinically significant by regional or intra-articular analgesia. However, their presence indicates that degenerative change has taken place and that even if the animal is apparently not lame at the time of examination, these changes are

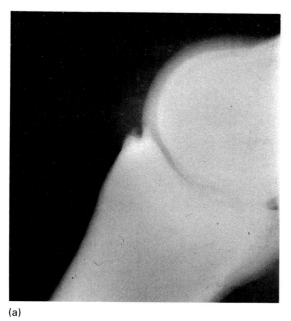

(a)

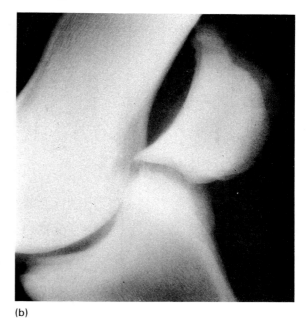

(b)

Fig. 4.20 (a) Obvious periarticular osteophytes visible on a dorsoproximal 1st phalanx. (b) Sesamoids showing massive new bone deposition at their proximal and distal margins. Most cases show more subtle changes.

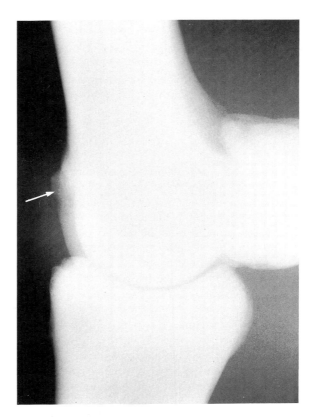

Fig. 4.21 Demineralization and irregularity of the mid-sagittal ridge (arrowed). There are also changes on the dorsoproximal aspect of the 1st phalanx and the proximal sesamoids.

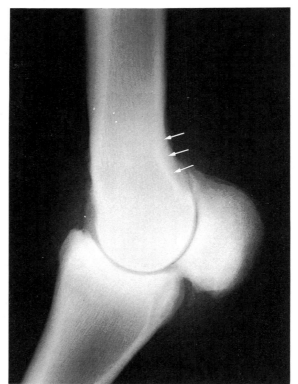

Fig. 4.22 A case of advanced degenerative joint disease showing a palmar concavity in the distal cannon.

present, are irreversible and have the potential to result in lameness at some future date. They must not be simply dismissed as irrelevant!

Fetlock DJD in association with other joint problems

Changes of DJD are often seen in the fetlock associated with similar lesions in the PIP, DIP and small tarsal joints and with clinical navicular disease. The aetiology of these lesions is in doubt, but the fact that they are associated with pain and are part of complex distal limb polyarthritis syndrome has been shown repeatedly by selective nerve block and intra-articular anaesthesia (Wyn-Jones 1986 unpublished data). Quite extensive lesions are seen in young adults and are likely to complicate and confuse both the diagnosis and treatment of navicular disease.

Treatment (for greater detail, see section on DJD, p. 273)

The efficacy of long term results of any treatment will be related to the duration and severity of the joint changes. In this context, absence of radiographic signs does *not* mean absence of pathological change, only absence of *bony* change. *NB* the pathological sequelae of advanced osteoarthritis are, by and large, irreversible; also, the coexistence of pathological processes elsewhere may make individual joint therapy inappropriate or futile.

Main types of treatment are

1 Removal of the initiating cause — e.g. overwork, chip fractures, infection, etc.

2 Rest — this is the most beneficial therapy in early cases and should be for a period of 3–4 weeks followed by a gradual introduction of walking exercise.

3 Systemic therapy. This is of little value unless NSAIDs such as phenylbutazone are being used for their *analgesic* effects in multiple joint or intractable individual joint problems.

4 Intra-articular therapy.

(a) Corticosteroid — its potential anti-inflammatory effects will produce a rapid diminution of clinical signs. However, its side effects (see section on anti-inflammatory drugs, p. 279) are considerable, especially the temptation to put the animal back to work too soon following the rapid clinical improvement. Informed opinion suggests that it is indicated in very few cases of DJD.

(b) Hyaluronic acid — sodium hyaluronate. Clinical evidence suggests that hyaluronic acid is superior to corticosteroid for the treatment of DJD in that healing processes are unaffected or promoted rather than suppressed. Its effects, however, are not consistent and become less predictable and satisfactory with increasing severity of the disease.

Many dose rates and injection protocols have been suggested but there is no basis for disagreeing fundamentally with the recommendations of the commercial suppliers.

(c) Glycosaminoglycan polysulphate. Used in man and the horse both in Europe and USA.

Chip fractures of the MCP articulation

Dorsoproximal 1st phalanx fractures are caused by hyperextension of the fetlock joint. They present in the acute phase as a sudden onset lameness with varying degrees of joint capsule distension, increased pain on joint flexion and discomfort on palpation of the site. They may also be seen radiographically during investigation of chronic lameness (Fig. 4.23) and then their clinical significance may be in doubt. Some are said to be separate centres of ossification but there is unfortunately no sure way of distinguishing radiographically between them; the presence of an apparent fracture 'bed' is not sufficient evidence.

Separate ossification centres are often bilateral and incidental findings. If pain is localized to the fetlock, there is no other discernible cause and the lesion is unilateral, then there is grounds for suspicion that the lesion is significant.

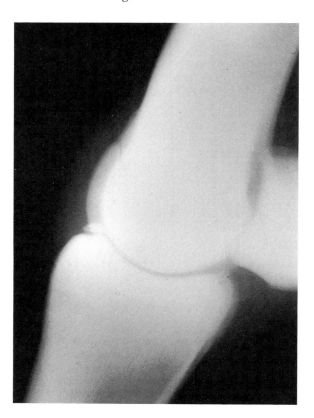

Fig. 4.23 A 'chip' fracture or separate ossification centre of dorsoproximal 1st phalanx.

Treatment

In the acute case, 3 months enforced rest with support bandaging of the fetlock is usually sufficent.

If the fragment is large or the cause of recurrent bouts of lameness, removal is indicated. Arthroscopically aided surgery is the ideal; however, arthrotomy can be performed, although there is some increased risk of post-operative osteoarthritis, periarticular new bone growth and reduced joint movement. Identification of the affected side by carefully marked oblique films is essential to ensure the arthrotomy is made on the correct side of the digital extensor tendon, (usually medial).

Avulsion fractures of the proximopalmar margin of the 1st phalanx (Fig. 4.24), at the insertion of the short distal sesamoidean ligaments occur principally in the hind legs of trotters (Petterson and Ryden 1982).

They affect predominantly the medial aspect of the 1st phalanx, are best visualized on a well-penetrated, conventional dorsopalmar radiograph and on judiciously angled obliques. Because of the considerable concavity of the proximopalmar 1st phalanx contour they do not show up well on straight or flexed lateral views.

They are a cause of lameness and although a conservative approach has been recommended by some authors, surgical removal is a more certain method of treatment. The somewhat difficult approach is via an incision in the proximal palmar pouch, with the fetlock then being placed in hyperflexion to facilitate access to the fragment between the palmar metacarpal condyle and the sesamoids.

Other intra-articular chip fractures can occur and cause pain and lameness. Their presence initiates degenerative change within the joint and they should be removed. Early detection of these fractures is

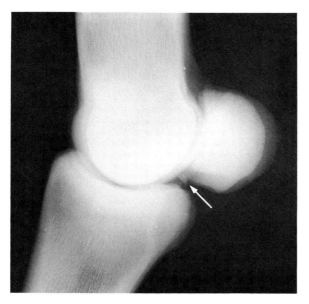

Fig. 4.24 An avulsion fracture of the proximopalmar margin of the 1st phalanx. Unusually, it shows up well on this slightly obliqued lateromedial projection.

essential if DJD is not to be a significant feature. *This means radiography at an early stage.* As a guideline — if conservative therapy has not produced dramatic improvement within *1 week* of the onset of lameness then the joint must be radiographed.

Suggested further reading

Pettersson H and Ryden G (1982) Avulsion fractures of the caudoproximal extremity of the 1st phalanx. *Eq Vet J* **14**(4), 333–5.

The proximal sesamoids

The proximal sesamoids are sesamoid bones formed *within* the suspensory ligament; their dorsal cartilages form some 30–40% of the distal articulation of the fetlock, and they *cannot* be considered in isolation from either ligaments or joint.

The proximal suspensory ligament blends with the sloping abaxial face of the bones, and its pull is transmitted on by the numerous ligaments which arise from the entire base of the sesamoid bones and run distally to the 1st and 2nd phalanx. The axial faces of the bones are the origin of the intersesamoidean ligament. They are therefore buried in ligamentous tissue and have only the cartilage-covered articular face visible. (see Figs. 4.18c and d).

Sesamoiditis

Sesamoiditis is a bad name since it simply means inflammation of the sesamoid. However, it is widely used to signify the lesions produced by tearing of either proximal or distal suspensory ligament fibres of the ligament/bone interface, with or without avulsion fractures. Inflammatory change principally affects the ligament and bone, often with effects extending to associated structures such as collateral and annual ligaments, tendon sheath, the fetlock articulation and subcutaneous tissues.

Aetiology and pathogenesis

Aberrant or undue stress and strain on the suspensory apparatus can produce tearing of ligament fibres or avulsion fractures. The normal hyperextension of the fetlock joint, which occurs at speed or when landing from a jump, places an enormous load on these attachments. Injuries are more likely to occur in competition animals, especially if unfit, tired and uncoordinated.

Clinical signs

Clinical signs include acute onset of moderate to severe lameness with diffuse swelling around the sesamoid region and pain on palpation and manipulation. The swelling can take several hours to become noticeable. There may be distension of the fetlock joint capsule too. The animal will hold the fetlock in a semiflexed position and not allow it to descend to a normal level.

In chronically affected animals the swelling will be firm, painless and localized to the area of the sesamoid. Ligamentous thickening may be present proximal to the bone.

Diagnosis

In the acute injury local symptoms are a good indicator. However, radiography is *essential* to eliminate major sesamoid or other fractures. In the chronic case local evidence is not reliable; other causes of lameness may be present in the limb and selective nerve blocks must be used (ASNB followed by a palmar block). Radiography will frequently show new bone growth on the surface of the sesamoid bone, often radiating irregularly from the bone profile; (Figs. 4.25a and b) and calcification or ossification of the proximal and, less frequently, the distal sesamoidean ligaments. There may also be mottling of the bone opacity, in part caused by superimposed new bone, an increased coarseness of bone trabeculation and avulsion fractures.

Disuse osteopenia. In long standing, severely lame animals, which have refused to take proper weight on a limb for some time, 'granular' lucencies of the sesamoid bones become apparent. This would seem to be the first indication of a disuse osteopenia which eventually progresses to a stage where the sesamoids appear delicate and lace-like: 'ghost sesamoids' (Fig. 4.26).

Vascular channels. Some controversy exists as to the importance of vascular channels within sesamoids. They are seen in approximately 50% of cases. In normal animals they are small, well defined and fewer than four in number. With disease they are said to increase in numbers and size (see Fig. 4.25a). However, such variations may be seen occasionally in animals which are not lame, and clinical evidence

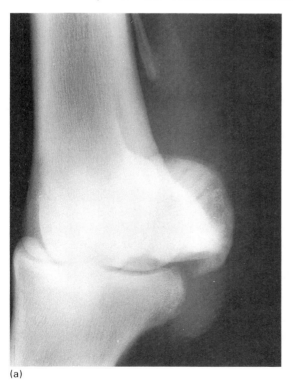

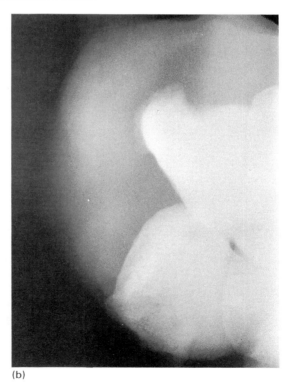

(a)   (b)

Fig. 4.25 (a) Very prominent vascular channels are seen in this sesamoid. There is also evidence of new bone growth around its periphery. (b) With the beam centre angled at 60° to the horizontal, this lateral to medial projection, centred on the sesamoids, shows clearly the new bone referred to in (a). The cassette is held under the sesamoids and at right angles to the beam centre.

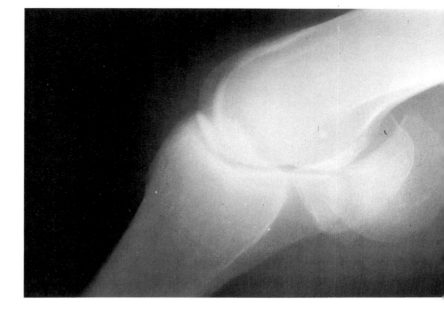

Fig. 4.26 'Ghost' sesamoids — a diffuse osteopenia caused by many months of severe lameness in this leg.

of pain must be present before they can be regarded as significant. Some regard these structures and their alteration in pathology as being akin to the changes occurring in the navicular bone, with bone ischaemia and histological evidence of arteriosclerosis and thrombosis.

Both new bone and avulsion fractures of the abaxial surfaces of the sesamoids can be difficult to visualize by standard techniques. A projection described by Palmer (1982) (Fig. 4.25b) is useful to visualize this area.

DJD change in the fetlock joint may also be present.

Treatment

The best first-aid treatment is a board cast (Fig. 4.27); it provides immediate support, pressure and relief from tension. For these early cases the only subsequent treatment of value is immobilization and rest. Ideally a cast should be applied from, and including, the hoof (see section on casting, p. 266) to just below the carpus, and left on for 2—3 weeks, then changed, or replaced by a heavy pressure bandage. Complete stable rest for 3—4 months is mandatory, followed by walking exercise in hand for a further 2—3 months before the animal is turned out. This too must be carefully managed to prevent the patient's initial exuberance from undoing the good work of the previous months.

Owners must be told unequivocally that these injuries are extremely serious and only time will allow complete healing. A minimum lay-off period of 12 months will give the animal the maximum chance of returning to work; less than this, and recurrence is a strong possibility.

No effective treatment, apart from rest to consolidate healing, is available for the chronic case. Repeated ligament fibre rupture and scar tissue disruption lead to further scarring and weakness of the

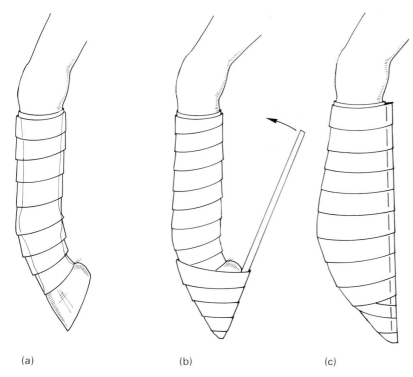

(a) (b) (c)

Fig. 4.27 Three stages in the application of a board cast: (a) A snug pressure bandage is applied to control swelling at the site. (b) A board, or flat piece of wood the same width as the hoof and long enough to extend to below the carpus is taped directly to the hoof with adhesive dressing. (c) The board is brought up to the palmar cannon and bound in place with more adhesive elastic dressing. This provides immobilization of the fetlock and a 'strut' to help the animal bear weight; especially useful during transportation.

suspensory apparatus. *NB* Raising the heel with a block is *contraindicated* — it does not reduce tension on the suspensory apparatus — it increases it because of the reduction in deep flexor tendon support for the fetlock.

Suggested further reading

Palmer SE (1982) Radiography of the abaxial surface of the proximal sesamoid bones of the horse. *J Am Vet Med Ass* **181**(3), 264–5.

Sesamoid fractures in the adult

Aetiology and pathogenesis

Sesamoid fractures principally occur as racing injuries — they are probably caused by the severe distractive forces that the suspensory ligaments exert on the bones during fetlock extension. Trauma, such as being struck by the ipsilateral hind toe, may also play a part. This must also be taken into account when assessing the prognosis.

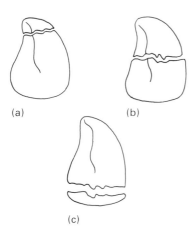

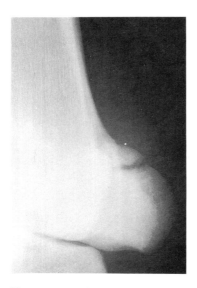

Fig. 4.28 Three types of common sesamoid body fracture: (a) apical; (b) mid-body; (c) basilar.

Fig. 4.29 A 45° DPLMO projection of an apical fracture in a lateral sesamoid. This fracture occurred one month prior to its referral for surgery. Removal of the fragment was difficult because of the extensive fibrous union, yet was necessary because of its misalignment at the articular surface.

Clinical signs

These will vary greatly depending on the location of the fracture whether one or both sesamoids are affected and whether any serious damage to the associated ligaments has occurred. Swelling can range from minimal, in cases of small apical fractures, to obvious in mid-body fractures, with associated fetlock joint and tendon sheath distension. Suspensory disruption can lead to hyperextension of the fetlock. In horses racing on circular tracks, the medial sesamoid on the outer leg is most often involved.

Diagnosis

Any animal showing signs of acute onset pain and swelling in this region should be radiographed early on in the clinical course. Three basic types of fracture may be seen (Fig. 4.28). The fractures will usually involve the articular surface.

Treatment

First aid treatment in any animal with a suspected or potential sesamoid fracture should consist of a heavy pressure bandage at least, and ideally a board cast (see Fig. 4.27).

Apical fractures carry a good prognosis if the fragments are removed *early* (Fig. 4.29). As a guide, fragments less than one third of the length of the sesamoid are amenable to surgery. Healing may take place without surgical intervention but will only carry a reasonable prognosis if the fragments are non-displaced and there are at least 8 months of inactivity; even so, most will heal only by fibrous union. The surgical approach is through the proximal palmar pouch of the joint capsule with the fetlock in hyperflexion. There must be a minimum of disruption to the suspensory ligaments as the fragment is removed.

Transverse, or mid-sesamoidean fractures can be successfully reduced and compressed by the lag-screw technique; again, *the earlier the surgery the better the chances of success*. The technique is made simple by using a special clamp (Synthes) which compresses the fragments and acts as a drill guide. Remember that any disruption of the sesamoid body will have damaged the main suspensory ligament insertions; therefore distracted fractures carry a poorer prognosis for a return to athletic soundness. Conservative treatment usually results in non-union of the fragments, considerable local reaction and fetlock DJD.

Basilar fractures have a *poor* prognosis. They usually involve the entire width of the bone and, because they have little abaxial support from the suspensory ligament insertion, will often be distracted, opening up a wedge-shaped gap.

Removal of the entire distal fragment is not feasible since it removes the origin of the distal sesamoidean ligaments as well. Compression fixation can be difficult because the distal fragment has little depth and may comminute under compressive forces. The fragments will usually heal by fibrous union but be susceptible to refracture, and will, by misalignment and callus formation, invariably produce DJD of the fetlock joint.

The use of cancellous bone grafts has been advocated to help bony union in those cases where the fragments have been distracted, and even in relatively uncomplicated cases as an aid to bone healing. Pulsing magnetic fields have also been used to stimulate fracture repair and are reported to have been effective in accelerating healing where mechanical stability has been achieved.

Sesamoid dehiscence

Fracture of both sesamoids, complete disruption of the distal sesamoidean ligaments at their origin or a combination of both result in sudden onset severe lameness or 'breakdown'. The leg will not bear weight and the fetlock can be hyperextended. Extensive swelling of the sesamoid region is present, and occasionally there may be open luxation of the joint. A common complication to this massive musculoskeletal injury is irreparable damage to the digital arteries, with consequent foot ischaemia.

First aid is by application of a board cast (see Fig. 4.27). Radiography is essential to detect sesamoid fractures.

Salvage for breeding purposes is all that can be hoped for with this condition and the only two treatments available are chronic casting, or fetlock joint arthrodesis. The latter is an extemely difficult technique requiring radical arthrotomy and subsequent compression fixation. Ischaemia and wound breakdown is a frequent complication to the surgery which, if successful, is, however, a better technique than casting. Ideally surgery should be delayed some 14 days to assess vascular integrity. During this time systemic antibiosis is mandatory and it is also suggested that the fetlock area itself be regularly treated with topical disinfectants such as Pevidine to minimize penetration of bacteria through the potentially avascular skin.

T-fracture of the sesamoids

Occasionally the basilar fractures are comminuted, having a vertical fracture line too. Internal fixation of these would be unwise, since the near vertical screw is likely to distract the vertical component of this fracture, and there is insufficient depth of bone to allow placement of a horizontal screw.

Axial fracture

Axial fracture occasionally occurs in association with lateral or medial third metacarpal condylar slab fractures. It may be overlain by the main cannon fracture and consequently missed on the straight dorsopalmar (DP) radiograph. Slightly oblique DPs are necessary to visualize it. Displacement is minimal and surgical repair is not usually indicated. It is thought that they probably heal without specific treatment.

Proximal sesamoid fractures in young foals

Young thoroughbred foals have been reported to have a relatively high incidence of proximal sesamoid fracture. The main aetiological factor is believed to be when the foal, usually under 2 months of age, gallops to exhaustion trying to follow its long legged dam (Ellis 1979). This often occurs when the pair are turned out for the first time and one of the suggested preventative measures is the provision of small 'nursery' paddocks.

The fractures may be simple and apical, mid-body or basilar or they may be comminuted; distraction may or may not be a feature. They involve the forelegs principally, can affect both sesamoids in one leg and both legs can be affected. Most animals are lame initially but the pain diminishes rapidly and some cases may be missed. Occasional foals are only mildly lame even at the outset.

Treatment is usually by pressure bandaging and box rest for 4 weeks or so. Chip and small apical or basilar fragments can be removed surgically with an improved prognosis. Comminuted fractures or those with large distracted fragments carry a poorer prognosis as do those cases where both legs are involved.

Suggested further reading

Bowman KF, Leitch M, Nunamaker DM, Fackelman GE, Tate Jr. LP, Park MI, Bales CL and Raker CW (1984) Complications during treatment of traumatic disruption of the suspensory apparatus in thoroughbred horses. *J Am Vet Med Ass* **184**(6), 706–15.

Ellis D (1979) Fracture of the proximal sesamoid bones in thoroughbred horses. *Eq Vet J* **11**(11), 48–52.

Fackelman GE and Nunamaker DM (1982) *Manual of Internal Fixation in the Horse*, pp. 53–5 and 80–5. Springer-Verlag, New York.

Grant BD (1982) The sesamoid bones In *Equine Medicine and Surgery* 3e RA Mansmann, ES McAllister and PW Pratt (Eds) American Veterinary Publications, vol 3, pp. 1066–71. Santa Barbara, California.

Haynes PF (1980) Diseases of the metacarpophalangeal joint and metacarpus. *Vet Clin North Am* (Large animal practice) **2**, 33–9.

Medina L and Wheat JD (1981) Bone grafting for the treatment of transverse sesamoid fractures in horses. *Proc 27th Ann Conv Am Ass Eq Prac* 345.

Spurlock GH and Gabel AA (1983) Apical fractures of the proximal sesamoid bones in 109 standardbred horses. *J Am Vet Med Ass* **183**(1), 76–9.

Constriction of the palmar or plantar annular ligament of the fetlock

Annular ligaments are tough fibrous bands which encircle joints and prevent the displacement of a tendon which would destroy its mechanical efficiency.

The palmar annular ligament of the fetlock is illustrated in Fig. 4.30a. Constriction can occur if either the annular ligament, or the structures lying within it, or both, are damaged. Low tendon rupture with consequent swelling can be a cause, as can wire cuts, puncture wounds or any infection in the area. The healing process results in fibrous thickening of tendon and/or the annular ligament; the latter, being inelastic, will not give way under the increased strain, but will

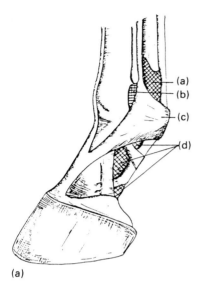

(a)

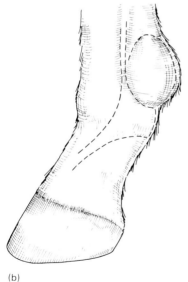

(b)

Fig. 4.30 (a) In this (a) is the digital sheath; (b) is the palmar pouch of the fetlock joint capsule; (c) is the annular ligament. (b) Diagrammatic illustration of the distended flexor sheath 'notched' by the encircling annular ligament.

'dig in' to the structures which it encircles. A greater number of horses, however, show no evidence of primary damage to the tendons or annular ligament, and Geering and Webbon (1984) suggest that the primary lesion is a chronic synovitis leading to sheath and ligament fibrosis but usually of unknown origin. They also observe that the firm fibrous 'adhesion' previously described between the annular ligament and the superficial flexor tendon (SFT) is a normal structure through which the latter receives some of its blood supply.

Clinical signs

The animal will present with a non-specific lameness in a fore or hind limb and possibly with a history of previous fetlock or tendon damage. There is almost always distension of the proximal digital flexor synovial sheath and the characteristic feature is a distinctive notching of the tendon sheath swelling as seen from the side (Fig. 4.30b). Occasionally the hair over the area will need to be clipped before this can be seen.

The lameness does not improve with rest and may become worse as the constriction will cause inflammatory change in the sheath and tendons with possible adhesion formation. Careful palpation will occasionally reveal a distinct notch in the SFT as it dips under the proximal annular ligament, along with thickening of the tendinous or ligamentous structures or both.

Diagnosis

Based on the clinical signs, the presence of the notch being especially important, and the response of the lameness to intrasheath local anaesthesia or, less specifically, a fetlock block preceded by a negative ASNB.

NB distal tendon strain which does not respond with a diminution of lameness over 3—4 months should be examined again for signs of annular ligament constriction.

Sesamoid injuries should be eliminated as a cause through radiographic examination.

Treatment

Surgical resection is the only effective treatment. An incision is made over the lateral edge of the SFT, caudal to the vessels and nerve. The incision is continued through the annular ligament and the underlying adherent tendon sheath for the whole of the ligament width. The sheath is not sutured; the subcutaneous tissues are coapted and the skin closed routinely. Pressure bandaging is maintained for several weeks, and exercise in hand is started 2—3 days post-operatively to restrict adhesion formation.

All cases show improvement after surgery, but the prognosis is most favourable in those animals where there is no significant tendon change.

Suggested further reading

Gerring EL and Webbon PM (1984) Fetlock annular ligament desmotomy: A report of 24 cases. *Eq Vet J* **16**(2), 113–16.

Conditions of the suspensory ligament

The suspensory ligament lies directly behind the 3rd metacarpal or metatarsal bone and between the 2nd and 4th (splint) bones. Its origin is the distal row of carpal bones and the proximal cannon bone. Although containing a variable amount of striped muscle tissue, especially in young animals, it is principally a simple band of elastic tendinous tissue until the junction of the middle and distal third of the cannon bone where it splits into a lateral and medial branch which insert on to the abaxial surfaces of the respective sesamoids. Its structural function is completed by the distal sesamoidean ligaments, which insert on the 1st and 2nd phalanx and by the extensor branches which leave the lateral and medial branches to course distally and join the common digital extensor.

Inflammatory change within a ligament is known as 'desmitis'.

Single branch desmitis

Probably the most common injury, single branch desmitis is usually seen in horses competing at speeds, though its frequency in long event horses is increasing, probably because of the fatigue factor. It affects the forelimbs more frequently than the hind.

Its cause is unequal loading of the fetlock whilst in extension, so that one branch bears the brunt of the strain. The predisposing factors are probably multiple but must include poor conformation, shoeing and course conditions, along with fatigue and incoordination. Under this type of excessive strain there is tearing and separation of ligament fibres, with haemorrhage and much inflammatory reaction.

Clinical signs

There may be a lag of an hour or so between the injury occurring and the onset of observable pain and swelling. The degree of lameness varies with the severity of the desmitis and may be minimal at the straight trot.

The affected branch will be thickened at its edge and rounded compared to the normal, sharply defined border. Palpation should be done both during weight bearing and with the leg in flexion, so relaxing the flexor structures. If recent, the site of injury will be painful and there will be diffuse periligamentous swelling. Pain can be evinced by deep palpation or, by making the animal stand on that one leg, or by trotting in deep, soft going. In the chronic case the branch will be obviously thicker but pain is unlikely on simple manipulation.

Diagnosis

Diagnosis is based on clinical signs and in the chronic case is supported by nerve block evidence. If the area is suspect, analgesia of the affected side alone will aid specificity.

Radiography is essential to rule out fractures of the sesamoid bone which can produce a similar clinical picture, and to examine the adjacent small metacarpal or metatarsal (splint) bone which is often fractured distally in association with the desmitis.

Bilateral branch desmitis

These injuries often involve complete or nearly complete separations of the ligament branches. They are catastrophic injuries with an extremely poor prognosis. There is usually a positional change with the fetlock sinking down on weight bearing; clinically it is similar to sesamoid dehiscence and rupture of the distal sesamoidean ligaments.

It can be distinguished from sesamoid fracture by radiography and by careful palpation, which may reveal the actual site of the tear.

In incomplete rupture there may be no positional change unless the opposite limb is lifted off the ground. However, swelling and thickening will be bilateral on the affected fetlock.

Desmitis of the main ligament body

Less common than single branch desmitis, desmitis of the main ligament body is, however, seen with increasing frequency. The common site is just proximal to the bifurcation and is often associated with splint bone fracture or periostitis.

In acute cases, pain and some swelling will be apparent, especially if the leg is flexed, though radiography is needed to assess splint bone integrity.

In chronic cases and ones with repeated injury, the swelling at the site is obvious and may make palpation of splint bones extremely difficult.

Treatment

Treatment of single branch, mild bilateral branch and main body desmitis should be concerned initially with compression, immobilization and rest.

Compression is probably the most effective way of minimizing the accumulation of intraligamentous haemorrhage and exudation, and preventing further disruption to the tissue microstructure. Therefore the most effective first aid is a firm pressure bandage applied as soon as possible and ideally in conjunction with a board cast (see Fig. 4.27).

The animal's future can then be considered and the owner warned of the poor prognosis. With complete rupture the animal is extremely unlikely to work in any capacity again but may be suitable for breeding; with partial rupture or single branch desmitis the outlook is brighter, but resumption of speed work is unlikely and will depend, of course, on the severity of the injury.

If further treatment is to be attempted then the owner must be warned of the long convalescence and the real dangers of a too early return to strenuous exercise.

If treatment is to be continued then the ideal is a plaster cast for some 6 weeks to ensure maximum immobilization (see section on casting), followed by a further 3–4 months of stall rest. At this time the animal will not be noticeably lame and owners must again be warned not to succumb to the temptation of turning the animal out. Thirty seconds of uncontrolled high spirits can ruin the work of months and, of course, the horse!

At 5–6 months post-injury, walking exercise can begin in earnest, and at 12–14 months further healing will be minimal. At this stage a *very gradual* reintroduction to work can be contemplated.

Note: injury to this region often receives inadequate work-up and may be simply diagnosed as 'tendon problems' or a 'swollen fetlock'. When they fail to return to soundness these horses ae radiographed and found to have a distal 'splint' fracture. This may be siezed on as the source of the continuing lameness and there is a temptation to resort to surgery (see section on metacarpal disease p. 97). This should be resisted as these fractures are rarely the source of pain, despite their frequent non-union, and it is usually an underlying desmitis which is the primary problem.

Treatment of traumatic disruption or severe bilateral branch desmitis of the suspensory ligament should only be undertaken after serious consideration of the very poor prognosis, even as a salvage procedure. Complications which are likely are: a compromise of blood flow to the distal limb; local infection; loss of stability of the fetlock joint with subsequent severe DJD and the development of weight bearing laminitis on the contralateral foreleg.

Immediately after injury external support should be provided, ideally with a board splint. Before further treatment is decided on, a period of several days should elapse to allow evaluation of local ischaemia, etc. During this time the animal should receive systemic antibiotics and the skin in the area of the disruption should be maintained in an aseptic condition. Further long term treatment will either be immobilization in a board splint or plaster cast or by arthrodesis of the fetlock. The latter is an extremely difficult technique and should not be contemplated by the inexperienced. However, in the right hands it can be successful but only as a salvage procedure.

Suggested further reading

Bowman KF, Leitch M, Nunamaker DM *et al* (1984) Complications during treatment of traumatic disruption of the suspensory apparatus in thoroughbred horses. *J Am Vet Med Ass* **184**(6), 706–15.

Mayer W and Raker CW (1980) Diseases of the suspensory apparatus. *Vet Clin North Am* (Large animal practice) **2**, 61–80.

Diseases of the metacarpi

The 2nd and 4th metacarpi (splint bones)

The 2nd and 4th metacarpi are vestiges of the 2nd and 4th digits. The 2nd or medial splint bone is usually 2–3 cm longer than the 4th or lateral and has a more extensive articulation at the carpus. Their distal extremities taper until some 1 cm from the end when they flare out into the so-called 'button'. These are palpable with variable ease in different animals. In young animals, a fibrous interosseous ligament unites the splint bones with the cannon; this ossifies progressively with age.

Radiography

Ideally fine-grain screen/film combinations should be used without a grid. Initial screening views should be 45° dorsopalmar lateromedial (DPLM), or dorsopalmar mediolateral (DPML), obliques with further projections as required. Exposures for splint bones will leave the cannon bone grossly underexposed! Longitudinal grooves in the splint bones and superimposition of portions of the cannon bone can give the artefactual impression of fracture lines. If in doubt radiograph the opposite leg! The angle of deviation of the distal splint bones away from the cannon may sometimes appear quite sharp; however there is much normal variation.

Periosteal new bone growth ('splints')

These occur most frequently on the medial or 2nd metacarpal and occasionally on the lateral aspect of the leg. They also occur on the hind limb. The periosteal irritation is caused by undue stresses on the insertions of the fibrous interosseous ligament between the 2nd and 3rd metacarpal bones. The 2nd metacarpal articulates in a direct weight bearing fashion with the 2nd carpal bone above it and the interosseous ligament between the 2nd and 3rd metacarpal bones therefore suffers greater stress than that between the 3rd and 4th metacarpal bones. 'Bench knee', or the more lateral placement of the cannon relative to the carpus, is said to exacerbate the problem. Ossification of the interosseous ligament is a normal ageing process so that the incidence of this condition diminishes with age.

Periosteal irritation can also be caused by direct trauma, usually from the opposing foot. Base narrow, toed out animals are more likely to interfere, although 'splints', as the bony enlargements are known, can be found in horses with a normal conformation.

Severe or repeated trauma can result in large accumulations of bone which may interfere with the suspensory ligament lying axially and are always a blemish.

Clinical signs

In the acute phase, the signs may be minimal. Some swelling can occur at the site (hot splint) and there will be variable pain on palpation. The animal may be mildly lame or show no gait deficit at all.

Chronic osseous change (cold splint) is seldom a source of lameness and is usually noted as a cosmetic blemish. Occasionally the bony mass will be felt to impinge on the suspensory ligament. However, if a lameness exists, the splint should not be incriminated unless other causes have been eliminated by careful use of regional anaesthesia.

Diagnosis and treatment

Acute

Local signs will suggest the diagnosis, especially in an animal with the appropriate conformational defect. If severe signs are present the site should be radiographed to eliminate fractures. Conservative treatment only is indicated with enforced rest for a minimum of 28 days and, most importantly, the application of a snug pressure bandage to disperse inflammatory exudates and haemorrhage. With this regime, subsequent bony swelling and blemishing should be minimal. Animals which repeatedly 'interfere' may be improved by removing some of the medial wall of the hoof just at the bearing solar surface and being fitted with shoes which have a narrow medial branch.

Chronic

Chronic bony swellings or 'cold splints' are not usually a cause of lameness, and other causes must be eliminated by nerve block examinations, etc. before this diagnosis is made. Most are presented as blemishes in show horses or because the presence of a swelling exacerbates the situation where one leg interferes with the other.

Many authorities have held that removal of 'splints' is a risky procedure in which post-operative reaction can create a lump as big as, or bigger, than the original. This is a minimal risk with the larger masses, though of course a possibility where very small splints are removed. The author's experience is that, with proper technique and after-care, most 'splints' can be removed with only minimal post-operative thickening at the site. The criteria adopted by the author for removal are that (a) the splint is interfering with the animal's 'raison d'être', i.e. showing *or* (b) it is a proven cause of lameness, *or* (c) it is, by its size, leading to interference from the other leg and promoting further trauma, *and* (d) the owners are made fully aware of the *possibility* of extensive post-operative reaction.

Surgical technique

Following the application of an Esmarch's bandage and tourniquet, a *gently* curved incision is made skirting the base of the mass. The skin and underlying fascia are retracted, exposing the periosteum-covered swelling. The periosteum is incised, again around the base of the swelling, and then elevated off the new bone. It will always be firmly adherent in the region of the junction between the 2nd and 3rd metacarpals and must sometimes be cut free. It is retracted caudally and a chisel used to remove the surplus new bone down to just *below* the normal level of the cortex of the cannon and splint bone. If the new bone extends over the suspensory ligament great care must be taken not to damage it or the neurovascular bundle which lies palmar to it. The area is flushed to remove bone chips and the periosteum laid down over the bare bone but *not* sutured. The fascia is coapted and the skin closed with subcuticular and then simple, interrupted sutures.

Post-operative pressure bandaging is vitally important to prevent subsequent swelling and it is maintained for at least 21 days. Strict rest is always enforced for at least 2 weeks.

It cannot be emphasized enough that firing or blistering *do not* reduce the eventual size of the bony swelling; rather they will, in all likelihood increase the reaction and therefore the bone deposition.

Prevention

There is little of practical benefit that can be done to prevent interfering, as this is usually due to established conformational defects. Ensuring that shoes fit properly and closely on the medial branch is essential and in intractable cases the use of interference boots should be considered. Tired or unfit animals have a much less co-ordinated gait and efforts should be made to avoid this state of affairs. Where splints exist and exacerbate the situation their removal should be seriously considered.

Where there is trauma to the interosseous ligament because of the over-exercise of young horses, a more appropriate training programme must be devised.

Fractures of the small metacarpal bones

Fractures of the small metacarpal bones are usually caused by direct trauma, especially interference or kicks and as a consequence to suspensory ligament injuries.

The small metacarpal bones are relatively unprotected by soft tissue and are exposed to trauma. They are also delicate in structure, especially at the distal end.

Distal fractures

Distal fractures, whilst they may be the result of direct external trauma, are now thought to be due mainly to stresses inflicted on the bone by the adjacent suspensory ligament. The bone may fracture in association with a suspensory branch rupture or, in an attempt to explain the large number of distal splint bone fractures found incidentally, it has been suggested that during hard exercise the suspensory ligament snaps back against the relatively fixed small metacarpal or metatarsal bones, rather like a released bow-string.

Non-union of these fractures is the rule. They are not usually a cause of lameness and any pain in the area is more likely to come from an associated suspensory ligament injury. They are occasionally comminuted, and, whilst often showing the characteristic 'elephant's foot' radiographic sign of non-union they occasionally show no sign at all of healing even after some considerable time. The appearance of the fracture line is therefore no real guide to its age.

Treatment

In the acute phase treatment is often tied up with the treatment of an associated suspensory ligament injury and in any event consists of nothing more than pressure bandaging and rest. The distal fragment should not be removed unless it can be proved conclusively by sensitive local anaesthesia that it is the cause of lameness. *NB* beware of inadvertently performing a palmar or palmar metacarpal block!

Proximal fractures

Proximal fractures are usually the result of considerable external force and are therefore often compound. Fractures may be comminuted and may enter the carpal or tarsal joints. In virtually all compound and some closed fractures, osteitis, sequestration and the formation of chronic drainage tracts are subsequent complications. The large collateral ligaments of the carpus have a major insertion into the heads of the 'splint' bones and proximal fractures can result in carpal instability.

Diagnosis is based on a sudden onset of lameness and local heat and swelling. The gait deficiency may not be marked except in fractures of the proximal third and those entering the carpus or tarsus, when lameness can be severe. In young animals especially, carpal instability may also be a feature. Radiography is essential whenever fractures are suspected or when a chronic drainage tract is presented for investigation. *NB* radiographs of normal splint bones occasionally show longitudinal lucent lines which may be mistaken for fractures; they will have no overlying heat or swelling and in longer term cases no associated periosteal reaction. Sometimes the pattern of new bone produced by the periosteal reaction to interosseous ligament irritation will give rise to an apparent radiolucent line which can mimic a fracture. These must be carefully evaluated, especially if the degree of lameness does not suggest a fracture.

Periosteal reaction in early cases will be absent and fracture lines clean-edged. In older cases the latter become indistinct, and aggressive, rough periosteal new bone will be seen. In chronic or healed cases the periosteal new bone will have a smooth outline tapering to normal bone. Where septic osteitis is present and with good quality radiographs the new bone is often seen to have the pallisade appearance characteristic of the equine periosteal reaction to infection. A sequestrum and involucrum are often recognizable (Figs. 4.31a and b).

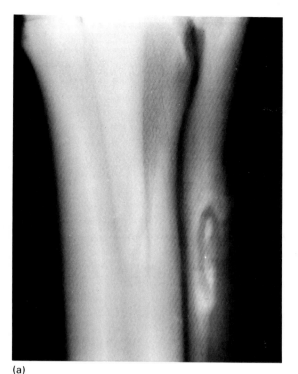
(a)

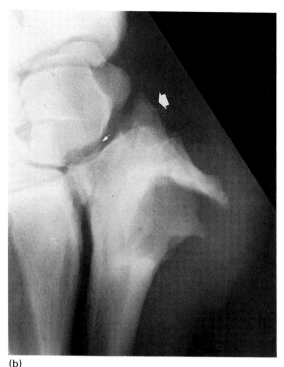
(b)

Fig. 4.31 (a) A classical involucrum and sequestrum in a 2nd metacarpal bone. (b) Extensive new bone formation as a result of chronic septic osteitis in a 4th metatarsal bone. Note the new bone in the insertion of the calcaneometatarsal ligament (large arrow) and evidence of degenerative joint disease in the articulation with the 4th tarsal bone (small arrow). This joint communicates with the tarsometatarsal articulation.

Treatment

Non-compound fractures of the middle portion of the small metacarpal or tarsal bones will respond to conservative treatment. Pressure bandaging and enforced rest will allow healing to occur, the cannon acting as an effective splint.

Fractures of the thicker proximal third often need internal fixation to prevent carpal instability. The technique is to lag-screw the proximal fragment of the splint bone back on to the 3rd metacarpal or cannon bone using, ideally, ASIF (Association for the study of Internal Fixation) type screws. Larger diameter screws should be used with great care as their insertion may weaken and further fracture the splint bone fragment.

The reader is strongly recommended to study the anatomy and relationships of this area on a macerated specimen before embarking on this procedure — it is time well spent!

Check radiographs should be taken 3 months post-operatively and the fixation evaluated for signs of screw loosening. This is manifest by radiolucency around the head and threads, and if present is an indication to remove the screw.

Compound fractures are treated conservatively for the first few weeks by pressure bandaging and antibiotic therapy. The use of internal fixation in the face of infection should be avoided if at all possible; septic osteitis, draining tracts at the operative site and screw loosening are almost inevitable results. Severe fracture of the proximal splint bone may, however, occasionally require internal fixation despite these risks. Infection of a fracture site usually results in a non-union with associated osteitis and often sequestrum formation. When infection has become localized following the conservative therapy, surgery can be performed to remove the infected portion of the splint bone.

The leg is exanguinated with an Esmarch's bandage, and a gently curving incision is made around the base of the infected mass. The skin, including the drainage tract, is elevated; fibrosis often renders the fascial and periosteal layers unrecognizable and this usually has to be done by sharp dissection. The fracture area is easily recognizable by the reaction and purplish granulation tissue, and is removed with a chisel (Figs. 4.32a and b).

Only a portion of the splint bone need be removed and the healthy distal fragment should be left *intact*; it will survive, and only a relatively small skin incision need be made. *All traces* of infected bone and soft tissue are removed and the wound is closed by suturing only the proximal 75%; part-suturing ensures good drainage of the area. If the wound is completely closed infection is entrapped and wound breakdown is assured. Pressure bandaging and 3−4 months rest complete the treatment.

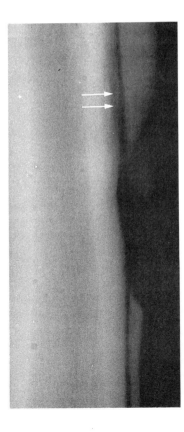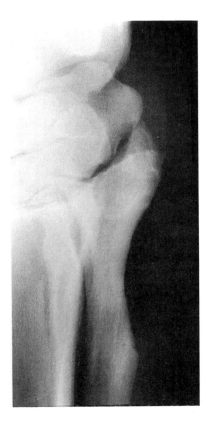

Fig. 4.32 (a) The septic osteitis seen in Fig. 4.31a has been removed at surgery. Note that the distal portion of the small metacarpal bone has been left *in situ*. The linear lucency (arrowed) in the cortical bone of the cannon could indicate residual osteitis which might prevent healing. (b) The same bone seen in Fig. 4.31b following surgery. Removal of the infected bone and overlying fibrous tissue mass created a large amount of dead space which took several weeks to granulate.

Suggested further reading

Allen D and White NA (1982) Management of proximal splint fractures and exostoses in the horse. *Proc 28th Ann Conv Am Ass Eq Prac* 89—95.

Moens Y, Verschooten F, De Moor A and Wouters L (1980) Bone sequestration as a consequence of limb wounds in the horse. *Vet Radiol* **21**, 40.

Diseases of the 3rd metacarpal and metatarsal (cannon) bones

Fractures

Slab fractures of the lateral condyle are common racing injuries. They are an important differential to other fetlock conditions, especially since non-displaced examples do not produce very obvious clinical signs. All acute injuries to the metacarpophalangeal articulation should be radiographed at a *very early stage*.

Fracture fixation will be dealt with under a separate heading. (see section on fracture fixation, p. 253)

The 'bucked shin' complex

When a young horse is first exposed to enforced exercise, the internal structure of the bone, especially the slender cannon, undergoes extensive remodelling to accommodate the new stresses. If the bone adaptation cannot keep pace with the demands made on it, i.e. in animals trained too fast and too hard, the result may be the metacarpal condition known as 'bucked shins'.

The pathogenesis is related to microfracture of the dorsal cortex with development of periosteal irritation and new bone. The fractures are typical of those produced by compression and are similar to stress fractures in man.

Clinical signs

Visible lameness is often minimal and this is due in some part to the frequent bilateral involvement. In animals competing in an anti-clockwise direction the predominant lameness is often on the left leg and vice versa. A fall off in performance may be the first sign noticed. There is often some swelling in the mid-metacarpal region and pressure in these areas will elicit a marked pain response.

Radiographs must be of high quality to demonstrate early lesions. There is often only a small amount of change at the site and periosteal reaction will be minimal. Fine-grain screen/film combinations will aid visualization, as will bright light illumination. In good quality films the periosteal reaction will be seen to be finely pallisaded. In more chronic cases of 2—3 months duration, the new bone is much more obvious and well organized. The microfractures are not visible to conventional radiography; complex techniques such as Xeroradiography are needed to demonstrate them.

Treatment

As with many other race track injuries, the treatment for these injuries range from the sensible to the bizarre. There is no logic nor benefit in any treatment other than the rational one of rest, supplemented by pressure bandaging in the early stages and followed by a return to work in 2—3 weeks time at a *slower* rate.

Cortical fissure fractures

Older horses, 3 years and over, presenting with either an acute or chronic shin disease must be examined carfully to determine whether they have a dorsal, cortical fissure fracture. The leg distribution is as in the 'bucked shin' syndrome, though the fractures are usually on the dorsolateral aspect of the cannon at the junction of the middle and lower thirds. The fracture line runs at 30—40° to the long axis of the metacarpus and courses proximally. Occasionally it exists over a longer length producing a 'saucer' fracture.

Clinical signs

Recent fractures will cause marked local pain, some swelling and lameness which will diminish with chronicity and rest. Diagnosis is by local signs and by radiography. Good quality and high definition radiographs are essential and several projections centred on the site and varying slightly in obliquity may be necessary before the fracture is well visualized. These projections must be used again for subsequent monitoring of fracture healing. Periosteal and endosteal new bone will impair the clarity of the fracture line which must be searched for carefully.

Treatment

Pressure bandaging and rest is recommended in acute and non-extensive lesions. Four weeks of rest should be followed by a very slow return to work. A too rapid return to exercise will result in relapse. Serial radiographic examinations are advisable and extension of the fracture is a signal for a further rest period or surgical inter-vention. Several techniques have been used; one involves lag-screw compression of the fracture line (Fig. 4.33). The technique is not easy, and although it accelerates healing there is a significant proportion of cases in which refracture distal to the screw occurs 6—12 months after resumption of heavy work. Other methods which have been tried include drilling holes across the fracture line in the hope that dowels of bone will eventually traverse and stabilize it. More recently some workers have expressed optimism about the effect of pulsing magnetic field therapy on these fractures. However, this optimism must be tempered by the fact that others have shown no measurable effect on fracture healing. The underlying pathology of stress fractures of the dorsal metacarpal cortex is, as yet, not fully understood by any means. More effective treatment must await a more thorough understanding

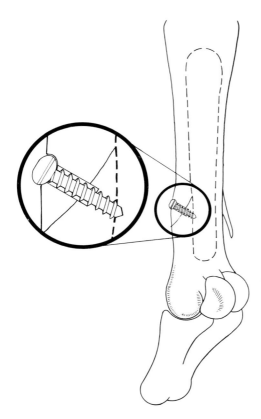

Fig. 4.33 The location of a saucer-shaped cortical fracture. The lateral splint is omitted for clarity. The insert shows detail of how the screw is inserted lag fashion through the cortex biting only in cortical bone deep to the fracture line. The screw must not cross the medullary cavity (shown dotted).

of the condition. However, the most effective therapy will always be prevention, through better training methods which prepare youngsters more thoroughly and an awareness of the risks of forcing totally immature animals into high stress athletic situations.

Suggested further reading

Auer JA, Burch GE and Hall P (1983) A review of pulsing electromagnetic field therapy and its possible application to horses. *Eq Vet J* **15**(4), 354−60.
Norwood G (1979) The bucked shin complex. *Proc Am Assoc Eq Prac* **25**, 88−97.

5: Conditions of the Upper Forelimb

Conditions of the carpus

Anatomy

The carpus or more popularly 'the knee' is a composite of three joints. The radiocarpal, a ginglymus or hinge joint is the most mobile, opening to some 90°. The intercarpal is a similar type of joint and opens some 70°. The carpometacarpal is an arthrodial joint and does *not* open at all. The fibrous joint capsule is common to all these articulations. Dorsally it forms the dorsal carpal ligament and forms fibrous canals for the extensor tendons, whilst its palmar part is thick and dense, smoothes out the irregularities of the palmar carpus and forms the dorsal surface of the carpal canal. It continues distally as the infracarpal check ligament.

The synovial membrane forms three sacs, one for each articulation. The radiocarpal has a separate sac, but the intercarpal and the carpometacarpal communicate between the 3rd and the 4th carpal bones.

The carpal complex is spanned by two large abaxial ligaments, one medial, one lateral, running from the radius to the lateral and medial cannon and splint bones. The 1st carpal bone, where it exists, is embedded in the distal end of the medial ligament.

Radiography

Fine-grain screen/film combinations should be used without a grid except in the largest of breeds. The conventional dorsopalmar (DP) and lateral projections are barely adequate to assess the joint and, at the very least, two DP obliques should be taken. (In the dorso palmar lateromedial oblique (DPLMO) the accessory carpal is visible, in the DPMLO it is superimposed on to the carpal bones.) In addition, the flexed lateral view, though sometimes difficult to take if the animal resists flexion, can provide useful information about joint margins, and skyline views of the carpal bones will often reveal unsuspected marginal fractures (Fig. 5.1).

Remember that the dorsal carpal surface is greatly convex and that small lesions will only show on direct tangential projections. The beam should also be centred on the appropriate joints and the beam centre must be at right angles to the long axis of the leg otherwise the superimposition is most confusing.

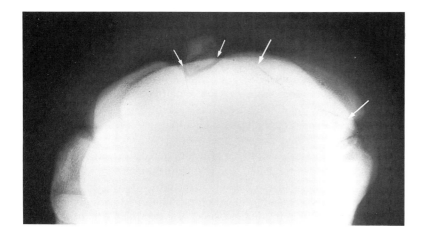

Fig. 5.1 Skyline view of the distal row of carpal bones showing an hitherto unsuspected fracture of the 3rd carpal bone (small arrows) in addition to the larger slab fracture (large arrows).

Potential artefacts

The 1st carpal bone is present in many horses and in small proportion the 5th is also visible; these should not be confused with chip fractures. The distal radius is also a site where artefacts can lead to misdiagnosis; its lateral extremity is, in fact, the distal vestigial ulna and in the young animal the separate ossification centre and intervening cartilage is occasionally diagnosed as a fracture or cyst. Even in the adult, small radiolucent areas can persist to mark the rudimentary division between radius and ulna. The large depression in the centre of the distal caudal radius will always appear as a lucent area, and again is occasionally misdiagnosed as a cyst or area of pathological lucency. In some DP films the aggregated mass of flexor tendons at the level of distal radius create a well defined 4−5 cm wide linear opacity superimposed on the lateral portion of the distal radius, and the vestigial ulna may be seen, if calcified, especially in some DPLMO views, as a thin, curvilinear opacity in the same general position.

Contrast radiography

This is extremely useful to determine the origin of sinus tracks, synovial fistulae and fluid distensions of unknown origins.

Biomechanics and general considerations

When the carpus is non-weight bearing the component bones fit loosely together allowing some transverse movement and substantial rotation. Flexion should be easy, non-painful and the heel should touch the elbow easily. Failure to achieve this indicates some pathological process. When the limb is weight bearing, the complex of radius, carpal bones and metacarpi come together to form a rigid strut; at maximal load they interlock perfectly.

Conformation variations are important in the pathogenesis of carpal disease since they will disrupt the normal loading pattern of the joint and lead to abnormal stresses and strains. Common abnormalities are where the carpal bones are set more palmar than normal in relation to the mid-line of the radius, 'back in the knee', carpus valgus or 'knock knees', carpus varus, or 'bowed knees', or where the carpal bones are more medially placed relative to the radius, the so-called 'bench knee'.

As the carpus snaps from its loose state to the rigid state of weight bearing, the conformation of the joints concentrates the impact stresses on the dorsal aspect of the bones. This increases with speed and the associated progressive hyperextension of the carpus. Fatigue compounds the effect as does the conformational abnormality known as 'back in the knees'. Repeated uneven loading results in marginal and slab fractures and leads to degenerative joint disease.

The economic necessities of running immature, hurriedly prepared animals in high speed competition is another factor leading to the high incidence of carpal disease. In Europe, the practice of racing on turf on courses with gentle right and left turns mitigates these effects somewhat. In countries which race on tight circuits and artificial track surfaces there is a high prevalence of carpal injuries in young animals.

Clinical examination of the carpus

At slow speeds, carpal disease does not produce a gait abnormality with any discernible characteristic features. At greater speed one may get an impression of reduced carpal flexion.

Animals with high stepping gaits can show an obvious limitation in knee flexion and jumping horses an unusual degree of clumsiness. Carpal flexion tests will usually produce an exacerbation of lameness though this must persist for more than three or four strides to be significant.

Swelling, pain on palpation and flexion and occasionally heat are the earliest signs of carpal disease both after acute external trauma or athletic injury.

Palpation should try and establish which structures are damaged, whether swelling is in the extra-articular soft tissues, or due to distended synovial sacs or both. If the margins of the joints are palpable, then consistent pain over a specific area may indicate a marginal fracture and, as a general rule, this is easier the earlier the examination is carried out.

Flexion of the carpus may be restricted, initially by inflammatory swelling and pain, later by post-trauma fibrosis which thickens the joint capsule and subcutaneous tissues and can bind the extensor tendons through adhesions.

Swelling and pain in the palmar aspect along with carpal canal distension may indicate a fractured accessory carpal bone.

In certain cases intra-articular anaesthesia should be considered. The two proximal joints are easily palpated, even through fibrous tissue, and the technique is a simple one (see section on intra-articular anaesthesia). *NB* never inject through known or potentially infected tissues.

In chronic cases there may be well defined, non-painful swellings with or without generalized thickening, and with or without synovial sac distension and restruction of movement. The presence of these abnormalities does not, in itself, mean that they are significant in causing lameness. Regional or intra-articular anaesthesia must be used to exclude other causes and confirm carpal pathology, especially before surgery is contemplated.

Degenerative joint disease (osteoarthritis)

Degenerative joint disease (DJD) is the inevitable sequel to *all* intra-articular pathological processes. In the carpus it commonly follows sudden, acute trauma, with intra-articular fracture, or chronic repetitive trauma to immature or confromationally abnormal joints. Degenerative joint disease is the name given to the complex of pathological processes involving joint capsule, synovial membrane, cartilage and bone in both degenerative and proliferative changes. There are many theories as to the pathogenesis but the end result is fibrosis of synovial membrane and joint capsule which together can limit flexion. Cartilage thinning with alterations in its chemical composition and periarticular bone proliferation produces marginal osteophytes. These are not single tooth-like projections as may be wrongly inferred from radiographs, but a marginal lip of bone around most, or all, of the joint rim. They are not the cause of lameness in themselves but merely a radiographically recognizable sign of disease. Occasionally they will become very large and may fracture (see section on degenerative joint disease, p. 273).

Clinical signs

There may be some signs of external trauma such as skin and sub-cutaneous thickening and scarring but in horses suffering from concussion-induced disease there may be nothing apart from some joint distension. In chronic cases a generalized thickening of the joint capsule and chronic synovial distension can be appreciated especially if both legs are compared; there *may* be reduced flexion too.

Diagnosis

Diagnosis is based on clinical signs only in early cases, though synovial fluids analysis will show an increased cell count and reduced viscosity. In young animals, recent hard work and evidence of improper preparation will provide support for the diagnosis. Radiographic changes will not become apparent for several months, and then only on good quality radiographs exposed for joint margins. These are squaring, or 'lipping' of joint margins, best seen in the DP projections, progressing to frank, 'beak-like' osteophytes in later cases. There may also be increased prominence of the insertion of the synovial joint capsule in the centre of the proximal row of carpal bones in lateral views. Cartilage, or subchondral bone changes are not recognizable until the disease is far advanced.

Treatment (see also chapter 10)

First and most important is to stop athletic exercise, taking the animal out of training or racing, etc. Box rest, with daily walking in hand allows for subsidence of inflammation but maintains joint flexibility; frequent passive knee flexion is also useful to prevent stiffness. Externally applied therapy should be restricted to the application of pressure from bandaging or a tailored, elastic, carpal support stocking. 'Blisters', etc. are a waste of time and can make matters worse by increasing dorsal cutaneous fibrosis and thereby reducing flexibility.

Intra-articular corticosteroids have been advocated and they do reduce inflammation dramatically. Their great danger is that, in the short term, they reduce the ability of the joint to withstand stress, and as the clinical signs improve so quickly, these animals are often put back to work too soon and accelerated joint damage takes place. If an animal is injected with corticosteroid, at least 4–6 months must be allowed for healing before it is reintroduced to hard work.

Movement of joints in non-load bearing structures has been shown to improve cartilage quality and therefore swimming should be theoretically beneficial. However, bones are not subject to much stress with this form of exercise and may become relatively osteopenic, therefore a period of conventional training must elapse before hard exercise is started.

The intra-articular injection of hyaluronic acid as its sodium salt has been shown to benefit cases of degenerative joint disease. It, along with rest and a controlled return to activity is a logical treatment for osteoarthritis which is uncomplicated by fractures or other injuries. Although it requires aseptic techniques for injection and may cause a transient post-injection aggravation of signs as do the corticosteroids, it is rapid in its anti-inflammatory affect and does not produce, with multiple injections, anything analogous to the well described steroid arthropathy.

In recent years a new compound, polysulphated glycosaminoglycan, has become available and is advocated for the treatment of DJD. Its great advantage is that it is reported to promote cartilage healing. However, it has some drawbacks and its efficacy in practice may be limited by cost and the need for repeated intra-articular injections.

Carpal chip fractures

Hyperextension at speed leads to the dorsal edges of the small carpal bones being subject to enormous compressive loading, see Fig. 5.2. In the USA, where all racing is anticlockwise; the lateral aspect of the left carpus, and medial aspect of the right are most often involved. It is the dorsal articular margins of the distal radius, proximal intermediate, distal radial and proximal 3rd carpal bones which are most commonly affected. Aggravating factors are immaturity, unfitness, or extended exercise leading to fatigue along with conformational defects such as 'back in the knees'.

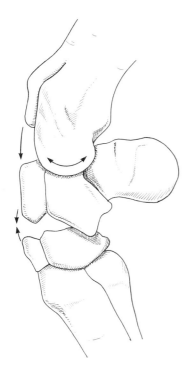

Fig. 5.2 Diagrammatic illustration of how the bones of the carpus move relative to one another during flexion. The arrows illustrate how the dorsal margins of the carpal bones impact upon each other during extension.

Clinical signs

Early signs, including lameness, may be minimal, but there is usually a degree of synovial sac distension and some pain; the gait deficiency is not characteristic and a nerve block work-up may be needed.

Early radiography of suspect knees is imperative since the prognosis deteriorates rapidly if exercise is not curtailed immediately or if surgery is delayed. The long term result of any intra-articular fracture is osteoarthritis of varying degree but this can be minimized by early diagnosis and treatment. The importance of oblique views of the carpus is stressed in Fig. 5.3.

Treatment

Conservative therapy is indicated only if the fracture fragment is not displaced and one is certain that the animal will be rested until healing has taken place. Treatment is box rest, with exercise 'in hand', starting gradually and increasing over several months. A minimum of 6 months lay off is essential, as well as a radiographic confirmation of healing, before training restarts.

Displaced or loose chips should be removed surgically as early as possible. Delay leads to the establishment of DJD which is minimal at

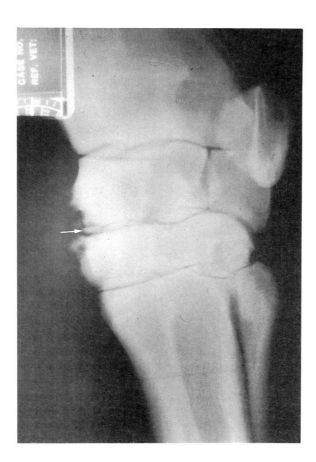

Fig. 5.3 A DPLMO projection clearly showing a small chip fracture of the radial carpal bone (arrowed) with much associated periarticular new bone formation on both sides of the joint. *NB* this lesion was not visible on a straight lateromedial projection.

first, but progresses over the months and years to incapacitate the patient.

Surgical removal of fracture fragments and curettage of defects in the carpus must be done under conditions of strict asepsis. Ideally, surgery should be done under arthroscopic control. With this technique interference with the structure of the joint is minimal since only two or three small puncture wounds are created. The constant high pressure stream of electrolyte solution used to distend the joint effectively washes out any debris and post-operative reaction and convalescent time is much reduced compared to that which follows arthrotomy.

Prior to surgery the position of the fragment must be determined accurately using oblique radiographic projections. For arthrotomy the horse is placed with the affected side of the carpus uppermost. A C-shaped incision is made over the fracture site and the skin and subcutaneous fascia reflected together. A straight incision is then made as close to the fracture site as possible but avoiding the sheaths of the extensor carpi radialis and common digital extensor tendons. Self-retaining retractors are used to open the incision in the fibrous joint capsule and the fragment located and removed. It should be prised out of its bed and any fibrous attachments severed. Although partial flexion of the joints can help this procedure, especially if the incision is not directly over the fragment, it unfortunately also tautens the tissues on the dorsal surface including the wound edges, and can make access more difficult. The fracture bed, surrounding new bone and any 'kissing' lesions on the opposing bone should be curetted or chiselled away and any synovial proliferations removed with scissors. Following irrigation with at least 2 litres of sterile Hartmann's solution the joint is closed by suturing the fibrous capsule. The synovial membrane need not be sutured even if it can be identified clearly. The loose fascia is coapted and the skin edges apposed by a continuous suture through the subcutaneous tissue and deeper layers of the skin. Finally the skin is closed with simple, interrupted non-absorbable sutures. The instillation of 20 mg hyaluronic acid as the sodium salt into the joint during closure has been shown to reduce post-surgery reaction and new bone formation (Auer 1980).

Post-operative management consists of snug pressure bandaging for 2−3 weeks, taking care not to cause bandage rubs over the medial distal radius and accessory carpal bone, with box rest. After the first 3−4 days small amounts of hand walking can be allowed, increasing over 2−3 months. At this time the horse can be turned out, preferably in a small field or paddock, and, for the first few times, only after a long period of walking in hand to take the edge off its exuberance.

Six months post-operatively the animal should be ready to go back into training.

Carpal slab fractures

These are fractures which extend across the face of one of the carpal bones and roughly parallel to it. They usually reach from one articulation to the other and, in the carpus, it is the 3rd bone which is most often affected. Smaller marginal chip fractures may also be present, also fractures in the sagittal plant.

Aetiology and pathogenesis

Carpal slab fracture is an injury of the fast gaited horse. It is likely that intra-articular stresses create initially a fissure fracture. The clinical signs at this stage will be minor and the fissure may progress to a full fracture immediately or, if not recognized, during subsequent exercise. There would seem to be a definite relationship between the occurrence of slab fractures and the intra-articular use of corticosteroids.

Clinical signs

Fissure fractures will show as a non-specific, low grade lameness whose onset may be either during, or some hours after, fast exercise. There is a variable amount of joint distension; and it may be confined to the radiocarpal or intercarpal joints or affect both if the fracture is across the upper row of carpal bones. The distal intercarpal joint capsule is tight and will not distend. When fissures progress to slab fracture there is severe pain and marked lameness with unmistakable joint distension: pain is evinced on palpation and flexion of the joint.

Diagnosis

The signs of fissure fractures are not characteristic and diagnosis is only by careful and good quality radiography. The fissure and non-displaced slab fractures are difficult to see unless the beam passes along the fracture line, so several tangential views may be required; even then, normal bony margins can produce confusing vertical lucencies (Fig. 5.4). Skyline views (see Fig. 5.1) will show fracture lines and other sagittal fractures. The whole radiographic examination may therefore be somewhat extensive, but it is worthwhile. Fissure or non-displaced fractures are treatable, with a good prognosis; displacement of the slab which could occur with further exercise substantially reduces the chance of a successful outcome.

A useful rule of thumb is that if clinical signs indicate the possibility of intra-articular bone damage, radiographic examination should be thorough enough to either confirm or completely exclude that possibility.

Care should be used when using intra-articular anaesthesia in these animals, as with any case of suspect fracture. Uncontrolled exercise without the restraint of pain can lead to further osseous or articular damage.

Treatment

The treatment of choice for slab fractures is undoubtedly internal fixation. The size of the slab in most cases precludes its removal. The technique for lag screw fixation is described under the section on fractures. If treated early the prognosis for non-displaced fractures is

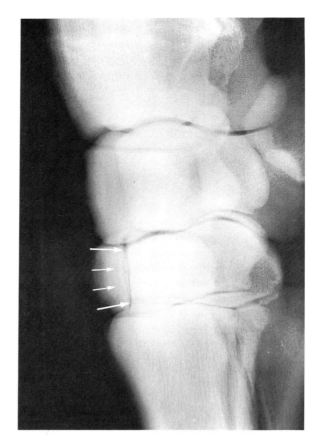

Fig. 5.4 A DPLMO taken at about 20° from the straight lateromedial projection showing a non-displaced fracture of the 3rd carpal bone (large arrows). In the normal horse this projection will often show a vertical line at this site — this is the dorsal border of either the 2nd or 4th bone depending on the angulation and should not be misdiagnosed. It is barely visible in this picture (small arrows).

good. In cases where diagnosis or treatment has been delayed, DJD will inevitably be present and will probably prevent a return to full working ability.

Sagittal fractures of the 3rd carpal bone do occur and are only well visualized on skyline views. The prognosis is poor since they are not amenable to internal fixation and results of conservative therapy are disappointing.

Multiple carpal fracture

Each case of multiple carpal fracture must be carefully evaluated radiographically. Individual fractures may be amenable to fixation and varying degrees of carpal arthrodesis is possible. However, if multiple repairable fractures are present, other small fragments, many undetectable or inaccessible, will usually be present too; their presence will compromise full recovery. In very severe cases pan-carpal arthrodesis should be considered, although it is extremely difficult surgery. The animal will be fit only as a pet or for breeding purposes.

Fracture of the accessory carpal bone

The accessory carpal bone fractures in a characteristic manner; the main fracture line being vertical and running along the vertical groove which lies on the outside of the bone and accommodates the ulnaris lateralis tendon. This groove also coincides with the thinnest portion of the bone (Fig. 5.5). The fractures are often comminuted and occasionally with multiple fragments (Fig. 5.6).

The aetiology of the fracture is uncertain though it has been suggested that overloading of the limb with the carpus in slight flexion may be the cause. The author believes that hyperextension of the carpus coupled with a sideways compressive effect from the taut annular ligament may also be an effective disruptive force. The fact that this injury tends to occur early in a race at a time of maximum acceleration and late on in long races when tiredness supervenes, could support both views. A third theory is that the two muscles inserting on the proximal border of the accessory bone, the ulnaris lateralis and the flexor carpi ulnaris, having separate innervations, radial and ulnar nerves respectively, may begin to contract out of phase in a fatigued animal, cause unequal loading and lead to fracture.

Clinical signs

The onset of lameness is usually immediate on fracturing; lameness is severe, the leg being held in a neutral, non-weight bearing, toe-tipping position at rest. Within an hour or so swelling of the area is apparent and of course there is pain on palpation or manipulation of the area. The gentle medial concavity of the accessory bone forms the lateral wall of the carpal canal or tunnel and, therefore, fractures will affect the carpal synovial sheath resulting in synovitis and distension. In animals where fracture has occurred some time previously, the synovial distension can be the most obvious sign of problems in this area.

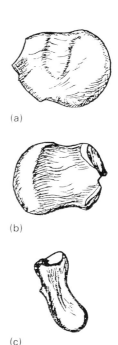

(a)

(b)

(c)

Fig. 5.5 Three views of an accessory carpal bone. (a) Lateral side showing groove for ulnaris lateralis tendon; (b) medial view showing its medial concavity; (c) proximal view.

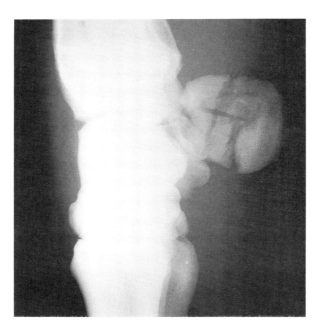

Fig. 5.6 A comminuted accessory carpal fracture.

Treatment

Conservative and surgical therapy would seem to meet with about equal success in returning animals to work but this may be the result of the technical difficulties involved in the surgery. Conservative treatment is pressure bandaging for 6–8 weeks with box rest continuing for a total of 5–6 months; unrestricted activity must not be allowed for 8 months. In the early stages, tube casts (see section on casting, see Fig. 4.27) can be used to minimize movements; in theory they are preferable to bandaging since they will not compress the palmar fragment inwards towards the carpal canal and they prevent the distracting effects on the fragments of carpal flexion.

Surgical treatment is feasible only in the simple, vertical fractures and consists of lag-screwing the palmar fragment on to the dorsal one. It is technically difficult to do because of the curved nature of the bone and its central waist (Fig. 5.5c). The screw will either invade the carpal canal or emerge out of the lateral side of the dorsal fragment if even slightly misdirected. Only one screw can be placed.

If internal fixation is feasible and successfully carried out, its benefits will be: stabilization of the palmar fragment preventing it from rotating inwards towards the canal; encouragement of bone healing and minimizing callus and obviating the necessity for very prolonged bandaging with its attendant risks of pressure rubs and not inconsiderable expense. If the facilities and expertise are available it is the treatment of choice in selected cases.

Avulsion fractures of the accessory carpal bone

Avulsion fractures occur on the proximal and occasionally the distal border. They lie within the tendons of insertion or the ligamentous origins and they respond well to a rest period of some 8 or 9 months.

Carpal canal (tunnel) syndrome

Fractures of the accessory carpal bone, or rarely, other trauma leads to fibrosis of the posterior annular ligament, thickening of flexor tendons within the canal, a synovitis and damage to associated vessels and nerves.

Clinical signs

There is lameness of varying severity and quite marked resentment of carpal flexion. Thickening and induration of the area are palpable, as is the bulging of the carpal sheath between the common digital extensor and ulnaris lateralis tendons. If these signs are present the carpus should be radiographed to establish whether a fracture is present.

Treatment

Drainage of the sheath gives only very temporary relief. Intrasheath injection of corticosteroids will prolong this relief but will not alter the root of the problem. Removal of an elliptical strip of annular ligament up to 1 cm wide through a 12—15 cm skin incision centred on the accessory carpal bone and palmar to the cephalic vein relieves the compression on the canal and adhesions within the canal can be freed at the same time. The subcutaneous fascia and skin are closed and the leg wrapped in a snug pressure bandage. Five to 6 weeks box rest is indicated before a return to work can be contemplated, although the presence of a recent accessory carpal fracture may lengthen this period.

Fluid carpal swellings (hygromas)

Apart from the joint and carpal sheath distensions already mentioned the carpus can display a variety of acquired fluid-filled swellings.

Hygromas originate as extensions of tendon sheaths, herniations of synovial structures and organized seromas. They are probably traumatic in origin though, in their chronic state, are not usually locally painful; they will, however, sometimes cause lameness through limitation of flexion. This is often due to associated fibrosis of the dorsal fibrous capsule and possibly adhesions between tendons and these sheaths.

The site of the hygromas may sometimes give an indication of its origins but the simple technique of contrast injection followed by radiography will give the answer in most cases (*NB* remember to evaluate joints, etc. by prior plain films).

The contrast agent, which must be water soluble and sterile, is injected with the same regard to asepsis as with any intra-articular puncture; 20—30 ml is not excessive and gives good contrast. Five minutes walking will ensure that it disperses to the limits of the cavity. In some cases enormous synovial proliferation will give the lining of the cavity a plicated or rugal appearance.

Treatment

Traditionally the treatment of all synovial swellings has been aspiration and pressure bandaging with or without corticosteroid injection. The results are disappointing since the distension returns rapidly once pressure is removed. In fact no treatment will ever restore the knee to its original appearance and optimistic owners must be warned of this. Surgery is often the best hope for non-recurrence, but not all cases are amenable; the surgery is difficult and traumatic and post-operative swelling and scarring can compound pre-existing fibrous deformity. In addition, the carpus, because of its range of movement, is an area renowned for poor wound healing, and pressure bandaging can itself give rise to problems with rubs especially over the accessory carpal bone.

If despite these factors, extirpation is chosen, the procedure must be done under general anaesthesia. Initially, the synovial swelling should *not* be evacuated as its distension helps identify its margins. An Ensmarch's bandage and a tourniquet simplify the procedure and should be used if at all possible.

Often these structures have no definable wall or sac but are apparently fluid-filled cavities within fibrous tissue. If a connection to the parent synovial structure can be identified it should be carefully sutured to prevent further leakage. Dead space is a major problem and if the skin flap is large, poor vascularization of the wound margins may compromise healing. The latter can be overcome to an extent by leaving the skin attached to a good thickness of subcutaneous tissue as the skin flap is dissected free, and the former by suturing the proximal 80% of the wound only to provide drainage. The author prefers this method to the use of drains which can be difficult to maintain. Similarly, the author prefers pressure bandaging in the early stages to the casting which is recommended by some surgeons.

Whatever technique is used, wound breakdown and recurrence of the hygroma are significant risks and substantial post-operative fibrosis is certain.

Acute carpal trauma

The carpus is very prone to trauma: clinicians know only too well the animal that has slid on its knees along an asphalt road or dirt track or has ploughed knees first into an immovable obstacle. Carpal trauma is not an inconsiderable risk in any procedure where a horse is restrained with its foreleg up, e.g. when performing nerve blocks the odd animal occasionally collapses without warning on to its knees. Fortunately, severe damage is rare unless the ground surface is gravelled or rough but it is an added reason, if any is needed, for care with such procedures.

Injuries fall into two broad categories: those where the skin remains intact and those with full thickness breaks. Where there is no skin break, treatment should be to remove any pieces of grit, etc. embedded in the skin, cleansing of the area and the application of a pressure bandage as soon as possible. Pressure dissipates any extravasated or inflammatory fluid and prevents further accumulation, it will even control haemorrhage if applied soon enough. Antibiotic and antitetanus therapy is essential since opportunist blood-borne organisms can colonize inflamed or damaged tissues and because of the possibility of small undetectable puncture wounds being present.

The virtues of pressure bandaging do not end with the acute case; even in long standing lesions one can obtain a substantial reduction in the size of a knee by the judicious application of pressure. Pressure should be kept on for at least 10 days but in the later stages the initial rest should be punctuated by some walking in hand and some physiotherapy. Physiotherapy comprises manual knee flexion during bandage changes to discourage adhesion formation. It is also good indicator of recovery, becoming easier and less resented with time. Slacking of pressure and return to work must be gradual over several days — a sudden removal of bandages and the freedom of the wide open spaces is a recipe for a certain resurgence of swelling and stiffness.

Little or no improvement in pain, stiffness and lameness over the first week is a strong indication to radiograph the knee.

Many cases of carpal trauma present with full thickness skin wounds of varying severity. The nature of the trauma means that they are frequently contaminated, often with gravel or grit. There may be penetration of tendon sheath or, rarely, joint capsule and a discharge of synovial fluid. This can be quite copious and will clot into yellow stalactites, rather like candle wax drips, below the wound.

Treatment

These cases must be treated vigorously! If they are not, extensive carpal fibrosis will result, with septic tenosynovitis and synovial fistulae a distinct possibility.

First aid is important in these animals and again consists of the application of pressure to reduce haemorrhage and exudation into the tissues; in the short term it can be crudely applied with any makeshift bandage but professional attention must follow soon.

Major wounds should be dealt with under general anaesthesia, if at all possible. After debridement, and the surgeon must be careful not to remove too much subcutaneous fascia in his enthusiasm, the wounds can be sutured. Dead space, exudation and drainage are problems, especially in an area of constant movement such as this, and are best solved by part suturing. As a rough guide $2/3 - 3/4$ of any wound may be closed leaving the most dependant part open for a length of at least $1-2$ cm. Treated like this, most will heal; completely sutured wounds will usually break down. Skin flaps are common, V-shaped ones can have both arms closed, one completely, one partially. Inverted Vs can be similarly closed but it may be necessary to deliberately extend one arm to give drainage to the inevitable pocket of dead space. Unless obviously damaged beyond redemption skin flaps should be given the benefit of the doubt and not cut off. Nature is a far more able judge of what will and will not survive. Small wounds should not be sutured but allowed to granulate and epithelialize under the control of the external pressure. They are not likely to become exuberant though this development can be easily treated by resection and grafting if necessary.

Synovial fistulae can be difficult to deal with. They usually arise from the dorsal tendon sheaths and rarely from the joint capsule. In early cases, their investigation with probes, fingers, etc. should be circumspect as it is likely that such interference will introduce infection. Synovial flow will often maintain the sterility of the sheath or joint and, under the influence of pressure, the fistula will usually seal itself or eventually close with granulation tissue. The temptation to find the aperture and suture it should also be resisted as this too will introduce infection and foreign material. Antibiotic therapy in these animals must be broad spectrum, vigorous and prolonged: *10 days* is the minimum.

Established chronic fistulae are likely to be infected producing turbid, flocculent synovial fluid. Their origin can be discovered using contrast radiography, the contrast medium being injected through a catheter inserted into the fistula. It is likely to be one of the tendon sheaths and the treatment of choice is irrigation. An indwelling catheter can be inserted into the fistula followed by frequent and copious irrigation performed over 5–6 days. Pressure bandaging and antibiotic therapy are also used. Other more radical treatments are curettage of the sheath followed by irrigation and the surgical creation of a second fistula of the proximal end of the sheath with the insertion of an irrigation catheter. Again, pressure bandaging and antibiotic therapy are essential adjuncts.

Despite intensive therapy some fistulae are refractory and persist along with increasing swelling, fibrosis and stiffness. The author has experience of some cases where the tendon itself was infected and partially necrotic; in one case there was tendon rupture. Complete extirpation of the sheath can be considered but it is difficult surgery with much residual reaction and fibrosis. The prognosis with these cases is poor.

Chronic swollen carpi

Occasionally the clinician is presented with a swollen knee which has a long history of neglect or mismanagement. Even after some months, active inflammatory change can be present as indicated by pain on palpation and manipulation, heat and a radiographic appearance

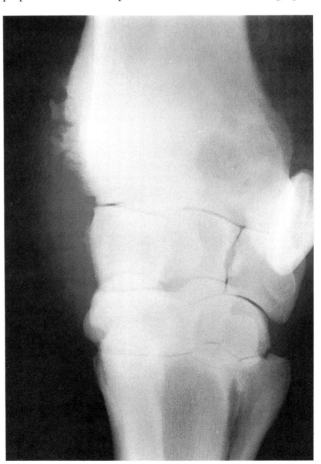

Fig. 5.7 A DPLMO projection demonstrating chronic long term bony change on the dorsomedial and dorsal carpus. The new bone is well organized yet still retains a palisaded appearance in the superficial layers. Periarticular remodelling indicates degenerative joint disease of the radiocarpal joint.

of widespread periosteal reaction of the active palisaded type — characteristic of chronic, low grade infection (Fig. 5.7).

These cases will usually respond well to *prolonged* courses (2—3 weeks) of a broad spectrum antibiotic, or antibiotic combination, in association with careful pressure bandaging. Within the first few days there will be a dramatic reduction in size of the knee with a smaller but significant diminution over the remaining 2 weeks or so. They must be box rested during the treatment regime and for 2—3 months subsequently. However, daily walking *in hand* and manipulation of the carpus is also important to promote carpal flexibility. The knee will never be normal again and some restriction in flexion is inevitable but this simple technique enables many animals to be salvaged and eventually to perform at a reasonable athletic level.

Suggested further reading

Auer JA (1980) Equine lameness: diseases of the carpus. *Vet Clin North Am* (Large Animal Practice) **2**, 81—90.
McIlwraith CW (1983) Arthroscopic surgery — athletic and developmental lesions. *Proc 29th Ann Conv Am Ass Eq Prac* 103—17.
Selway SJ (1983) Arthroscopic surgery — the carpal and fetlock joints. *Proc 29th Ann Conv Am Ass Eq Prac* 95—102.

The Radius

Abnormalities of growth plate

See section on juvenile limb deformities, p. 198.

Fractures of the radius

See section on Fractures, chapter 9.

Fissure fractures of the radius

The animal presents with a non-characteristic lameness of the affected leg and a history of sudden onset. There may be a little swelling and pain on palpation of the forearm, more evident distally, to indicate the site of the problem. The small number of cases seen by the author were referrals of some weeks duration and the distinctive radiographic feature was a diffuse aggressive periosteal reaction along the fracture margins. The cracks are difficult to see except on high quality films and the exact cause of the fracture is often uncertain. The swelling and periosteal reaction could equally well be signs of a localized cellulitis. The presence of a wound, the response to antibiotic therapy, or the complete absence of a discernible fracture line would be factors pointing in that direction.

Treatment

If the position of fracture plane cannot be determined accurately, internal fixation carries the risk that screws or plates may be wrongly placed and weaken the fracture line. There is also the considerable risk of complete fracture during anaesthetic recovery. If the fracture can be mapped then internal fixation is the treatment of choice, though with 6—9 months rest (albeit with the constant worry of complete fracture) healing will take place without surgical interference. In these cases analgesics are contraindicated as they can encourage greater weight bearing.

The elbow region

Olecranon bursitis 'capped elbow' 'shoe boil'

These terms are used to describe any swelling at the point of the elbow. The cause is invariably trauma either from the shoe of the ipsilateral forefoot during recumbency or the ipsilateral hind foot of high gaited trotting horses. In the former case the development of the condition is likely to be over a period of time and may be associated with another disability which causes the horse to remain lying for long periods. Shoes with long heels or caulks are also a cause. Trauma from hind shoes at speed can result in major wounds to the elbow or severe, repetitive blows to the area.

Clinical signs

The results of acute severe trauma will be a diffuse, hot, painful swelling of the area with the possibility of skin lacerations. Infection can be introduced through unnoticed puncture wounds and in these cases the symptoms will worsen over several days. Lameness is variable but will in general parallel the severity of local signs. Non-infected cases will show improvement of local signs with rest.

More chronic, low grade trauma can result in no more than localized skin thickening and hair loss but more typically the condition develops as a fluctuant swelling at the point of the elbow. Initially this is due to seroma or haematoma formation, but, if the cause is not removed, a chronic, fibrous, acquired bursitis develops.

Diagnosis

Lesions in the elbow region should always give rise to the suspicion of trauma from feet but swellings over the elbow can be due to ulnar or olecranon fractures or conditions of the elbow joint, although confusions with the latter is unlikely. Radiography is important to eliminate both major fractures or bone damage associated with the capped elbow syndrome.

Treatment

Acute lacerated injuries must be dealt with promptly with the decision to debride and complete or, more sensibly, part suture the wound being made on general surgical principles. Bandaging of the area is not really feasible and so treatment is usually restricted to antibiotic cover in those cases where infection is suspect, and *removing the cause*. If recumbency is the cause, further trauma is prevented by cross tying, removal of the shoe, or fitting of a 'sausage boot'. Failing that, temporary bandaging of the foot over a thick padding base will have the same effect initially.

Wounds caused by hind feet are allowed to heal by not using the animal and then prevented by using an elbow protector fitted to the harness.

Where the swelling does not diminish with conservative treatment, its presence makes matters worse thereafter. Surgical removal of the mass can be performed and is done through a C-shaped incision. Occasionally the fibrous walled bursa will 'shell out' but excision in this region where there is extensive movement always leaves dead space and healing problems. It is virtually impossible to apply pressure to the site and post-operative swelling is a major feature. Again, part suturing allowing dependant drainage can be useful and, if temperament allows, the animal should be cross tied for 8–10 days after surgery.

Long term prevention in animals who lie for long periods is by fitting of a sausage boot when the animal is not being worked.

The elbow joint

The elbow is a ginglymus or hinge joint. The distal humerus forms one side of the joint while the radius and ulna combine to form the glenoid or semilinear notch into which the humerus fits.

There is only one direction of movement, flexion and extension over an arc of some 55–60°; the axis of movement is slightly oblique so that flexion moves the forearm laterally.

The radius and ulna are held tightly together by the interosseous ligament of the forearm both proximal and distal to the interosseous space. This distal portion ossifies and the two bones fuse before adulthood. By this time, however, growth at the proximal radial growth plate has ceased and the relationship of the radius and ulna at the elbow is not affected.

The joint capsule is tightly applied except caudally and distensions are not easy to see or feel. Mild distension may escape notice entirely and even gross swelling can be missed unless both elbows are palpated or viewed simultaneously from in front. Even then, inequalities caused by one leg being weight bearing and the other not can be confusing.

Elbow luxation

Reported rarely in horses but should be suspected where there is severe trauma to the elbow region and subsequent major distortion. It is occasionally seen in association with an ulnar fracture (Monteggia fracture).

Clinical signs

Lateral or medial luxations cause the leg to be held in semiflexion; mobility is severely restricted and resented. The elbow appears wide when viewed from in front. Caudal luxations cause the leg to appear short, as the proximal radius and ulna are displaced behind the distal humerus. Cranial luxation will, in a high percentage of cases, be accompanied by ulnar fracture.

Diagnosis

Local signs and radiography. The latter is essential to check for fractures of the ulna or the presence of chips at the articular margin.

Treatment

Reduction can only be under general anaesthesia and muscle relaxation may be necessary. The reductions are difficult. Medial and lateral luxations are best reduced by putting the elbow into hyperextension and attempting to use the anconeal process as a fulcrum, positioning it behind the distal humerus and levering the humeral condyles upwards and into the mid-line where they can fall back into the glenoid.

Fractures of the ulna and olecranon

Aetiology and pathogenesis

Caused by direct trauma from kicks or traffic accidents; also by avulsion of the olecranon as a result of triceps pull. This can happen if an animal, usually when fatigued, slips with a foreleg stretched out in front.

Clinical signs

There is usually a sudden onset of severe lameness. The affected leg is held with all the joints slightly flexed and the toe resting on the ground. A characteristic feature is the animal's understandable reluctance to exert any triceps pull on the olecranon; this results in a typical 'dropped elbow' stance which is also seen in radial paralysis and in some cases of post-anaesthetic ischaemic myopathies. Some animals, however, can bear weight on the leg reasonably well. This is probably a function of the position of the fracture and the intactness of the distal glenoid which, with the leg upright takes most of the stress of weight bearing.

There is variable swelling in the area of the elbow and there may be none detectable for the first hour or so. The amount of crepitus also varies with comminution and the degree of instability.

Diagnosis

Olecranon fractures are often missed, firstly because they tend not to produce severe local signs and secondly, being uncommon, they are not consciously looked for. An initial examination which does not detect the fractures may not be repeated, as rest for a week or so will often produce an improvement in gait. Further examination is often delayed until the rate of improvement slows and stops and it is a worrying fact that most olecranon fractures seen at the University of Liverpool Equine Hospital were over 10 weeks old when first referred.

As with all fractures, early diagnosis and treatment are essential. Any sudden onset, severe lameness should raise strong suspicions of a fracture and the leg examined minutely from top to toe. Accurate diagnosis through clinical signs alone is not always possible but such an examination should produce sufficient evidence of pain, local swelling, resentment to manipulation and occasionally crepitus, to indicate an urgent need for radiography. *NB* always compare with the other side!

Radiography

Fortunately, penetration of the relatively slim ulna and olecranon is within the capability of most practice X-ray sets. The diagnostic projection is the straight lateromedial and to achieve it the leg must be pulled gently out in front to extend both shoulder and elbow. This is invariably resented at first but can usually be done in the standing animal with a little patience. The cassette is pushed into the axilla and the exposure made.

The ulna most commonly fractures into the semilunar notch (Fig. 5.8). All grades of comminution are possible with the fracture involving the ulnar shaft and the olecranon. In young animals avulsion of the proximal ulnar apophysis is possible.

Craniocaudal projections are useful, especially if comminution is present and they will also reveal fragment misalignment and any damage to the humeral condyle. In long-standing fractures, the joint margins should be scrutinized for osteophytes which would indicate a DJD.

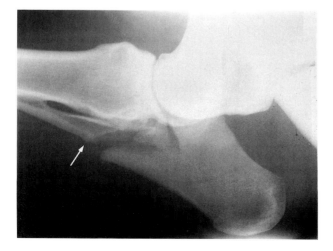

Fig. 5.8 An ulnar fracture. Note how the fracture has become distracted as a result of extensor traction. New bone at the fragment margins (arrowed) indicates that this is not a recent fracture.

Treatment

In those fractures involving the ulna shaft the results of *early* surgical treatment are excellent. In fractures involving the semilunar notch and in olecranon fractures with a low level of comminution it is, without doubt, the treatment of choice. The operation consists of the reduction and compression of the fracture through the application of a dynamic compression plate to the caudal or tension band side of the ulna.

Most descriptions of the surgical technique advise laying the animal on its side with the affected limb uppermost. An alternative, which the author has found to offer easier access, is to have the animal in dorsal recumbency with the elbow flexed and the carpus extended to its limits. Another advantage is that the weight of the lower limb ensures good apposition between the radius and humerus, and ensures that when the fracture gap is closed by applying compression to the caudal surface of the ulna, this apposition is reinforced; also that the deeper layers of the ulnar fracture are adequately compressed.

The ulna is approached via a caudal incision between the heads of ulnaris lateralis and the ulnar head of the deep digital flexor muscle. The fracture line is exposed, and if necessary, the fragments are aligned manually. Where the fracture has been present for many weeks, as is often the case, fibrous tissue and callus will be present, making perfect reduction impossible. If the callus is large enough to prevent snug apposition of the plate it can be chiselled flat, although no attempt need be made to clean the fracture line: the non-union will ossify once stabilized and compressed. A narrow compression plate of ASIF (Association for the Study of Internal Fixation) design is contoured to fit the curve of the ulna; the proximal portion has to be twisted slightly to allow it to seat snugly. With very proximal fractures, the plate can actually be shaped around the blunt proximal end of the ulna. Some surgeons, rather than twist and contour the plate will chisel away the caudal ulna so that it presents only a flat surface to the plate.

The plate is used to compress the fracture using standard ASIF techniques. In most cases the fracture gap is too large to be closed completely by the compressive action of the plate alone. A tension device will have to be used, though this is not a problem because of the good distal access to the caudal radius. Points to watch are that no screw enters the elbow joint; that screws in the olecranon need to be angled to follow its concave cross-section and that in young animals they must be of the cancellous type, and that, again in immature patients, care must be taken not to span the proximal radial physis and restrict its growth. In adults the plates should be left in place if they cause no problems. In immature animals they may be removed after some 3–4 months if there is any worry about interference with differential growth.

The wound can initially be covered by a pressure bandage or a simple 'Stent' bandage if no great swelling is anticipated. The post-operative management of the case should be box rest for 2–3 months with walking exercise in hand commencing early in this period and increasing steadily in amount.

The immediate post-operative reduction in lameness is impressive and the long term outlook is good. Even in long standing, untreated cases the author has found the technique very worthwhile. In early cases the area should be carefully checked for skin penetration. In long haired animals the superficial wounds inflicted by kicks can pass unnoticed until the animal is clipped. If any are found, surgery should be delayed and antibiotic therapy started. Conservative treatment should be considered only in those cases where the fracture is non-distracted and non-articular. It should consist of absolute box rest for no less than 8 weeks. There is an obvious risk of the fracture distracting and this is likely to occur as the animal rises; if its temperament allows then cross tying will prevent this. In animals with severely comminuted fractures the level of comminution may preclude internal fixation, and if they are to be salvaged for breeding purposes conservative treatment is the only alternative. The complications of conservative treatment of these fractures are: DJD of the elbow joint, with or without non-union of the fracture, resulting in pain and swelling; atrophy of the triceps mass; flexural contractures of the carpus and fetlock; angular deformities of the opposite limb in young animals and, of course, permanent disability.

Septic arthritis of the elbow

Septic arthritis of the elbow is an uncommon condition, but it is seen often enough to warrant inclusion here. Occasionally the result of foreign body penetration or known trauma, it is more commonly of unknown origin.

The symptoms will be a lameness increasing in severity over several days to a stage where the animal bears weight only reluctantly. There is usually detectable swelling and pain on pressure and manipulation. There is commonly the development of a discharging sinus at or around the protruberance of the lateral condyle of the humerus. This may be either as a result of direct penetration from sharp objects at the time of initial wounding, or by necrosis of contused tissues subsequenlty. The sinus may discharge purulent fluid initially with necrotic ligamentous tissue as the nidus for the infection. Later penetration of the joint capsule will result in the discharge of turbid infected synovial fluid.

Diagnosis

In cases where there is a discharging sinus at this site, the diagnosis should be fairly self-evident. However, it is possible for the discharge to be purulent and not synovial fluid yet the joint still be infected. In these cases, and in those without an obvious wound, aspiration of joint fluid will be necessary to achieve a diagnosis.

Turbidity or flocculence suggest infection and a high white cell count will confirm this (see section on septic arthritis above).

Treatment is by joint lavage (see also section on septic arthritis above) coupled, in appropriate cases, with surgical debridement of any necrotic tissue around the sinus tract. The size of the resultant tissue defect can be large and cause concern over healing. However, given time and regular cleansing most cases heal well without further interference even when the joint is exposed! *NB* parenteral antibiotics used alone without local treatment are useless and waste valuable time.

Cases diagnosed early and treated vigorously carry a relatively good prognosis. Established infection causes irreversible joint damage!

Suggested further reading

Edwards GB and Vaughan LC (1978) Infective arthritis of the elbow joint in horses. *Vet Record* **103**, 227–9.

The humerus

Humeral fracture

Humeral fracture is a rare occurrence in the adult although more common in foals, in most cases due to trauma from the dam.

Diagnosis is based on a sudden onset of complete lack of function of the distal limb which will usually be trailed behind as the animal walks. Overriding of fragments is common and the leg may appear shorter. The overlying muscle masses can prevent adequate examination of the area but pain and swelling are usually severe enough to pinpoint the problem area. Crepitus can usually be felt or heard on manipulation and its audibility is often increased by pressing ones ear or a stethoscope to the area of the tuberosity. If still in doubt a simple sound conduction test can be done. With a stethoscope on the humeral tuberosity the cannon bone is tapped sharply with a piece of wood; sound travels well in the intact leg and can be clearly heard. In the other limb, the fracture interrupts conduction and only a dull sound is transmitted. Although not infallible, it can be a useful additional pointer and along with crepitus is something a dubious owner can appreciate. This may be an important factor where adequate X-ray facilities are not at hand because, bearing in mind the virtually hopeless prognosis with fractured humerus in the adult, the veterinary surgeon may decide upon immediate euthanasia rather than subject the animal to a harrowing journey to the nearest referral centre.

In small ponies and foals treatment may be considered, though the likelihood of success is not good. A conservative regime of 3–4 months box rest is associated with some considerable pain but may result in healing although the subsequent distortion of the limb due to fragment overriding and flexural contracture of the carpus may be unacceptable. In addition, the immature animal is likely to develop angular deformities or weight bearing laminitis of the contralateral limb. Finally, fracture of the humerus caries a high risk of radial nerve damage. The presence of radial paralysis can be difficult to assess immediately post-fracture because of limb posture and because perineural inflammatory change may produce as effective a paralysis, albeit temporary, as nerve severance. Assessment of sensory deinnervation is not reliable, especially in the immediate post-fracture period.

The use of a 'Thomas extension splint' may provide some rigidity and some weight bearing ability for the leg — provided it is well fitting. A loose or badly fitted device may exacerbate the leverage on the fracture and can make matters worse.

In young foals and small ponies, internal fixation can be considered. Radiography is a prerequisite and should be done under general anaesthesia so that the leg can be manipulated and drawn forward to avoid superimposition of the thoracic inlet and other limb.

The fractures are usually spiral or oblique and may involve the proximal or distal physis. There is always considerable overriding which makes reduction at surgery difficult and, in cases of longer standing, well nigh impossible. Other surgical problems are the short length of bone coupled with the wide medullary cavity, and in young foals, relatively thin cortices.

The simplest method of fixation is the use of multiple or stack pinning techniques where as many Steinmann pins as it takes to fill the narrowest part of the medullary cavity are inserted in the conventional 'retrograde' manner. The advantages of this method are (a) the use of conventional implants, (b) good stability — in all directions including the rotational plane, and (c) a reduced tendency for the implants to drift distally as can happen with a large, heavy solid pin.

Other techniques are the use of 'clover leaf nails' which are hollow pins of large diameter and with a clover leaf cross-section. They are light, give good stability in all directions but, although inserted in the usual retrograde manner, can be difficult to use without specialized ancillary equipment. Unfortunately they cannot be cut to length, so a large stock of different sizes must be maintained. This is usually impracticable and limits their usefulness in large animal orthopaedics.

The squat, irregular shape of the equine humerus makes it a difficult bone to plate and virtually impossible to double plate; the presence of the radial nerve also adds to the difficulties of the surgeon! There is a high incidence of implant failure following single plate application even when the strong broad ASIF dynamic compression plates are used and unless the fracture configuration allows double plating other techniques should be considered first.

A final point to be considered is that of post-operative infection. Repair of humeral fractures is only a realistic proposition in the smallest, and, therefore, usually the youngest patients. Regrettably, the incidence of post-operative complication following fracture fixation in neonates is high, with the foals being reluctant to stand and suckle. Prolonged recumbency, nutritional deprivation, even for a short time and immunological incompetence are all factors which encourage and create a high incidence of enteritis, along with systemic and local surgical site infections.

In these cases the animal's immunological status must be measured, or if this is not practicable, assumed to be low. Every effort should be made to make good deficiencies with, for example, plasma transfusions. It *must* also be realized that post-operative attention to feeding and nursing is as important as the actual surgical technique. However, in those foals which overcome these difficulties, healing is rapid and the prognosis for a return to athletic soundness can be good.

Suggested further reading

Bramlage LR (1983) The status of internal fixation of long bone fractures in the horse. *Proc 29th Conv Am Ass Eq Prac* 119–23.

Milne DW and Turner AS (1979) *An Atlas of Surgical Approaches to the Bones of the Horse*. WB Saunders, Philadelphia.

Denny HR (1976) The surgical treatment of fractures of the olecranon in the horse *Eq Vet J* **8**(1), 20–5.

Fackelman GE and Nunamaker DM (1982) *Manual of Internal Fixation in the Horse*. Springer Verlag, Berlin.

The shoulder region

Introduction

Pathological conditions affecting the shoulder region of the horse are *rare*. However, the diagnosis of 'shoulder lameness' is frequently made, usually, and regrettably, in the absence of any logical diagnostic work-up. The term 'shoulder lameness' implying a specific condition with specific symptoms and pathogenesis, is, of course, meaningless but it has unfortunately, through repetition, acquired respectability and has become a convenient label for undiagnosed lameness.

Examination of the shoulder region

Occasionally, obvious local signs will draw attention to the shoulder region on the initial examination. However, if these are not present then the shoulder should only be implicated as a site of pathology when the much commoner distal limb problems have been excluded by careful clinical examination and nerve blocks.

Much has been made of characteristic gait abnormalities as a method of diagnosing pain in the shoulder region: unfortunately, none is particularly reliable especially in those cases where the lameness is less than severe. Generally, pain arising from proximal limb joints will cause an animal to restrict flexion of the affected articulation and resort to circumduction of the leg in order to advance it; therefore 'throwing a leg out' *may* be an indication of upper leg pain. Fixation of the scapulohumeral joint may also occur in an effort to minimize discomfort. This can be difficult to appreciate and the clinician must specifically watch for it and also compare the movement to the opposite side: again it becomes easier the more severe the lameness and the slower the trot. On the lunge the characteristic head nod is present and the lameness is usually worse when the affected leg is on the inside of the circle.

If present, asymmetry of shape is one of the better indications of pathology in the shoulder region. With the animal standing as 'square' as possible, i.e. taking weight evenly on both forelimbs, the suspect area should be viewed from all angles and compared to the opposite side: the best comparative view is had by kneeling in front of the forelegs, if animal's temperament allows, and silhouetting both shoulders against the sky (Fig. 5.9).

The clinician must be careful not to confuse swelling with an

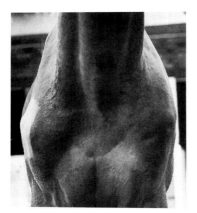

Fig. 5.9 A 'worms-eye' view of the disparity between the outline of the scapulohumeral joints in a horse suffering from right sided suprascapular paralysis ('sweeney').

accentuated prominence of the proximal humerus caused by disuse or neurogenic atrophy of surrounding musculature. Atrophy or 'wasting' of scapular muscles is a consistent feature of shoulder pain and disease of several weeks duration. The triceps and cranial upper limb muscle masses can suffer too, though principally in long standing elbow problems. A point worth noting is that atrophy of the supra-scapular muscle masses is *not* a feature of lameness originating from the lower limb although *minor* atrophy can occasionally be seen in *severe long standing* cases.

The traditional way of exacerbating pain thought to be originating in the shoulder is to extend the entire limb. This is done by standing in front of the leg, grasping it, and leaning backwards. The severity of the animal's reaction is taken as an indication of severity of the pain elicited. This method is somewhat non-specific as it also extends the elbow and the other joints and the reaction to this unusual manoeuvre is also largely dependant on the animal's temperament.

A rather more specific, though still crude, method is to abduct the limb slowly, grasping it by the forearm and elbow, holding it abducted for 30 seconds and then trotting the animal away. The elbow is not stressed to such a great extent and the involuntary worsening of a lameness is a better guide than an acute pain reaction.

Intra-articular anaesthesia

See section on regional and intra-articular anaesthesia, pp. 15—22.

Radiology of the shoulder region

The advent of rare-earth screen/film combinations has placed this area into the realms of 'standing' or erect radiography. With moderately powerful mobile type generators even large animals need not be anaesthetized.

The animal is positioned so that the cassette lies lateral to and slightly above and cranial to the point of the affected shoulder, the leg is then slowly and carefully drawn forward to position the scapulo-humeral joint in front of the cassette: even animals with extremely painful lesions will tolerate this if it is done slowly. Another advantage of rare-earth screen/film combinations is that, as no grid is necessary in most cases, accurate alignment of tube and cassette is not needed. This means that a slightly oblique craniocaudal, mediolateral oblique can be used making it unnecessary to pull the shoulder out too far.

The rapidly tapering thickness of the region makes two exposures necessary for full evaluation; a relatively low power one to show detail of the projecting cranial portion of the articulation, and a second, with a much higher exposure value, to visualize the caudal portion which is overlain by thick pectoral and brachial musculature.

With very large animals, a grid is necessary. Careful adjustment of beam and grid are essential and the long exposure times inevitably required with most generators mean that time and money is saved by conducting the examination with the animal under general anaesthesia.

Conditions of the scapulohumeral articulation (shoulder)

Bicipital bursitis

Trauma to the point of the shoulder can damage the tendon of origin of biceps brachialis which, after arising from the tuber scapulae, courses forward and downwards through the bicipital groove on the proximal humerus just cranial to the humeral head. The movement of this tendon over the intertuberal groove is facilitated by the large bicipital bursa which may also suffer damage.

Clinical signs

Symptoms include a sudden onset of severe lameness or, in cases of septic bursitis, an increase in severity to non-weight bearing over 2–3 days. The animal is reluctant to stand on the leg and in more severe cases may absolutely refuse to do so. This is because the 'biceps' is one of the extensors of the shoulder and forms, via lacertus fibrosus, an attachment to extensor carpi radialis and hence is part of the 'stay apparatus' of the forelimb.

Active extension of the shoulder will also cause pain and in most cases, the leg will be dragged behind and not advanced (Fig. 5.10).

Swelling of the region is often not noticeable.

Diagnosis

There may be few or no local signs, so lower limb causes must be ruled out initially. Local pain with pressure over the intertuberal groove and manipulation, especially flexion of the scapulohumeral joint and extension of the elbow, will indicate that there is pain in the region. Elimination of shoulder and scapular conditions by negative radiographic findings and normal scapulohumeral joint synovial fluid analysis will then tend to concentrate interest on the bursa. Paracentesis

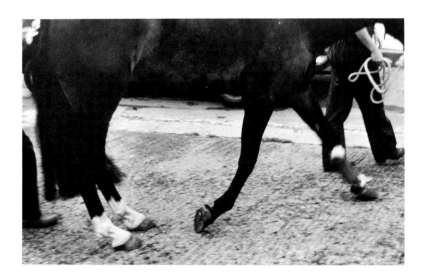

Fig. 5.10 The typical leg carriage of a horse with a right sided, septic, bicipital bursitis.

of the bursa is possible especially if it is distended, though it is never a simple task. After the skin over the point of the shoulder is anaesthetized the shoulder is held in as flexed a state as the animal will allow; this tenses the bursa and makes penetration easier. A 6–8 cm (2½–3″) needle is inserted over the intertuberal groove and, applying suction to an attached syringe, the area is probed. On penetrating the bursa, fluid enters the syringe.

Treatment

Traumatic bursitis without the presence of infection will respond to rest — a minimum of 3 months box confinement being necessary followed by a further 6 months or so of restricted exercise. Even then the risk of a relapse is substantial. Steroid therapy should be used with extreme care as the risk of subsequent osseous metaplasia is high. The author has experienced one case of septic bursitis which recovered fully after surgical exposure and drainage of the sheath followed by irrigation through an indwelling catheter for 7 days. Systemic antibiosis alone produced only mild and temporary remission. Generally, however, the prognosis in these cases must be extremely guarded.

Osteochondrosis of the shoulder joint

Osteochondrosis of the shoulder joint, and its sequel osteochondritis dissecans (OCD), is a clinical entity in horses and must be considered when evaluating a case of lameness originating in the shoulder region of a young animal. In the UK the condition is traditionally associated with young heavy horses, but in recent surveys, thoroughbreds have figured prominently. There is a sex incidence, with males predominating.

Aetiology and pathogenesis

See section on osteochondrosis, p. 194.

Clinical signs

Most horses present with a history of intermittent lameness. The onset is insidious and the severity is variable with a high proportion being bilaterally affected. Occasionally owners will associate the onset of lameness, or an exacerbation of mild lameness, with some traumatic episode. Those lame on a single leg show a typical foreleg lameness gait at the trot, with 'nodding' or dipping of the head as the unaffected leg takes weight. Sometimes the clinician can see that the shoulder is being held in a flexed position through all phases of the stride, otherwise the gait is not remarkable. If bilaterally affected, the foreleg gait will be stilted or 'pottery' and it will be similar to any other bilateral lower limb lameness. The lameness tends to worsen with exercise. There may be pain when the shoulder joint is flexed, extended or abducted and deep pressure over the shoulder will often cause a persistent pain reaction. In those cases which have been lame for some time there can be atrophy of the supra and infraspinatus muscles and the heel of the foot elongates to create a 'boxy' hoof.

Diagnosis

If muscle atrophy is not a feature and fixation of the shoulder joint is not recognized then it will be a negative response to nerve blocks and absence of pathology in the lower limb which focuses attention on the shoulder. Even if local signs indicate scapulohumeral involvement, it is wise to eliminate the lower limb in this way before concentrating on the shoulder. Pain on manipulation and pressure and an exacerbation of the lameness following manipulation should point to the presence of pathology but it is intra-articular anaesthesia which will provide solid evidence (see section on regional anaesthesia, pp. 15–22).

Radiography is necessary before a positive diagnosis can be made. Two types of changes can be seen: firstly an alteration in the contour of the humeral head and occasionally the scapular glenoid so that they take on a flattened appearance, especially in the caudal half of their contour; and secondly, those changes characteristic of degenerative joint disease. The latter are principally periarticular bone spur formation and are seen usually at the caudal border of the humeral head and less often at the cranial border of the glenoid. In established cases, heavy sclerosis of the humeral head around the primary bone deficit is also visible; this may mask the lucency of the latter and any subchondral cysts which may be present. Unlike the situation in the dog, loose intra-articular bodies or 'joint mice' are not a feature of the condition in the horse.

When reading the films the clinician must remember that he is viewing only one profile of the joint and this is dependant on the angulation of the main beam, also, that articular cartilage defects will not be visible on non-contrast films.

In early cases, the minimal changes may go undetected in less than optimum quality films. In these instances better quality radiographs may be taken under general anaesthesia or the animal re-radiographed later.

NB where positive evidence of osteochondrosis is found it is wise to radiograph the other leg; the changes are often bilateral.

Treatment

Two factors mitigate against successful surgical treatment. Firstly, the almost inevitable presence of degenerative joint disease which would compromise the result of any surgery and secondly, the difficulty of the surgical approach.

There are few reports of surgical management of shoulder OCD in the horse but some suggest that there is occasionally a dramatic response.

Two surgical approaches are suggested. Mason and MacLean (1977) approach the joint by transecting the teres minor muscle followed by a vertical incision in the joint capsule while Schmidt, Dueland and Vaughan (1975) transect the infraspinatus tendon insertion followed by a 5 cm curved incision through the joint capsule. The defect is identified and cartilage flaps and devitalized bone is curretted away. Following irrigation the joint is closed.

Conservative management seems to have mixed results. One survey (Nyack *et al* 1981) indicates that animals with minor lesions, if subjected to many months rest and a reduction in dietary intake, can become sound enough to be used as pleasure horses or breeding animals. The advisability of using these horses for breeding purposes is open to question, although it is likely that only the tendency towards rapid growth is inherited and this of course can be managed by dietary restrictions.

The use of corticosteroids is not indicated; they give only temporary relief and may encourage, during that time, overexertion and further damage.

Suggested further reading

Dyson S (1986) Diagnostic techniques in the investigation of shoulder lameness. *Eq Vet J* **18**(1), 25–8.
Dyson S (1986) Shoulder lameness in horses: an analysis of 58 suspected cases. *Eq Vet J* **18**(1), 29–36.
Mason TA and MacLean AA (1977) Osteochondrosis of the head of the humerus in two foals. *Eq Vet J* **9**, 189–91.
Nyack B, Morgan JP, Pool R and Meagher D (1981) Osteochondrosis of the shoulder joint of the horse. *Cornell Vet* **71**, 149–63.
Schmidt GR, Dueland R and Vaughan JT (1975) Osteochondrosis dissecans of the equine shoulder joint. *Vet Med Small Anim Clin* **70**, 542–7.

Fractures of the scapula

General considerations

The scapula or 'shoulder blade' is a flat plate of bone, triangular in shape lying against the cranial thoracic wall; distally it articulates with the humerus. The articular surface or glenoid is a shallow concavity whose surface area is much smaller than the head of the humerus. The scapula is surrounded and well protected by musculature apart from its craniodistal portion, the supraglenoid tuberosity, which is vulnerable to trauma, forming, as it does, the 'point of the shoulder'.

The supraglenoid tuberosity and the cranial part of the glenoid form as two separate ossification centres which fuse, firstly together, and then as a block with the body of the scapula. This fusion is complete by 12 months. In the adult the site of fusion is marked by a medial indentation of the glenoid, the 'glenoid notch'. The supraglenoid tuberosity is the origin of two muscles; biceps brachii laterally and coracobrachialis medially.

Aetiology and pathogenesis

The initiating factor in all fractures is undoubtedly trauma. There is usually a history of a fall, a collision with a gate post or, as in several cases seen by the author, a history of an acute onset of lameness immediately on landing from a jump. Many fractures, even in the adult, follow the approximate line where the supraglenoid tuberosity and the cranial portion of the glenoid fused with the main body of the scapula. It is suggested that this fusion creates a weak point which persists for some time and predisposes to fracture at this site (Dyson 1985). It has also been suggested that the frequency of fracture at this point in adults is due to damage to the site which may have occurred possibly years previously. This view is supported by the occasional animal which has shown supra and infraspinatus muscle atrophy before the acute onset of lameness, and by the finding in some horses of radiographic changes, including ossification of the biceps tendon, too well established to have developed in the time interval between the onset of lameness and the examination. An equally plausible theory is that the glenoid notch, which is sometimes quite deep, is an intrinsic weak point in the distal scapula.

Clinical signs

Although it might not be seen in those animals out at pasture, there is a sudden onset of severe lameness; usually following some type of trauma or violent activity. Initially there is some swelling at the site and, of course, pain on manipulation or pressure. The severity of the lameness soon abates so that a week or so after the onset the animal may be walking reasonably well. Within a month even animals with intra-articular fractures can be walking virtually sound although 2—3/10th lameness persists at the trot. This improvement is not maintained however, and many months later this will be the picture presented to the clinician. There is always some degree of muscle atrophy and in later weeks an impression of swelling in the region can be heightened by an increased prominence of the point of the shoulder due to the atrophy. The latter is variable in extent and different muscles are affected; supra and infraspinatus are the most common but the pectorals and triceps may be involved too.

In the acute phase the animals will not trot, and it is inhumane to force them; later, lunging will worsen the lameness, and one report suggests that the exacerbation is greater when the affected leg is on the outside of the circle (Dyson 1985).

If the fracture line extends to affect the suprascapular nerve where it crosses the cranial border of the scapula some 12—15 cm from the glenoid, neurogenic atrophy can compound the problem. In these cases, atrophy of the supra and infraspinatus muscles is very rapid and instability of the shoulder develops. This shows as a transient abduction of the scapulo-humeral joint during the weight bearing phase of the stride.

Diagnosis

The sudden onset of a severe lameness should, in itself, suggest a traumatic origin and raise the possibility of a fracture. When trauma is known to have occurred in the form of a fall, collision or an awkward landing from a jump then a fracture should be high on the list of likely diagnoses. In these circumstances, pain and swelling should indicate that the shoulder region is involved; if not, then a clinical examination of the remainder of the limb should eliminate other causes. Radiography is usually needed to reach a definite diagnosis. This can be done standing, though drawing the leg forward to bring the shoulder clear of the chest can be difficult especially in early cases where the pain is severe; even then a slow steady pull will usually be tolerated.

Intra-articular anaesthesia is often not helpful, even in intra-articular fractures. There can be some reduction in pain, but the rest of the fracture line is also extremely painful and is not affected by the anaesthesia.

Treatment

There is little chance that an animal which suffers a fracture of the scapula will ever be fit for athletic purposes again. There are sporadic reports of some cases either recovering spontaneously or after surgical fixation, but in general the prognosis is very poor. Intra-articular fractures inevitably lead to degenerative change in the joint (omarthritis) and chronic pain. This fact must be pointed out to owners who are often encouraged by the improvement in lameness seen in the first few weeks following fracture.

In very young animals fractured tuber scapulae can sometimes be reattached using cancellous ASIF screws, but in the older animal this type of fixation cannot withstand the pull of biceps and the other muscles. Some fractures can be plated but access is difficult and the bone itself, being, in most parts, only a thin plate, offers very poor holding for screws; there is also the risk of damage to the suprascapular nerve.

Resection of the supraglenoid tuberosity as a treatment for fractures of the tuberosity has been performed with the muscles supposedly reattaching to the parent scapula (Leitch 1977). Its value for routine treatment is doubtful.

Conservative treatment is box rest for a minimum of 6 months, after which it is likely that most animals, other than those which have suffered a transverse mid-neck fracture where the outlook is more guarded, will be fit for breeding purposes. If in doubt, seek specialist advice!

Suggested further reading

Dyson S (1985) Sixteen fractures of the shoulder region in the horse. *Eq Vet J* **17**(2), 104–10.

Omarthritis (osteoarthritis of the scapulohumeral joint)

Omarthritis is the sequel to most conditions affecting the joint; fractures, joint trauma and osteochondrosis being the principle instigating factors.

The clinical signs will tend to be the same whatever the initial cause, except that osteochondrosis may superimpose its own symptomatology on that of the degenerative condition.

Uncomplicated cases will present as a non-specific lameness of variable severity and intermittent nature, at least initially. Unless local signs, such as muscle wasting, are present, then diagnosis is usually by elimination of lower limb conditions by clinical examination and especially nerve blocks. Intra-articular anaesthesia is extremely valuable with a marked reduction in the severity of lameness though not necessarily abolition of all the signs. At the same time synovial fluid can be taken for laboratory examination.

Radiography is extremely valuable, but good quality films are necessary to see the osteophytes at the articular margin, especially in early cases. Radiography under general anaesthesia is preferable so that the leg can be drawn well forward and the caudal portion of the joint well visualized. The osteophytes are seen principally on the caudal aspect of the humeral head and less often on the cranial glenoid.

Steroids will cause only temporary remission and probably the treatment of choice is intra-articular injection of sodium hyaluronate (hyaluronic acid). The response is variable with the prognosis better in early cases. A return to lameness is inevitable at some stage and it is wise to inform owners of this before embarking on expensive therapy.

Suprascapular nerve paralysis ('sweeney' or 'shoulder slip')

(Sweeny is derived from the German word Schweine, meaning atrophy.)

The suprascapular nerve is a short but thick nerve. It arises from C6 and C7 in the brachial plexus and then courses laterally to turn sharply around the cranial edge of the scapula some 6–7 cm dorsal to the supraglenoid tubrosity (tuber scapulae) and into the supraspinous fossa. Here it innervates the supraspinatus muscle and then passes on over the spine of the scapula to innervate the infraspinatus.

Aetiology and pathogenesis

The nerve is vulnerable to trauma as it crosses over the front of the scapula. An impact at this point puts the nerve, in the American idiom, 'between a rock and a hard place'. Trauma can come from collisions with gate posts, door sides, kicks or in a more chronic way from the pressure of a badly fitting harness. The latter was the prime cause of the condition in the draught and, especially, the plough horses of days gone by.

Loss of nerve conduction leads to paralysis of the supra and infraspinatus muscles. The two muscles and their tendons of insertion provide the main lateral stability of this inherently unstable, shallow ball and socket articulation and their loss of function results in uncontrollable abduction of the shoulder joint. Deinnervation of the muscles for more than a few days also leads to a rapid neurogenic atrophy.

Clinical signs

Clinical signs include a rapidly progressive atrophy of the supra and infraspinatus muscles; the speed of its development being far in excess of that caused by even severe shoulder pathology. In addition there is usually a varying degree of instability in the scapulohumeral joint, usually manifest in a sharp outward rotation of the shoulder during the weight bearing phase of the stride (Fig. 5.11). In severe cases the point of the shoulder appears to abduct by up to 15 cm (6″) or so. The trauma may have caused additional pathology such as a scapular fracture and symptoms of pain and swelling may be super-imposed on the neurogenic atrophy. *NB* the suprascapular nerve is motor only and therefore the paralysis does not result in a loss of sensation.

Diagnosis

The first sign of atrophy will be an increased prominence of the scapular spine compared to the other side. The presence of other clinical signs such as pain on pressure and manipulation must be looked for and if these are present the shoulder should be radio-graphed. (The clinician should take care not to confuse the increased prominence of the point of the shoulder which results from the atrophy, with a pathological swelling.) In the absence of other lesions, severe atrophy of the supra and infraspinatus muscles is virtually certain to have been the result of nerve damage. Where other lesions coexist, the rapid development of the atrophy and its profound nature will indicate that there is likely to be a nerve paralysis in addition. Instability of the shoulder joint in association with a developing atrophy is, in the absence of major fractures, virtually pathognomonic of suprascapular nerve paralysis.

Treatment

Adams (1974) suggests that removal of a 3 × 2 cm piece of the leading edge of the scapula where the nerve crosses might lead to a re-establish-ment of function. No evidence exists as to the efficacy of this treatment but no other is available.

Prognosis is far more important in these cases and unfortunately, as in all instances of nerve paralysis, is extremely difficult. Nerve conduction is an all-or-none phenomenon and minor perineural in-flammatory change and complete nerve severance may produce intially the same degree of paralysis. Only time will tell! If there is no return of function within 2 weeks or so, the outlook is grave. However, most clinicians will give these animals a month or 6 weeks before advocating euthanasia though, where instability is present, the distress caused to animal and owner may precipitate an early decision as to its fate.

Suggested further reading

Adams OR (1974) *Lameness in Horses* 3e. Lea and Febiger, Philadelphia.

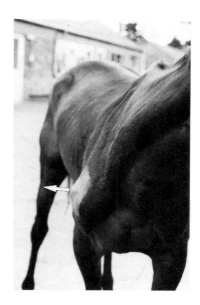

Fig. 5.11 The same horse as in Fig. 5.10 showing the characteristic abduction of the shoulder during the weight bearing phase of the stride.

6: Conditions of the Upper Hind Limb

The hock joint

Introduction and anatomy

The hock joint is a complex of many large and small joints: only one has any significant range of movement, and this, the tibiotarsal (tarsocrural) articulation, provides all of the flexor mobility of the hock. The others are bound together by strong ligaments and play no part in the bending of the joint. The tibiotarsal articulation is a ginglymus or sliding hinge joint, one of nature's ways of providing a great range of unidirectional movement within a single joint. It is important that the hock is thought of in terms of a complex structure and not simply as 'the hock'. It is a fund of pathological changes, each affecting different regions, and if the hock is not thought of in terms of its constituent parts, understanding these conditions can be difficult.

Figure 6.1 illustrates some of the clinically important structures of the hock. Individual details will be discussed under the appropriate condition headings (see also section on nerve blocks and intra-articular anaesthesia of the hock, pp. 9–22).

Physical examination

'Hock lameness' is a totally non-specific term; it does not describe a condition but merely identifies the hock region as a source of pain, and hence a gait abnormality. Beyond this umbrella term lies a profusion of individual conditions, any of which will produce a 'hock lameness'.

Pain arising from the hock region does not produce a specific or characteristic gait abnormality (see section on the recognition of lameness, p. 3). As a rule, pain in the hock region will be exacerbated by flexion but any movement which stresses the joint, for example flexion of the fetlock, may do the same. The mechanism here is probably that fetlock flexion exerts a corresponding extensor tendon pull, the latter are closely bound to the dorsolateral aspect of the joint and during fetlock flexion they can be felt to stand out from the dorsum of the hock. Presumably, in doing so, they cause strain or stress to the dorsal ligaments, joint capsules, etc. of the articulation. Illustrating this is that some cases of tarsal osteoarthritis (spavin) will be lamer following fetlock flexion than hock flexion.

Some physical abnormality, generally swelling, may indicate a possible source of pathology. However, in some cases of tarsal osteoarthritis or spavin for example, the hock may appear perfectly normal.

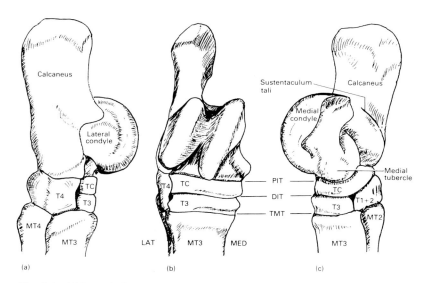

Fig. 6.1 (a) Lateral, (b) dorsal and (c) medial views of the hock. Note the pronounced angulation of the condyles of the talus. The lateral has a hooked distal extremity — the medial is larger and extends to the body of the talus distally. The 1st and 2nd tarsal bones are sometimes fused, sometimes separate.

Under these circumstances a four-point or fetlock block should be done, followed by lunging or further flexion tests. A persisting lameness indicates a more proximal pain source and narrows the diagnostic field substantially. Further attempts at regional anaesthesia are frustrated by the lack of specificity and the difficulty of assessing tibial and peroneal nerve blocks (see p. 14). Intra-articular anaesthesia is useful but it is a sad fact that the temperament of many British horses and the ineffectual handling abilities of many amateur owners make these techniques difficult and dangerous for all concerned and often completely impossible. This applies especially to the distal intertarsal and tarsometatarsal blocks which can be difficult to perform correctly and require very accurate technique. Where this is the case elimination of the stifle as the source of the problem will allow concentration of the hock. Statistically, stifle problems are not a common cause of lameness except in a narrow group of young thoroughbreds and then usually with some external evidence.

If a swelling is present, it is important to discover exactly which structures are involved and not to lump all such abnormalities under the misleading and meaningless term 'swollen hock'. Rather, palpation and a knowledge of anatomy should enable the clinician to decide whether the swelling is subcutaneous, or a distension of the tibio-tarsal joint capsule for example. Recognition of which structures are involved in a pathological process is a simple but major step towards reliable diagnosis, treatment and prognosis.

Radiographic examination

It is an old fashioned concept that a hock can be fully investigated through the two traditional lateromedial and dorsoplantar views. Most pathological change is identified on the profile surfaces of this solid bony mass and it is usually the projection tangential to the lesion that demonstrates it best. There are an unlimited number of possible tangents and the lateromedial and dorsoplantar are but two. There is no reason why these should form part of an evaluation if they are not considered necessary and are not the views which are likely to show a suspect lesion to best advantage.

Grids are unnecessary for all but the largest or most grossly swollen hock. Fine-grain screen/film combinations will give the best results, and rare-earth screen/film combinations will allow a much reduced exposure time. A light beam diaphragm is of enormous value for centring the beam and for restricting its size. In addition to reducing scatter, restricting beam size will allow four, or even six images to be made on a standard 36 × 24 cm cassette. An additional benefit of examining only a small area is that shorter focal/film distances can be used without significant distortion but with a great reduction in intensity, and hence exposure time.

Even when high quality radiographs have been taken, interpretation is still a problem. One of the best aids is a set of prepared bones which can be used, especially in angled tangential views, to identify the multitude of articular facets and the profusion of 'lumps and bumps'. Anybody who studies hock radiographs is well advised to spend some time preparing such a specimen.

Tarsal osteoarthritis ('spavin')

Background note

The word 'spavin' has an 'etymologically dubious' origin in the old French word 'espavain' (*Oxford English Dictionary*) and is defined as a disease of the horse's hock joint. With the greater clinical under-standing of the various conditions that has come over the past few years the term has now become insufficiently precise, even when qualified by adjectives such as bone, occult or blood, and has been supplanted by less romantic though scientifically more accurate terminology.

Aetiology and pathogenesis

Spavin is a condition of insidious onset which affects horses and ponies of all types and of all ages, apart from the very young.

Its incidence seems to bear little relation to the type or amount of work done, many animals which are little more than pets presenting with advanced disease. Several surveys indicate that trotters and pacers may suffer an unusually high incidence of the condition and at an especially young age; however, it is sufficiently widespread in the general equine population to be high on the list of differentials in any animal presenting with hind limb lameness.

The condition is essentially an osteoarthritis of the three, immobile distal joints of the hock, the proximal and distal intertarsal (PIT and

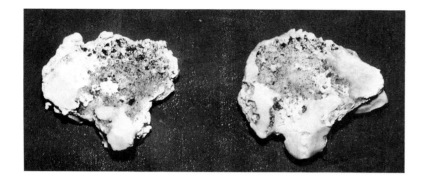

Fig. 6.2 The mating surfaces of the central and 3rd tarsal bones of a horse with long standing lesions of tarsal osteoarthritis (spavin).

DIT), and the tarsometatarsal (TMT) joints. It is *often* bilateral. It results in the usual pathological changes of cartilage degeneration, subchondral bone lysis, periarticular bone proliferation and synovial and fibrous joint capsular changes. Its rate of progression varies greatly and while there is a loose relationship between this and the amount of work done by the animal there are sufficient aberrant cases of apparently rapid development in pets and slow, insidious progression in hard working animals to prevent any sweeping generalizations.

Many theories have been advanced as to the aetiology of the condition, again the diversity in its presentation suggests that no individual theory is wholly correct and that it is most likely multifactoral.

Conformation has been suggested as the most important factor with trauma playing a secondary role (Adams 1974). A sickle hock, i.e. where the tibia and cannon make a more acute angle than normal, and a cow hock, where the hocks are close together when viewed from behind, are the two aberrations which are said to predispose to tarsal osteoarthritis by increasing the stresses on the hock, especially on the medial aspect. Shear stresses caused by sudden acceleration and deceleration and the inability of the relatively flat intertarsal and tarsometatarsal joints to resist these forces, have also been implicated (Gabel 1979); the same author has suggested that the unusual gait characteristics imposed on trotters and pacers may account for the high incidence in these types.

However credible in individual instances, these explanations do not account for the many cases seen in hunters, hacks and ponies where there is no discernible conformational or gait aberration and the level of stress is low because of the undemanding nature of the work. The truth is that there is no simple explanation and it is likely that other factors such as rapid growth, osteochondrosis, irregular and intermittent exercise regimes all play a part.

The early signs are those of classical degenerative joint disease (see section on DJD, p. 273). There is much subchondral bone lysis as the disease progresses and much periarticular new bone production. Figure 6.2 shows the disarticulated mating surfaces of the central and 3rd tarsal bones from a long standing case indicating the degree of bone destruction which can occur without fusion. Figure 6.3 is the contralateral hock from the same horse showing extensive and typical new bone formation at the periphery of the TMT joint. This new bone

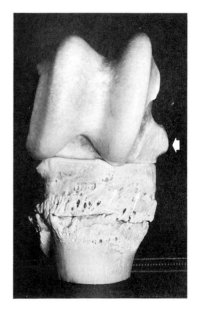

Fig. 6.3 The contralateral hock of the same horse as in Fig. 6.2 showing fusion of the central and 3rd tarsal bones and extensive new bone around the TMT joint. Note how much of the new bone is angled in the general direction of the medial tubercle of the talus (large arrow), suggesting that much of it lies within the insertion of the fan-liked dorsal ligament.

is made up of the periarticular osteophytes of DJD and enthesiophytes which seem to arise at the insertion of the large dorsal ligament. This runs from the medial tubercle of the talus to insert on the dorsal and dorsomedial aspects of the 3rd tarsal bone and the proximal cannon. Occasionally these enthesiophytes are the only lesions to be seen on radiography. Figure 6.3 also shows that periarticular lesions can extend to the dorsolateral aspect of the joints, also an apparent fusion of the central and 3rd tarsal bones. Fusion such as this has been thought to occur as a sequel to long standing disease, and formerly conservative treatment was aimed at maintaining the animal until such time as this occurred. However, in this case and in many others the arthrodesis, usually of the central tarsal (TC) and 3rd tarsal (T3) bones seems to have taken place in the absence of significant periarticular change. This would seem unusual in the light of the extensive change which can occur without fusion (see Fig. 6.2), and raises the question of whether this feature of the disease may not be a sequel to very early pathology, e.g. neonatal interruptions to the vasculature and enchondral ossification at the site, or even central or 3rd tarsal compression-type fracture.

Clinical signs

According to classical teaching, the animal with tarsal osteoarthritis presented with a swelling on the medial aspect of the distal hock. This manifestation, the so-called 'bone spavin' is now a relative rarity. When horses worked for a living and riding was not a pleasure pursuit lameness was tolerated; indeed there was little of value that could be done for such animals anyway. Paradoxically it is the advent of riding as a leisure pursuit and constant competition at all levels which has produced a more critical attitude in owners (and their friends). This means that lame animals, or those showing poor performance are now referred earlier in the disease course when pathological change is not extensive.

Not all cases of tarsal osteoarthritis will present as being lame on one hind leg; rather the owner will complain of one of a number of different problems, some rather amorphous. Among them are 'loss of impulsion', 'awkward on its diagonals', 'going unlevel', 'loss of jumping ability', 'unwillingness or even refusal to jump', a general 'fall off in performance', 'constant reduction in marks for dressage performances' and so on. To confuse the issue further they often present already labelled as 'shoulder or hip lameness', 'kidney problems' or most commonly as 'back cases'! It is important when being confronted with this type of prediagnosis by an apparently knowledgeable owner to conduct a full, impartial examination but at the same time to explain why one is disregarding their opinion.

Some cases actually present as lame in one leg but even in these, careful questioning will often reveal a fall off in performance in the period leading up to the onset of lameness. This is because the lameness at the trot was initially not sufficiently great to be apparent to an inexperienced person, or the lameness was bilaterally symmetrical and only became obvious when one side progressed, or when the animal was observed by a relatively experienced person, for example a dressage judge.

Most cases of tarsal osteoarthritis will have no bony lump at the 'site of spavin'. Occasionally, however, there will be a firm, pain-free swelling on the dorsomedial aspect of the distal hock, and infrequently the swelling may be large (the so-called 'Jack-spavin'), bilateral and associated with severe lamenes. This variation seems frequently to run a peracute course and usually affects predominantly the proximal intertarsal joint. The PIT joint capsule communicates with the tibio-tarsal joint and in these animals there is often mild distension of the latter.

The level of lameness in other cases is variable, some horses being so slightly lame as to be undetectable by the clinician on the straight trot. A fairly consistent feature is catching of the toe ('toe dragging' or 'trailing') and a consequent wearing of the shoe at the toe (Fig. 6.4).

Diagnosis

Diagnosis consists initially of establishing whether the animal is lame in one, or more legs. This is done by observing it at the straight trot and on the lunge (see section on diagnosis of lameness); the use of hip markers being extremely useful for both the clinician and the owner. This should be followed by flexion tests and it is worth reiterating that fetlock flexion tests can exacerbate a case of tarsal osteoarthritis. A physical examination of the limb may reveal a swelling at the dorsomedial aspect of the distal hock but more likely not. Care is necessary not to confuse the bulge of the dorsal metatarsal vein (the so called 'blood spavin') as it crosses the site, with the firm swelling of new bone production. There may also be wear of the shoe or hoof at the toe. It would be very unusual to find any noticeable degree of muscle atrophy in a case of tarsal osteoarthritis. Finally, this preliminary examination should eliminate the small possibility of spinal problems by assessing the range of movements of the patient's back.

Having established that the animal is lame on one or both hind legs, the next step is to pin-point the source of pain. A four-point nerve block above the fetlock will anaesthetize most of that joint and below, and will, in most cases, following further flexion tests and evaluation at the trot, eliminate or confirm the importance of this area. It must be remembered, however, that the animal may have more than one pain source and a partial improvement may not be the result of poor nerve block technique: in this context careful testing of skin desensitization is important!

At this stage having eliminated the distal limb there is a high statistical probability that the pain source is in the hock. Apart from foals where osteochondrosis is a problem, and thoroughbreds with their subchondral cysts, the stifle is not a common source of pathology and usually, when it is present, there is some physical indication such as joint capsular distension. Hip problems are also rare and are usually accompanied by some degree of gluteal muscle wastage. Nevertheless, the remainder of the hind limb should be carefully examined to eliminate these possibilities.

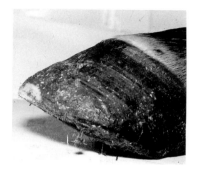

Fig. 6.4 Wear at the tip of a hoof caused by 'toe dragging' or 'toe trailing'.

The next step is ideally intra-articular anaesthesia of the TMT and DIT joints. These are the two articulations most commonly involved in the disease process and any improvement in the lameness or response to flexion after these blocks must hold some significance. If the fetlock has not been previously anaesthetized some care must be taken in interpretation of the TMT and DIT blocks, diffusion of local anaesthetic solution can sometimes affect the nerve trunks supplying the dorsal cannon fetlock and pastern region, and lesions here may be anaesthetized with confusing results. Again, careful checks on skin desensitization are necessary. In addition to this complication the blocks are not easy to perform, especially if the animal is unco-operative. Of the two the TMT block is easier and should be tried if possible (see section on nerve blocks, p. 20). Blocking of the PIT joint on its own is not often indicated but can be done via the tarsocrural joint capsule with which it communicates.

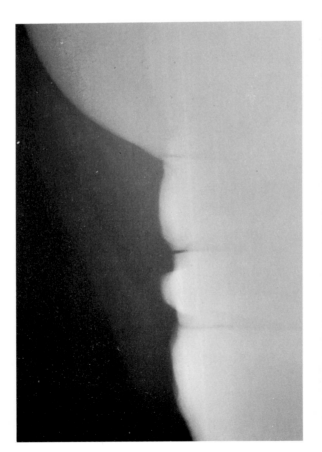 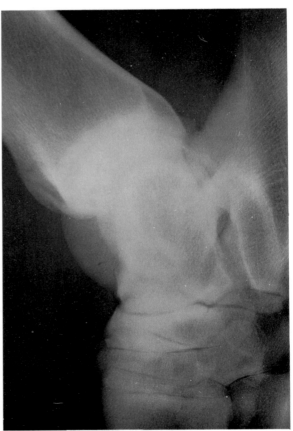

Fig. 6.5 (left)   The joint margin is clearly viewed on this accurately centred DPLMO projection.

Fig. 6.6 (right)   Radiographs such as this should not be used in the evaluation of suspect cases of tarsal osteoarthritis (spavin). Centering the beam too high has resulted in distortion of the relevant joint lines and over exposure has rendered their borders indistinct.

Tibial and peroneal blocks have major drawbacks and in general contribute little to the diagnosis of tarsal osteoarthritis. Some authorities believe that cunean bursitis contributes substantially to the pain and would include anaesthesia of the bursa in their diagnostic work-up. This can be a difficult block to perform in other than a very quiet animal and in general the author has not found it necessary. Even the protagonists of the technique admit that there is always a concurrent tarsal osteoarthritis and it is probably better to concentrate on that aspect of the disease.

Radiographic examination

Tarsal osteoarthritis *cannot* be diagnosed with any accuracy on poor quality or badly positioned radiographs. Severe and gross changes may be identified on such plates but pathology of such magnitude is rare nowadays, rather the clinician is looking for more subtle changes. The lesions of tarsal osteoarthritis are seen principally at the joint margins and cannot be identified convincingly unless those edges are seen clearly (Fig. 6.5). High definition radiographs are essential, but so is accurate positioning: Any degree of superimposition prevents recognition of change and radiographs such as shown in Fig. 6.6, although of good quality, are not diagnostic.

The lesions can be found *anywhere* along the dorsal hemicircumference of the PIT, DIT and TMT joints. Therefore, for full evaluation at least three tangents are necessary, the PDLMO, the LM, the 45° DPLMO and ideally the DP too. Threre is no need to expose the complete hock and light beam diaphragms allow 'coning down' to the area of interest which, even in the largest horse, is no more than some 5 × 5 cm. At least four such views can be obtained on one medium sized cassette. The undulant nature of the dorsal margins of the joints means that for each tangent the beam centre must be aligned at a slightly different angle to the mid-axis of the leg to avoid superimposition of the margins (Fig. 6.7). With practise this is not difficult to achieve although the tendency for the animal to rest and part flex the painful joint (Fig. 6.8) can make estimation of these angles somewhat tricky at times. Lifting a foreleg in these situations does not improve matters, usually causing the animal to fidget as its takes full weight on its painful leg.

If circumstances limit the number of views that can be taken, the lateromedial and the 45° DPLMO are the ones most likely to reveal pathological change; the DP is the least useful, superimposition of 1st and 2nd tarsal bones (T1 and T2), and the normally uneven border of the 3rd tarsal bone making interpretation difficult with this projection.

The characteristic radiographic changes of tarsal osteoarthritis are new bone production at the articular margin varying in extent from a 'squaring' of the edge to frank osteophyte production (Figs. 6.9a and b). Large osteophytes, or, more correctly enthesiophytes, are often seen at the insertion of the large dorsal ligament and distal to it on the dorsal cannon bone as well (Fig. 6.10). Irregularity of the subchondral bone margin is seen in early cases, progressing to an obvious irregularity with subchondral lysis and a narrowing of the lucent cartilage

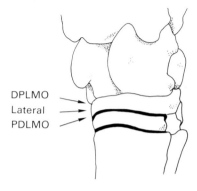

DPLMO
Lateral
PDLMO

Fig. 6.7 Illustration of the angulation relative to the horizontal of the main beam centre when making the various projections of the articular margins of the DIT and TMT joints. For simplicity, the average angulation should be 5° up or down.

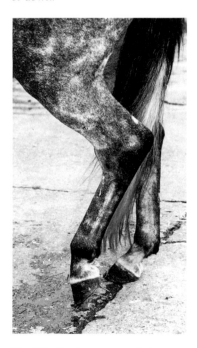

Fig. 6.8 Resting stance of a horse with a painful limb condition such as tarsal osteoarthritis (spavin).

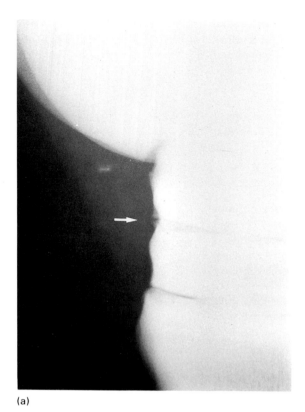

(a)

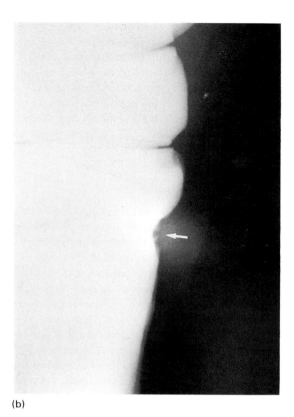

(b)

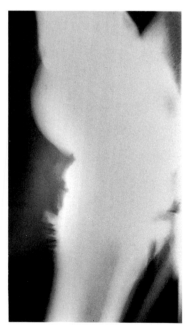

Fig. 6.10 Large periarticular enthesiophytes and palisaded exostoses on the dorsal cannon bone.

Fig. 6.9 Periarticular osteophytes at the periphery of (a) the DIT joint and (b) the TMT joint. In both instances the lameness exhibited by the animals improved to normality following intra-articular anaesthesia.

line. The converse, i.e. widening of the joint line, has been described as one of the changes seen radiographically in tarsal osteoarthritis: this is *not* a reality, but an artefact caused by poor quality films not permitting differentiation between the articular cartilage lucency and that of the subchondral lysis. Occasionally an absence of discernible joint line indicates natural ankylosis of a joint. The changes are often exaggerated in some cases of PIT involvement, there being obvious subchondral change and aggressive periarticular new bone (Fig. 6.11).

In many instances the radiological diagnosis is self evident. However, it must be remembered that evidence gained radiographically must be taken in conjunction with that of the clinical examination and some cases where changes are minor require the incontrovertible evidence of local analgesia before an unequivocal diagnosis can be made.

There are of course those cases where even after extensive investigation no firm decision can be made. Under these circumstances the author feels that it is pointless to recommend rest then re-examination as it is only work which is likely to exacerbate the signs of a level where positive identification is possible. Normal work under the palliative influence of phenylbutazone or some other anti-inflammatory agent is far more likely to produce diagnostic results in 3–4 months time and provided other lesions, to which exercise would be detrimental, have not been identified there is little harm in this and the eventual prognosis is not worsened.

Treatment

In the absence of any effective alternative treatment, a long period of rest has been the most frequently advocated mode of therapy for these cases. The hope was that time would allow either regression of pathology or natural ankylosis of the affected joints. Unfortunately it is the experience of the author and others that inactivity has little long term beneficial effect, the symptoms invariably reappearing as soon as the animal starts work again; also there is no doubt that natural arthrodesis does occur from time to time but it is not so common an occurrence that it can ever be relied on as a solution to an individual problem

There is therefore little point in resting an animal for 6 months or so in the hope of a permanent improvement, but every indication to carry on working under the influence of anti-inflammatory drugs, provided of course that these are effective in abolishing or substantially reducing the animal's pain levels. In practice it is rare that a drug such as phenylbutazone will completely abolish the discomfort and it may be that the work load or expectation of performance may have to be reduced. In addition, the rules of competition in many branches of equestrian sport proscribe the use of such drugs. Nevertheless a combination of reduced work and adequate medication can allow an animal which is not too badly affected to live a useful life. This course of action can also be used to advantage in cases where the initial diagnosis is equivocal; re-examination after 4−6 months of this regime will often show more positive radiographic changes and allow a definite diagnosis to be made.

Over the years several surgical techniques have flourished as the definitive treatment but then their popularity has waned as they were found to be ineffective. Pin-firing is probably the most ancient and presumably relies on the production of a massive inflammatory reaction on the dorsomedial aspect of the joint. This, in turn, might instigate the process of arthrodesis. However, bearing in mind the amount of cartilage destruction that is necessary to achieve this result with contemporary surgical techniques, it is unlikely that peripheral inflammatory reaction would do anything other than exacerbate the condition. Protagonists of pin-firing who counter this argument by insisting that the hot iron is inserted into the joints should bear in mind that the anatomy is such that not even a 25 gauge needle can be insinuated into these articulations in the living animal. It is also unlikely that the production of a pad of scar tissue would limit to any effective degree the small movement which takes place in these virtually immobile articulations and which result in pain in the diseased joints.

Wamberg's operation involved the creation of a diamond-shaped pattern of incisions in the subcutaneous fascia which enclosed the dorsomedial aspect of the hock, the so-called 'seat of spavin'. These

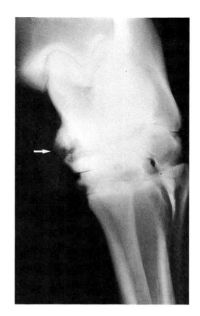

Fig. 6.11 Extensive periarticular new bone and subchondral cyst formation in this case where only the PIT joint is involved. The other hock joint in this horse was similarly involved.

were made through stab incisions in the skin and the technique presumably based any beneficial effect on partial deinnervation of the site.

Cunean tenotomy was another technique which relied partially on the creation of an inflammatory reaction on the medial aspect of the hock. The cunean tendon of insertion of tibialis anterior runs over the medial aspect of the hock and is lubricated in its passage by the cunean bursa. Although slightly variable in position it usually lies over the DIT and occasionally the TMT joints, and has been claimed by some authorities to become inflamed in cases of spavin; its ablation would therefore be a logical step in the control of pain. However, even if this bursa is inflamed there is always a concurrent osteoarthritis which is not affected by the surgery and which will continue to be a problem. Modern experience which suggests that bursal involvement is uncommon and probably of litle significance is borne out of the poor success rate of this technique.

The only consistently successful treatment for intertarsal osteoarthritis or spavin is surgical arthrodesis. Published reports (Edwards 1982; Wyn-Jones and May 1986) indicate that a return to functional normality can be expected in 80% of those cases where the distal two joints are affected and approximately 60% of those where the PIT is also involved. Both hocks can be operated on in those cases which are bilaterally affected. An interesting and consistent comment from owners is that following their eventual return to work these animals perform to a higher standard than they have ever been known to attain, adding weight to the author's belief that very many animals work and compete far below their potential because of unrecognized, chronic, low grade lameness.

The surgical technique for arthrodesis involves a 10 cm curvilinear incision on the dorsomedial aspect of the hock plantar and parallel to the dorsal metatarsal vein at the level of the affected joints. The author's technique is to incise subcutaneous fascia and the cunean tendon and expose the outer layer of the fibrous joint capsules; no part of the cunean tendon is resected. The joint edges cannot be seen as fibrous and ligamentous tissue smooths out all the irregularities of the bony profile. They are located in one of three ways: firstly by using a needle to locate, not the actual joint cavity, but the depressions in the bony outline at the bottom of which lie the articular margins. Once these depressions are located, a drill bit inserted into them tends to follow the path of least resistance, i.e. the joint lines. This technique is made easier by having a macerated bone specimen where it can be seen during surgery: the special relationships of this area are complex and this aid is extremely valuable. It is also a technique which is frustratingly difficult if much periarticular new bone is present as this prevents the easy location of these periarticular depressions. Secondly, intra-operative radiography can be useful though time consuming. Thirdly, and ideally, a fluoroscope/image intensifier system should be used. However, these must be used with care both from a radiation safety point of view and, more pragmatically, because they can compromise sterile technique if used carelessly. In addition the surgeon must realize that the articular margins curve in several directions and superimposition of joint lines can lead to problems with interpretation.

When the joints are located, the articular cartilage is destroyed by drilling down along the joint line. The author uses a 3.2 mm drill bit, and an air-powered drill. A hand-drill can be used although it is much harder work. The bit is inserted at two entry ports — each time in a slightly different direction to produce a radiating pattern of drill holes across the joint, many intersecting as the two fans of holes cross each other. Where the articulation is healthy the borings are dry and crisp and saline lubrication of the drill bit helps greatly. In diseased parts of the joint the borings are haemorrhagic and 'mushy' and lubrication is not necessary. The author has established a protocol whereby if either of the two distal joints appear radiographically affected, both are arthrodesed, the PIT being spared. If the latter is involved either alone or in combination with either or both the other two, all are drilled. Practically this seems to be a satisfactory solution to the problem of which joints to treat and is based on the facts that it is common to find the distal two joints affected without any sign of PIT involvement and uncommon to find the reverse; also that the post-operative progress of animals in which the PIT has been arthrodesed seems longer and, subjectively, more uncomfortable.

The use of stabilizing plates and lag screwing techniques has been tried but has not shown great benefit relative to the increased complexity of the surgery (Wyn-Jones and May 1985).

Post-operative discomfort is alleviated by both liberal use of analgesic drugs and early exercise. Walking in hand is started on the second post-operative day, starting at 2−3 minutes twice a day and increasing slowly. Many animals will not be lame at the walk 10−14 days later. At this stage the second leg can be operated on if necessary. Walking in hand continues, until 3 months later the animal will tolerate an unlimited amount. Then trotting exercise begins, again increasing in amount for 3 months until 6 months post-operatively, riding and training can be recommenced. It is important that *at no time* during this 6 month period should free exercise be allowed. A high proportion of the eventual failures of this operation can be attributed to an episode of violent exercise during these early months when convalescent animals were thoughtlessly turned out or escaped from their handler and when caught later were intractably lame on the affected leg. What happens is not certain but it is something that should be avoided!

Subsequent to surgery there is a sizable swelling on the medial aspect of the hock. This diminishes somewhat with time but never resolves completely. Surprisingly it does not seem to cause cosmetic embarrassment and owners comment favourably on how it often remains unnoticed even by experienced show judges!

Suggested further reading

Dewes HF (1982) The onset and consequences of tarsal bone fracture in foals. *NZ Vet J* **30**, 129−35.

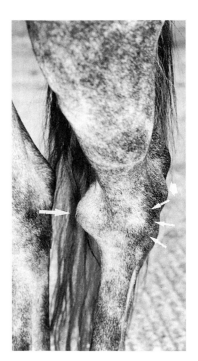

Fig. 6.12 Distension of the tibiotarsal joint capsule (bog spavin). Large arrow = dorsomedial; small arrows = dorsolateral; square arrow = plantarlateral outpouchings.

Edwards GB (1982) Surgical arthrodesis for the treatment of bone spavin in 20 horses. *Eq Vet J* **14**, 117–21.

Gabel AA (1982) Prevention, diagnosis and treatment of inflammation of the distal hock. *Proc Am Ass Eq Prac* **28**, 287–98.

Wyn-Jones G and May SA (1986) Surgical arthrodesis for the treatment of osteoarthrosis of the proximal intertarsal, distal intertarsal and tarsometatarsal joints in 30 horses: a comparison of four different techniques. *Eq Vet J* **18**(1), 59–64.

Conditions leading to distension of the tibiotarsal (tarsocrural) joint capsule ('bog spavin')

The tibiotarsal joint is voluminous, catering for a large range of movement. Its joint capsule is not normally distended and therefore not visible; however, intra-articular structures such as the condyles of the talus are easily palpable and in thin skinned animals various colateral ligaments and tendon sheaths can also be identified. When distended, the joint capsule protrudes between the restraining periarticular structures in four characteristic pouches (Fig. 6.12). The largest and most prominent is located dorsomedially, with a smaller one dorsolaterally and one each side of the joint just dorsal to the tuber calcis. The latter pair are often mistaken for a distension of the deep flexor tendon sheath which actually lies above and behind the site of the joint outpouchings. (This distinction is not helped by confusion engendered by the colloquial terminology of articular and tendinous thoroughpin for joint and tendon sheath distensions respectively.)

It is clearly important to distinguish true tibiotarsal joint distension from other swellings of the hock region. Cellulitis, or a more fibrous reaction following chronic infection, will produce generalized periarticular thickening and oedema; the result of venous or lymphatic drainage impairment will produce a similar result. The thickening will usually extend distally in the case of oedema and may do so in the case of infection if it is extensive or the inflammatory reaction itself compromises venous or lymphatic flow. Classically, oedema will 'pit' although sometimes very firm pressure is needed; acute cellulitis will produce a firm, non-pitting swelling which is painful on pressure and may feel decidely hot. A chronic reaction, on the other hand, will usually be relatively pain-free when squeezed and may pit somewhat; however there will be an underlying fibrous thickening which cannot be dispersed by simple pressure and good quality radiographs will often show *extra-articular* periosteal new bone formation. Superimposed on any of these can, of course, be a joint capsule distension caused by concurrent articular pathology.

Joint capsular distension is recognized by swellings having a 'fluid-filled feel' in the characteristic positions — dorsomedially and dorsolaterally and on both sides of the plantar joint margin. The acid test is to see if the fluid contents can be pushed from one distension to another. In some cases their collapse and filling is quite visible, but it is usually better appreciated by palpation at the appropriate sites. Where periarticular swelling is present it can be difficult to determine whether there is joint distension too; fortunately, even if the hock is severely swollen, the transmission of a pressure wave from pouch to pouch can usually be felt.

Osteochodritis dissecans (OCD) of the tibiotarsal joint

OCD is one of the most common joint lesions occuring almost exclusively in young, rapidly growing animals. Although the condition has been recorded in most joints in the body, the hock and stifle are the two articulations most commonly affected clinically. The distribution between hock and stifle would appear to vary on a geographical basis though this is probably dependent on the type of horse prevalent in any area. In Swedish standardbred trotters, hock lesions prevail while the 'warm bloods' show a much higher incidence of stifle lesions. In the UK most of the clinical cases of hock OCD encountered by the author are in the heavier breeds, particularly the Shire, possibly reflecting on the relative paucity of standardbreds, while the stifle lesions have been seen primarily in the thoroughbreds and their crosses.

Aetiology and pathogenesis

(see section on osteochondrosis for detailed account p. 194.)

A disease of young stock, OCD is seen virtually exclusively in well managed, rapidly growing animals. The current trends towards producing large, rounded, showable and saleable animals at a young age and, especially in draught breeds, the pressure on breeders to produce larger and larger animals is, no doubt, largely to blame: under these circumstances there is a failure of enchondral ossification (conversion of cartilage to bone). This results in the articular cartilage and underlying bone being insufficiently robust to stand up to normal wear and tear and a sudden movement can result in a separation of a section of subchondral bone along with its attached cartilage. There is a release of cartilage substance, etc. into the joint provoking an immediate inflammatory reaction, excess production of synovial fluid and consequent swelling of the joint capsule. The fact that the swelling can develop within a very short time and frequently follows strenuous exercise such as when a young animal is turned out, often leads to a misdiagnosis of a strain, sprain or simple trauma. Although trauma is of course the trigger factor, it is inherent weakness of poorly formed bone which is the underlying cause of the actual intra-articular injury.

There are two prime sites within the tibiotarsal joint to be affected by this condition. One is the cranial tip of the mid-sagittal ridge of the tibia; the other is the distal tip of the lateral condyle of the talus. Occasionally both sites are involved; more usually only one is affected. The lesions are frequently bilateral!

Clinical signs

Clinical signs include a sudden onset of a swelling of the tibiotarsal joint capsule accompanied by lameness. The severity of both the capsular distension and the lameness is very variable, as is their relationship. In a proportion of animals there may be no visible swelling of the joint, in others, no gait abnormality even after flexion tests, and, in some, despite radiographic changes being recognized, the animal shows no symptoms. This is probably due to there having been no cartilage rupture as yet. Generally the level of lameness is low, sometimes despite extensive swelling, and this is a useful diagnostic pointer. It is, of course, well to remember that bilateral pain will reduce the level of an individual leg lameness.

Diagnosis

The principal diagnostic features are that the patient is a young, usually under 2 years of age, well grown animal with a history of a sudden onset of tibiotarsal joint distension. There is usually only mild lameness at the trot and it is usually somewhat worsened by a flexion test. (In long standing cases or if animals are at pasture, the time of onset may not be known and the lameness may have subsided to minimal levels.) The clinician must also take care not to be swayed by stories of the animal being kicked. These are often just wishful thinking on the part of the owner to try and explain the symptoms and are especially attractive if the animal was turned out with other horses! There will also be no sign of periarticular reaction to indicate external trauma.

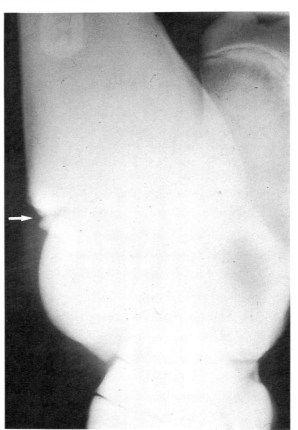

Fig. 6.13 Osteochondritis dissecans of the dorsal tip of the mid-sagittal ridge of the tibia.

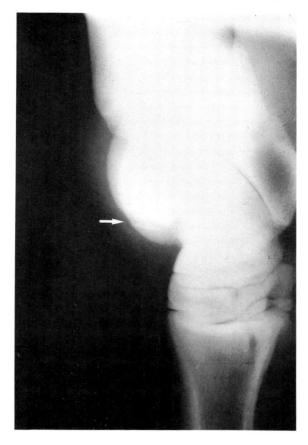

Fig. 6.14 A lateromedial projection showing fragmentation of the distal lateral condyle. In underpenetrated or poor quality radiographs the superimposition of the longer medial condyle of the talus can obscure the lesion.

Synovial fluid examination is unlikely to be helpful at this stage since these parameters commonly measured will show no changes specific for OC and will merely be characteristic of a non-septic synovitis. The presence of cartilage particles can be detected where there has been fragmentation but by this stage radiographic changes are usually present.

At this juncture the joint should be radiographed.

Radiography

Although there is some merit in a complete survey of the joint, especially if the condition is long-standing and degenerative disease is suspected, only two views are needed to evaluate the two common sites.

A well penetrated straight lateral projection is needed to show lesions on the distal dorsal tibia (Fig. 6.13) and while this can also be used to evaluate the lateral condyle tip (Fig. 6.14), superimposition of the medial condyle can mark smaller changes. The projection of choice in this case is the 45° PDLMO (Fig. 6.15) and lesions appear skylined

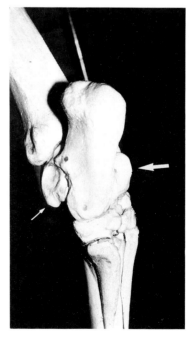

Fig. 6.15 The projection of choice (45° PDLMO) to visualize the lateral condyle of the talus (small arrow). In addition this projection allows evaluation of the rim of the sustentaculum tali (large arrow).

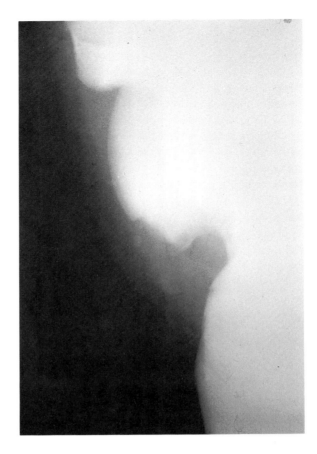

Fig. 6.16 A close-up of a 45°
PDLMO projection showing
fragmentation of the distal tip of
the lateral condyle of the talus.
Some osseous fragments are visible
within the pouch of the joint
capsule. This is a typical
osteochondritis dissecans lesion.

as shown in Fig. 6.16. Lesions appear as a fragmentation of the distal
condyle or a flattening of the condylar outline. Lesions of the tibia
appear as ununited fragments on the cranial aspect of the sagittal
ridge.

Treatment

Where lesions of osteochondrosis are discovered as an incidental
finding the treatment of choice is rest. In these cases it is likely that
although a subchondral defect is present, there has been no breach in
the surface cartilage and no leakage of material into the joint. In the
absence of stress, rupture of the cartilage envelope may not occur and
the defect will slowly ossify. Where joint distension and lameness are
present but lesions cannot be found on radiographic examination,
here too rest is indicated, although joint lavage can be used to assist
the reduction in swelling by mechanical removal of material toxic to
the synovial membrane. Where symptoms are present and a lesion is
identifiable, surgical removal of the fragments, curettage of the exposed
subchondral bone and subsequent lavage are indicated.

The choice of surgical approach depends on the location of the
OCD lesion, and on the equipment available. Ideally, surgery is best
performed with arthroscopic control. This results in minimum trauma

to the joint and a faster recovery time. However, since this technique is available to only a few, it will not be described in detail and interested readers should refer to the appropriate texts (see References, p. 292). In the absence of this specialized equipment and expertise, a wholly satisfactory result can be obtained with conventional arthrotomy. Whilst not difficult surgery it is *intra-articular* surgery and should not be undertaken unless the strictest aseptic requirements can be met.

The distal lateral condyle of the talus is best approached through the 'window' which exists between the major extra-articular structures and through which the dorsolateral pouch of the joint capsule protrudes when distended. Its identification in poorly distended joints is helped by compression of the other pouches, principally the dorsomedial causing the unsupported lateral one to bulge. A 6–8 cm incision is made running parallel and slightly medial to the crest of the condyle and lateral to the long digital extensor tendon; fascial layers are incised until the fibrous capsule and synovial membrane are penetrated. Care must be taken to preserve all ligamentous or tendinous structures, and this necessity tends to limit the distal extent of the deep incision. The lesion can be palpated and partially visualized through the incision and the end of the condyle must be curetted until smooth. Try to leave the remaining cartilage rim standing vertical to the subchondral bone; a sloping cartilage surface will not heal! Sometimes the bony fragments are large, well attached, and will not come away unless vigorously elevated. However, the rule must be that all fragments, however well attached, have to be removed. Occasionally too the cartilage appears intact and a flap is not immediately obvious. Again, the rule is that, if there is a radiological lesion (and one is operating on the correct leg) then the cartilage should be probed. It will then usually become obvious that it is unsupported and breaking through will reveal one or more loose subchondral fragments.

The joint is then copiously irrigated with Hartmann's or Ringers solution to remove any fragments, and the wound closed. Most surgical textbooks dictate the layers to be sutured. Unfortunately their identification is difficult especially since the effect of flushing fluid is to change the appearance of all periarticular tissues to a pale, washed out, soggy pink colour. The author prefers 2/0 or 3/0 Vicryl suture swaged on to a small, half-circle, *cutting* needle. Simple continuous sutures are entirely adequate but it is important to create as many sutured layers as possible between the joint cavity and skin, in this way a seal is virtually assured. For a good cosmetic effect the skin is closed firstly by a subcuticular pattern followed by simple interrupted sutures. The hock is kept bandaged for 2–3 weeks subsequently. At no time should corticosteroids be used in the joint although there is a good theoretical indication for the post-operative use of intra-articular sodium hyaluronate.

Lesions of the cranial distal tibia are approached through an incision placed some 3–4 cm proximal to the one already described and placed just lateral to the long digital extensor tendon. The dorsal tibial vein passes along the lateral aspect of this tendon, the dorsal tibial artery and the deep peroneal (fibular) nerve deep to it. Lateral branches of these vessels have usually to be ligated as the incision progresses and care must be taken not to damage them whilst retracting the wound edge: slight flexion of the joint slackens the wound edge to make access to the joint easier. As with the lateral condylar lesions, the defect is often hidden under intact cartilage, though probing will reveal a loose fragment contained within the cartilage envelope. Following fragment removal curettage must be carried out carefully so as not to damage the surface of the talus. Joint lavage is again an essential precursor to closure of the wound which should be by the same principles outlined above. An additional complication is provided by the large vessels lying on the periphery of the wound and care must be taken not to transfix them with the suture needle! Otherwise, immediate post-operative aftercare is pressure bandaging and a rest period of some 3–4 weeks followed by gentle walking exercise increasing in amounts over a further 4–5 months or so. It is difficult to predict when the capsular swelling will diminish but its persistence beyond 3–4 months would suggest that further investigation of the joint is advisable.

Definite figures on the efficacy of surgery are difficult to obtain, though a study on Swedish standardbreds indicates that surgically treated animals perform better than their conservatively treated counterparts but neither group do as well as non-affected animals (Hoppe 1984). The author's experience, principally with heavier horses, indicates that surgical curettage is effective in treating the condition and eliminating the blemish of the distended joint capsule.

Prevention

See section on osteochondrosis, p. 194.

Suggested further reading

De Moor A, Verschooten F, Desmet P and Steenhaut M (1972) Osteochondritis dissecans of the tibiotarsal joint in the horse. *Eq Vet J* **4** 139–43.
Stromberg B and Rejno S (1978) Osteochondrosis in the horse I. A clinical and radiological investigation of osteochondritis dissecans of the knee and hock joint. *Acta Radiol* **358**(Suppl), 139.
Hoppe F (1984) Radiological investigations of osteochondrosis dissecans of standardbred trotters and Swedish Warmblood horses. *Eq Vet J* **16**(5), 425–9.

Septic or infectious arthritis of the tibiotarsal joint

Aetiology and pathogenesis

The tibiotarsal joint is a common site for septic arthritis of systemic origin in the young; the navel/joint ill syndrome and its treatment is dealt with in a separate section (see p. 285). In the adult blood-borne infection is rare and most cases are caused by trauma in the form of puncture wounds or lacerations and occasionally as a sequel to needle puncture of the joint.

Clinical signs

The pathognomonic features of an infective arthritis in any articulation are a rapidly increasing joint distension and a *steady worsening* of lameness over several days to a point where the animal is no longer weight bearing. The experience of people who have had a septic arthritis is that it is excruciatingly painful. Much of the pain seems to be associated with the capsular distension so that if the initial trauma has left an open wound through which synovial fluid can escape, there can be minimal capsular swelling and a reduced, though still severe, level of lameness.

Diagnosis

The combination of capsular distension and a steadily worsening level of lameness should arouse grave suspicion that one is dealing with septic arthritis; this is especially so if it follows known trauma or arthrocentesis. The initial trauma may have resulted in lameness but, in general, pain arising from traumatic causes usually improves over the following days or, at the very least, stays at the same level. A worsening implies the superimposition of sepsis. It is, therefore, quite feasible to have, for example, an intra-articular fracture and sepsis coexisting and this must be borne in mind when evaluating this type of case. Puncture wounds may result in a sinus discharging synovial fluid, but blows to the hock usually disrupt tendon sheaths and not the capsule itself and so care must be taken to differentiate the origin of the discharge. If the capsule is distended then it is not likely to be the source of the synovial fluid; pressure on the capsule should cause an increased flow of fluid and failure to do so increases the likelihood that a tendon sheath is the culprit. Contrast radiography will provide a definite answer but there is a risk of introducing infection into a damaged but non-infected synovial structure. If it is deemed advisable that a catheter is inserted into the discharge point and 10–20 ml of a water soluble contrast agent is injected into the cavity. A cotton wool pad held against the sinus exit prevents too much reflux.

Aspiration of fluid from the joint cavity is an easy technique especially if the capsule is distended, and analysis of the fluid will show conclusively that infection is present. However, even this simple technique is not to be undertaken lightly as some thought must be given to the risk of introducing infection into a sterile joint, especially if soft tissue swelling suggests the possibility of a periarticular cellulitis.

Following suitable restraint and the creation of a subcutaneous bleb of local a relatively wide bore (16 g) needle is inserted into the dorsomedial pouch. Fluid should run out immediately but occasionally solid clots may obstruct the lumen and suction should be applied with a syringe. In infected joints the fluid is turbid and sometimes flocculant. Its white cell count is characteristically high, over 80,000 per mm^3 and mainly polymorphonuclear leucocytes. Culture of this fluid is surprisingly unrewarding unless taken directly into blood culture tubes or it is spun down and the solid plug of debris used on appropriate culture medium. A more rapid test is to stain a smear of this debris and look for bacteria.

In the early days of an infection, radiography will not help in the diagnosis of septic arthritis though it is useful to eliminate fractures, etc. Later, after 2 weeks or so aggressive spiculated new bone will begin to appear at ligamentous and capsular attachments and there may be evidence of subchondral or perichondral bone erosion. If a periarticular infection is present, aggressive palisaded periosteal new bone will be seen adjacent to capsular attachments.

Treatment

Treatment is by joint lavage: there is no effective alternative! Systemic antibiotics used alone are rarely effective. Acute infections may be controlled but chronic low grade infection almost always persists, and the by-products of infection, including various enzymes, superoxide radicals and tissue debris, remain within the joint stimulating self-perpetuating inflammatory changes.

Joint lavage or irrigation is a simple technique and used early is extremely effective. In its simplest form two needles are inserted into the affected joint as far apart as possible and large quantities of electrolyte solution are used to flush the joint cavity. The technique is best carried out under general anaesthesia. Large bore (14 g) needles ensure a good flow and catheter needles if available should be used in preference since solid needles can damage articular surfaces when the joint is manipulated. A minimum of 2, and ideally, 4 litres is run through, either using gravity or a push-pull system using a three-way tap and a 60 ml syringe with the electrolyte container acting as a reservoir connected to the three-way tap via a giving set. Hartmann's or Ringer's fluid should be used in preference to saline as their pH is more compatible with the intra-articular environment. The use of intra-articular antibiotics is not necessary, though the post-irrigation instillation of sodium hyaluronate or orgotein has therapeutic value. A much cheaper alternative is to perform a synovial fluid transfer, injecting 10–20 ml of clean synovial fluid aspirated from the stifle.

Two days post-irrigation the joint should be aspirated again when the cell count should have dropped markedly. Two or three irrigations are necessary to reduce the cell count to relatively normal levels and it is a good rule of thumb to irrigate at least once more than is considered absolutely necessary. Although expensive in terms of time and anaesthetic costs, the end results are worthwhile with many animals returning to full normality.

If diagnosis or treatment is delayed the prognosis is not so good. Solid material coalesces within the joint to form large aggregates which cannot be flushed and synovial and bony changes become irreversible. Irrigation through needles does not adequately clean out the joint cavity and infection within the solid material persists. In these cases an arthrotomy can be done through the dorsomedial or dosolateral pouches and the large, solid masses of accumulated debris removed manually and by irrigation. The wounds heal surprisingly well!

Systemic antibiotics are of course used in these cases, their effect being complementary to the removal of the debris. An antibiotic with a broad spectrum of action should be chosen if the organism is not identified. A combination of drugs such as penicillin and neomycin can be used to provide broad cover.

The ideal post-treatment exercise regime would involve non-weight bearing motion. However, this is not a practicable proposition with horses and a compromise should be made with an initial period of rest being followed by one of controlled exercise in hand as soon as pain and lameness fall to a reasonable level. Non-steroidal anti-inflammatory agents can be used to good effect but cortisone *must not* be given either locally or systemically in these cases.

Intra-articular fractures

Aetiology and pathogenesis

External trauma is the usual cause of intra-articular fractures with kicks from other horses, or hitting fences being most common. There is an instant onset of severe lameness in most cases with effusion into the joint and a consequent capsular swelling within an hour or so. Very occasionally, as with some fractures in other sites, the level of pain and lameness may be initially low but rises rapidly within a few hours. This can be misleading and where there is a history such as this, fractures should not be overlooked or a misdiagnosis of infection be made — the rate at which the level of pain and swelling increases is far too rapid for sepsis.

Diagnosis

An acute onset of lameness with either soft tissue or joint swelling should always raise suspicions of a fracture. In these circumstances radiographic examination should always be carried out sooner rather than later. While it is tempting to delay for a few weeks in the hope that the lesion is a soft tissue injury and will 'go away' with rest it must be re-emphasized that the difficulties of surgical treatment and the risks of permanent joint damage increase exponentially with time.

The X-ray examination should include sufficient views either to eliminate the possibility of fracture, or to delineate fully a fracture line and accurately position the fracture fragment(s) (Figs. 6.17, 6.18a and b, 6.19). The tibiotarsal joint is voluminous and fragments will often gravitate downwards and come to be in the dorsodistal pouch of the capsule at its communication with the proximal intertarsal joint.

Synovial fluid analysis will not be particularly helpful except to eliminate infection.

Treatment

Unless fracture fragments are large enough to be re-attached they should be removed, and, if feasible, the fracture bed curetted. Even

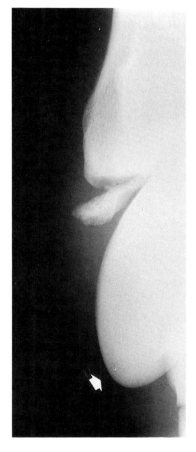

Fig. 6.17 This fracture on the lateral distal tibia shows clearly on this 45° PDLMO. (Arrowed is the protruberant lateral condyle of the talus.) The fragment was removed through an arthrotomy similar to the one described for approach to the lateral condyle.

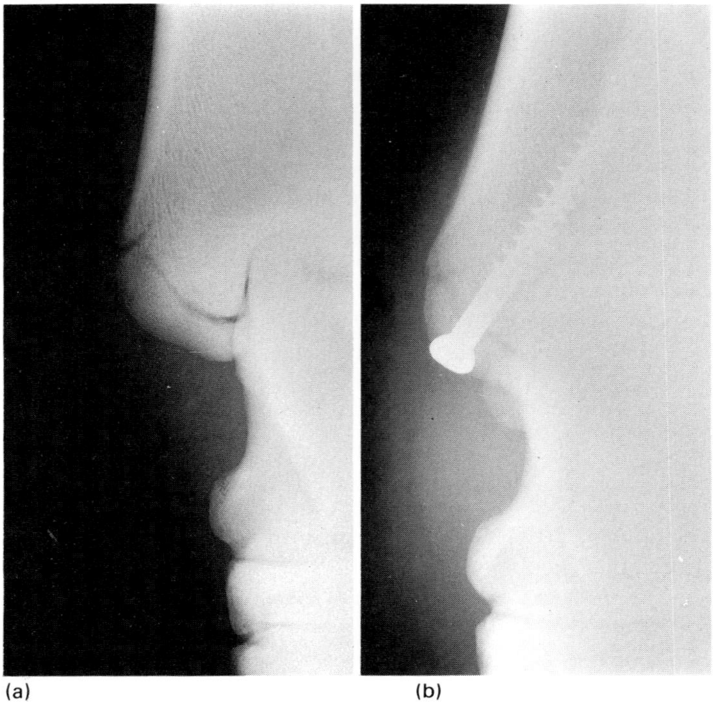

Fig. 6.18 (a) This fracture line was visualized best in a dorsoplantar projection. The fragment is large, non-displaced and an ideal candidate for internal fixation. (b) Compression fixation has been achieved with a single 6.5 mm cancellous bone screw. Care must be taken in this situation to avoid the screw impinging on the articulation.

(a)   (b)

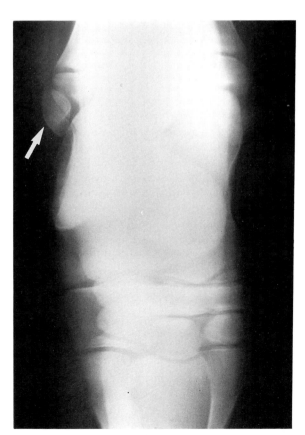

Fig. 6.19 The separate centre of ossification of the distal vestigial fibula (arrowed) must not be mistaken for a fracture fragment!

large fragments may be removed if the alternative is a dubious reduction and probable malalignment. The exception to this would be bone fragments at the origin or insertion of major ligaments. Fragment removal is carried out through arthrotomy incisions or under arthroscopic control. The position of the fragment must be accurately located first and the point of entry into the joint carefully prepared; despite the capacious joint capsule there is not much room for manoeuvre within it and incisions must be made as close to the fragment as possible. In many cases arthroscopy or manipulation under fluoroscopy and image intensification are the only feasible methods.

Major fractures of the talus and distal tibia do occur and are treated by careful reduction and compression using 'lag' techniques.

With all intra-articular fractures the prognosis must be guarded since degenerative joint disease is an almost inevitable sequel. Early diagnosis and treatment improve the odds substantially.

Post-operatively NSAIDs should be given with early walking in hand increasing in amounts over 3–4 months. At this point the animal should be turned out or 'roughed off' for a further 6 months or so.

Suggested further reading

Jackovljevic S, Gibbs C and Yeats J (1982) Traumatic fractures of the equine hock. A report of 13 cases. *Eq Vet J* **14**(1), 62–8.

Swellings of the plantar hock region

Distensions of the deep flexor tendon sheath

Anatomy, aetiology and pathogenesis

The three heads of the deep digital flexor unite into a common tendon of insertion. The superficial and deep heads unite at the level of the caudal distal tibia into a strong round tendon. This runs caudally and distally over the sustentaculum tali, i.e. medial to the tuber calcis, is joined by the medial head and the check ligament and continues to its insertion on the pedal bone. As it runs over the sustentaculum it becomes partly cartilaginous and is bound down to the surface of the bone by the strong flexor retinaculum. Its passage over the sustentaculum is lubricated by synovial fluid produced by an investing tarsal sheath. The latter begins about 5–7.5 cm proximal to the level of the medial malleolus and extends to about one quarter of the way down the metatarsus. Only proximal to the tuber calcis is the sheath free to expand and it is here that any swelling caused by increased secretion of synovial fluid within the sheath shows itself.

The cause of the increased secretion is usually trauma, resulting in damage to the tendon, the sheath and/or the sustentaculum itself. Roughening of its smooth surface either by fracture of the sustentacular rim or new bone growth leads to persistent irritation and inflammatory change as does any scarring and adhesion formation within the sheath.

Clinical signs

Distension of the tarsal sheath presents as a fluid-filled swelling in the groove between the Achilles tendon and the caudal tibia and it can be seen on both the lateral and medial side of the leg. Mild cases show a slightly elongated swelling, paralleling the long axis of the tibia but further filling gives the distension a dumb bell-like appearance with the narrow isthmus lying beneath the Achilles tendon.

The animal can be variably lame depending on the extent and chronicity of the originating trauma and they usually respond positively to a hock flexion test.

In chronic cases a period of rest will often result in a reduction in the size of the swelling but it will usually return to its previous size when exercise restarts.

Diagnosis

The diagnostic problem in cases of deep flexor tendon sheath distension is to distinguish a swelling of the tarsal sheath from a tibiotarsal joint distension and from the other fluid swellings which can occur at this site. The first is easily done; a sheath distension, the so called 'tendinous thoroughpin', has no connection with the tibiotarsal joint and can be distinguished from a plantar capsular distension, the 'articular thoroughpin', by the fact that pressure on it does not transmit a fluid pressure wave to the front of the hock. Similar pressure applied to the distended caudal joint capsule will be felt as an increase in tension in the dorsolateral and especially the dorsomedial pouches.

Other swellings, often indistinguishable on physical examination from a severe sheath distension, occur in the area and must be differentiated if treatment is envisaged. The most common are acquired cyst-like lesions which, since they have a connection with the sheath, must presumably have been caused by traumatic rupture of the sheath wall. The other type seen by the author is a distension, of unknown origin, of the gastrocnemius bursa which sits dorsal to the insertion of that muscle on the tuber calcis. Ideally a radiographic examination should comprise two stages; initial contrast radiography to establish the nature of the swelling, followed by a further examination of the sustentaculum if the lesion is seen to be a simple sheath distension. However, the initial contrast study can obscure detail of the sustentacular border and, if the plain study is not to be delayed until contrast is absorbed, it is usually performed first. Dorsoplantar and lateromedial views give little information on the state of the sustentaculum, but a 45° PDLMO (Figs. 6.15 and 6.20) show the gliding surface and the medial sustentacular rim. Fractures and new bone can be identified in this way. A skyline view of the tuber calcis and part of the sustentaculum can be obtained, even in the standing animal. A dorsoventral beam direction is used centred on the caudal aspect of a severely flexed hock (Fig. 6.21). Versatile equipment and a co-operative animal are needed otherwise the examination must be conducted under a general anaesthetic. If 20–30 ml of a water soluble contrast medium is injected in a sterile manner into a true sheath distension,

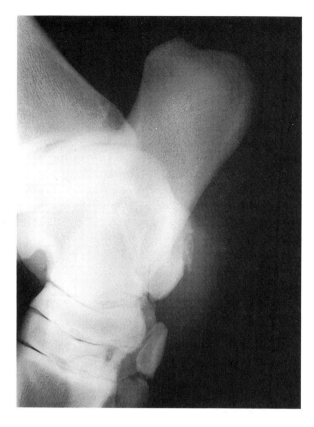

Fig. 6.20 A PDLMO projection showing a fracture of the medial rim of the sustentaculum.

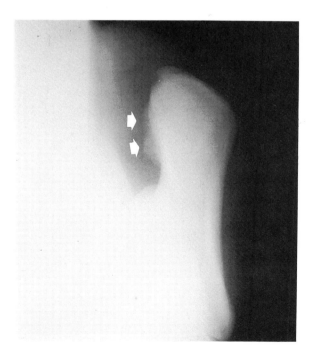

Fig. 6.21 A sky-line view of a tuber calcis showing new bone on its medial aspect (arrowed).

it rapidly extends down the length of the sheath especially if the leg is flexed a few times. This can be identified on a lateral projection. If the swelling has arisen as a result of a leak from the sheath entry of contrast into the main body of the sheath is delayed to an extent which depends on the size of the communication between them. If no contrast has passed within 15 minutes the animal should be lunged for 5–10 minutes and re-radiographed. Occasionally the slit is so small, or has such a one-way valvular action that only quite prolonged exercise can force a retrograde flow of fluid. If no passage of contrast occurs then it is likely that the swelling is due to bursal enlargement. In these investigations care must be taken to ensure good opacification of the fluid. Since the capacity of the distal sheath is small and hence the level of contrast is low good quality radiographs exposed for soft tissue are needed (Fig. 6.22). Occasionally the cyst wall is seen to have a corrugated, concertina-like appearance which seems to be due to massive synovial proliferation (Fig. 6.23).

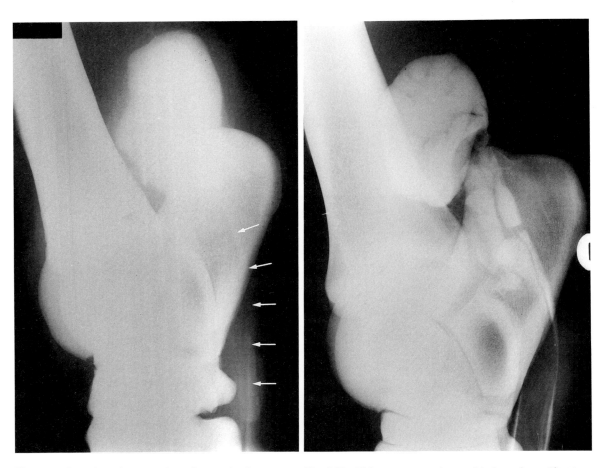

Fig. 6.22 Injection of contrast into the proximal synovial distension produced good opacification. However, only after 20 minutes of lunging did the distal sheath (arrowed) begin to opacify.

Fig. 6.23 This contrast study provided good opacification of the tendon sheath but, in addition, shows the multiple filling defects which are due to corrugation of the synovial cyst lining.

Treatment of these lesions is extremely unrewarding. Conservative therapy includes rest, aspiration of contents and injection of steroids in any combination. All these treatments result in only a transient reduction in size with an inevitable rapid resurgence as soon as exercise is started again. Frequent aspiration and steroid injection also carry a high risk of introducing infection.

Surgical treatment of simple sheath distension is only a valid proposition if there is some tangible abnormality of the sustentaculum with associated lameness. Removal of marginal fractures or even curettage of peripheral new bone is possible and the author has had some success with these techniques. However, tendon or sheath damage can never be completely repaired and the prognosis in these cases must be guarded. In those animals where the sheath distension is only cosmetic blemish and there is no lameness associated with it, the owner and the veterinary surgeon would be very well advised to leave well alone. Surgery of this area is fraught with difficulty as is the post-operative management with excessive movement and difficulty in maintaining pressure on the area making wound breakdown and post-operative swelling a great worry.

Occasionally some of the cystic or bursal distensions will reach a size whereby there is a mechanical hindrance to movement and an unacceptable blemish. Cysts such as these can be dissected free although again it is a major surgical exercise requiring an approach from both sides of the leg preferably with the animal in dorsal recumbency and the leg pulled into extension. If the dilatation has a connection with the DFT sheath, that must be identified and sealed otherwise fresh leakage will occur. The cysts are usually relatively thick walled with no distinct capsule and their inner surface is often thrown up into corrugations, dark brown to purple in colour. Again post-operative swelling and the likelihood of wound breakdown will prove to be a greater problem than the original surgery.

The author has seen several cases of trauma to the medial hock which has resulted in a marginal fracture of the sustentaculum coupled with a soft tissue wound discharging synovial fluid. Following positive identification of the synovial structure involved, i.e. the tendon sheath, by means of contrast radiography the lesions have been successfully treated. Curettage of the fracture site after fragment removal followed by twice daily irrigation of the tendon sheath via an indwelling small bore catheter passed distally to the termination of the sheath resulted in rapid healing of the cutaneous wound and, following removal of the catheter, spontaneous closure of the synovial sinus.

Suggested further reading

Edwards GB (1978) Changes in the sustentaculum tali associated with distension of the tarsal sheath (thoroughpin). *Eq Vet J* **10**(2), 97–100.

Capped hock

In the horse the superficial digital flexor muscle consists almost entirely of a strong tendon with little muscle fibre. It originates deep to the belly of the lateral head of the gastrocnemius and as it runs distally it winds around the tendon of the latter to lie superficially to it. Passing over the point of the tuber calcis it widens to form a cap-like structure then continues onwards to insert on the 1st and 2nd phalanx. In all horses there is a bursa between the superficial flexor tendon and that of gastrocnemius but in a proportion of animals there is also a superficial, subcutaneous bursa at the point of the hock.

Occasionally the bursa becomes distended and forms a floppy ball-like swelling over the point of the hock, the so-called capped hock. Often there is no known cause though sometimes the too tight application of bandages or other repetitive trauma precedes its formation.

The animals are rarely lame as a result of the lesion but it is a very noticeable blemish and owners usually ask for treatment for this reason.

As with other chronic synovial swellings treatment is usually disappointing and it is as well to explain this to owners at the outset. Conservative therapy of rest, aspiration of contents, or injection of steroids usually provides some temporary relief in mild cases but the size of the cavity does not seem to diminish, and further exercise causes it to distend once more. Where the distension is large there appears to be little elasticity in the skin or subcutaneous tissues and aspiration of the fluid produces an expanse of slack, very mobile skin which does not contract down and soon refills with fluid. Dimethyl Sulphoxide (DMSO) and similar preparations have little or no effect on these lesions and blistering and firing or both will be at best ineffective and more likely they will make matters worse by creating skin inflammation, infection and chronic thickening on top of the original swelling.

Owners often ask that the mass be removed as it would appear to be a relatively simple piece of surgery and offer a permanent solution. It must be explained very carefully that it is not the surgery itself, which is indeed fairly straightforward, but the post-operative management which presents great problems. The large dead space created at surgery, the necessity of creating a large skin flap, coupled with the great amount of relative movement in the area, beginning as early post-operatively as the anaesthetic recovery, leads to a very high incidence of wound breakdowns. Once this has happened the end result is likely to be far worse than the original capped hock. Even if wound breakdown does not occur the inevitable dead space fills with a certain amount of fluid creating a lesion almost indistinguishable from the original bursal enlargement.

In the case of show animals where an unblemished appearance is vital to their continuing existence surgical treatment may be unavoidable. The incision should be made lateral to the point of the hock with the leg in full extension: the bursa is dissected out, hopefully intact, being careful to leave as much subcutaneous tissue as possible so as to preserve the vascularity and viability of the flap. The leg is then flexed and the two skin edges matched together. Excess skin can be trimmed off the flap to reduce dead space but care must be taken not to remove too much or to end up with tucks and pleats of skin at the commisures of the wound. Subcuticular sutures should be used as well as simple interrupted cutaneous ones, and wound tension should be further reduced by the use of large tension sutures over a stent bandage. Pressure bandaging is essential, and an important point of post-operative management is to prevent the animal lying down for at least 2 weeks by cross tying. As in many other instances the animal's temperament and co-operation is all important.

Where cosmetic perfection is not paramount, the owner should be encouraged to come to terms with the blemish and accept it as such.

Curb (strain of the calcaneometatarsal ligament)

The term curb is usually used to describe the swelling produced by tearing and damage to the fibres of the calcaneometatarsal ligament at its insertion into the 4th tarsal and 4th metatarsal (lateral splint bone) and by the chronic sequelae to such an injury.

Some authors describe a congenital curb which is said to be a trait of some thoroughbred lines. However, this is likely to be a description of a certain type of conformation where the head of the 4th metatarsal bone is especially prominent.

Curb is usually used to describe swellings at the junction of the tarsus and metatarsus but the calcaneometatarsal or long plantar ligament can be damaged and hence produce a swelling anywhere along its length or at its origin from the plantar surface of the tuber calcis.

Animals with excessively angled hocks, the so called 'sickle' or 'cow hocks' are said to be predisposed to the condition. There is little other than anecdotal evidence to support this relationship and probably too few horses with perfect conformation to produce a control group. However, since the function of the ligament is to transmit an extensor pull to the metatarsus it might be reasonable to expect that any deviation from a straight line might increase the strain on the insertion.

Clinical signs

Clinical signs are a sudden onset of a soft tissue swelling at the characteristic site on the plantar aspect of the tuber calcis. There is pain on palpation and lameness exacerbated by flexion; with time the lesion becomes firm and pain-free but the swelling remains.

Diagnosis

The diagnosis is made initially by recognition of a swelling on the plantar aspect of the tuber calcis seen best on viewing the leg in a lateromedial direction. If the lesion is at the head of the 4th metatarsal it will fall into the category of a curb; however, a swelling anywhere in this region can indicate damage to the calcaneometatarsal ligament. In chronic cases, where there has been damage to the origin or insertion of the ligament, new bone may be formed and can be recognized on X-ray examination.

Treatment

Logical treatment must be based on the fact that a curb is a ligamentous tear and the acceptance of the fact that there is little can be done to affect the course of the healing process. The most effective therapy is an early recognition of the condition and prevention of further damage by ensuring that the animal is rested completely for several months, also by minimizing the accumulation of inflammatory exudate and subsequent swelling by pressure bandaging as quickly as possible after the acute condition is recognized.

Chronic lesions where healing has taken place by scar tissue replacement of the damaged ligament and by associated new bone formation will not be affected by any therapy. The only factor to bear in mind is that scar tissue collagen does not mature completely for 12 months or more and the longer the animal is rested the less the risk of a recurrence. Enforcing this rest period will be made difficult by the fact that the animal will not be lame after a month or so but an explanation of the mechanism of tendon and ligament repair will usually help owners understand the problem.

The stifle joint

Introduction

The stifle is composed of two separate articulations, the femorotibial, which allows flexion to take place and the femoropatellar joint which is essentially a device to allow the extensor pull of the massive quadriceps muscle to be transmitted to the tibia via a sesamoid bone. This is the patella or 'kneecap' and the distal patellar ligaments, are, of course, essentially tendons of insertion. The femorotibial joint is one of the very few in the body to have menisci.

Details of the structure and intercommunication of the joint synovial capsules are given in the section on intra-articular anaesthesia (see p. 21) and for further anatomical study the reader is referred to the standard anatomy books.

Physical examination of the stifle

Studies have shown that pain originating in the stifle region does not produce a characteristic gait deficit or lameness; the pattern of rise and fall of the quarters is the same as for lameness of any other cause. In cases of severe pain, the animal may 'fix' or immobilize its stifle; however, even this can be difficult to see and be certain about and it is often little more than a subjective impression to add to a weight of other evidence usually gleaned from a physical examination of the leg.

The stifle is a joint which is difficult to assess for several reasons. Comparisons between left and right are difficult because it is not possible to palpate symmetrically; pressure on normal joints for some reason will often elicit an uncharacteristic reaction from even the quietest animal; well fleshed, otherwise normal ponies and horses often exhibit pendulous rolls just above the patella which become especially prominent if the leg is in extension and are often mistaken for distensions of the joint capsule or the results of patellar trauma. Manipulation of the articulation is usually difficult, both because of the bulk of the upper leg, and because the 'reciprocal apparatus' causes every other joint in the limb to flex in concert. This also removes much of the specificity of any flexion tests which may be carried out. Because of this there are only a few signs which are of significance and which can be relied upon as good clinical pointers.

One of the most frequently seen, and most reliable, indications of joint disease is distension of the infrapatellar joint capsule. This is seen as a smooth swelling lying between the patella and the proximal cranial tibia. It can often be seen from some distance and palpation confirms a variably tense fluid-filled distension which masks the normally clearly palpable outline of the three distal patellar ligaments. It indicates pathology of either the femoropatellar or medial femortibial joint capsules which communicate in 90% of cases and, in about 10% of horses the lateral femorotibial compartment as well.

Other signs are soft tissue swelling on the lateral aspect of the stifle or over the patella, both areas where normally only skin and some loose fascia overlies bone; occasionally sinuses, often discharging some distance from the stifle and, in long-standing cases, muscle atrophy. Disuse atrophy of the upper limb musculature is *not* a feature of lower limb problems. Wasting of the quadriceps is often a consequence of chronic stifle pain as is gluteal atrophy to a degree. However, the bulk of the quadriceps mass can vary considerably depending on the animal's stance and great care must be taken over the comparison with the other leg.

Synovial fluid analysis may be a help in certain cases and its recovery is relatively easy provided the joint capsules are distended. A sample taken from the infrapatellar pouch is, because of their communication virtually certain to reflect changes in either the femoropatellar or medial femorotibial compartments or both. The lateral compartment will usually have to be sampled separately and this can be difficult unless this too is distended.

Radiography

Lateromedial and oblique views of the cranial stifle are relatively simple to obtain even in the standing animal and structures can be well visualized by inserting a cassette medial to the stifle and pushing it up slightly into the fold of the flank. Grids are not needed and for best definition fine-grain conventional or rare-earth screen/film combinations should be used. A surprising degree of obliquity can be achieved without too much distortion and to project the lateral rim of the trochlear groove clear of the much larger medial one a lateromedial view angled a good 30−40° in the caudocranial direction is needed: most animals tolerate this examination quite well.

The examination of the complete stifle with both lateral and caudo-cranial projections is not so easy in the conscious patient and unless the generator is of sufficient power to allow fairly short exposure times it is a procedure best done under general anaesthesia. The use of rare-earth screen/film combinations will be of enormous value in the standing animal. Apart from being much 'faster' these screens and films are much less sensitive to low energy scattered radiation and good films can be achieved without a grid. A light beam diaphragm with the ability to cone-down is of great help, again to reduce scatter from extraneous tissue and as an aid to aiming the beam. Accurate centring of the beam can be difficult so it is worthwhile spending a few minutes working out the anatomy of the site before the examination and not adopting the 'point and press' system which invariably leads to poorly centred films. As with many other sharply tapering sites it is well-nigh impossible to visualize clearly the thin peripheral and the relatively much thicker central structures with one exposure and two are usually necessary for a full evaluation of the lateral stifle; one using a fine-grain, extremity type, film/screen combination for the patella and trochlea and a second, using a faster combination, for the body of the stifle. In smaller animals this may not be necessary as the discrepancy in width is not so marked.

Upwards fixation of the patella

Aetiology and pathogenesis

Although often casually referred to as patellar luxation, upwards fixation of the patella is not a true dislocation.

The troclea of the femur is bounded by two ridges, the lateral and medial. The latter is much the larger and there is a definite notch between its bulbous proximal end and the distal shaft of the femur. The patella, which is a sesamoid in the tendon of insertion of the quadriceps muscle, has a fibrocartilagenous medial extension which hooks over the medial ridge of the trochlea rather like a sitting man hooking his arm over the wing of an armchair (Figs. 6.24a and b). This extension, which Sisson and Grossman (1975) say is actually part of the medial ligament, blends into the latter on the medial side of the trochlea and then continues distally as the typical ligamentous structure to insert on to the tibial tuberosity with the middle and lateral ligaments.

When the leg is in full extension the patella rides to the top of the trochlea and falls into the notch to a degree which is probably governed by both conformation and the thickness of the fat pad which lies there. The locking of the patella into the notch forms an important constituent of the 'stay mechanism' which allows the horse to rest its hind legs. When it needs to flex the stifles the quadriceps first contracts to lift the patella clear of the notch and then relaxes to allow it to slide down the trochlea. Thus any factor which interferes with the co-ordination of this process can lead to the patella locking in the notch, an inability to flex the stifle and therefore, because of the reciprocal apparatus, the whole limb.

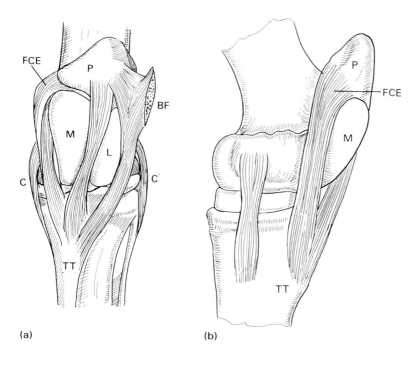

(a)　　　　　　　　(b)

Fig. 6.24 A diagrammatic illustration of (a) the cranial and (b) the medial aspects of the patella (P), the fibrocartilagenous extension (FCE) and the medial condyle (M). L = lateral condyle; BF = cut edge of biceps femoris; C and C' = medial and lateral femorotibital ligaments; TT = tibial tuberosity.

The conformational abnormality which is said to predispose to the condition is that of a 'straight hind leg' where there is a large angle between femur and tibia. Although attractive in theory it would be a very difficult association to quantify and the author has not noticed any such relationship. One of the factors which does seem to have a definite association with its onset is a loss of bodily condition. There is often the history of a period of weight loss for some reason, and the converse is certainly true that the frequency of locking can diminish or even stop altogether as a lean animal gains weight. The old name of 'straw cramp' suggests that in earlier days too the association with poor condition, i.e. animals fed on straw, had been made. The theory advanced is that weight loss brings with it a diminution in the size of the retropatellar fat pad, allowing the patella to seat further on to the top of the medial trochlear ridge. However, the clinician must be aware that this condition is not the prerogative of the thin horse; well-conditioned and even fat animals can show it!

A third plausible theory is that the locking is caused by poor co-ordination between flexors and extensors of the stifle. This theory is supported by the condition being seen more commonly in young animals and those used only spasmodically. It is rarely seen in the fit athlete.

Clinical signs

The clinical signs are classical and are caused by a sudden inability of the animal to flex its hind leg after the backward extension phase of its stride. This results in the leg pointing backwards in an extreme extensor rigidity. Locking can occur at any pace though usually at the walk or trot; most often it is noticed first when an animal moves off from a standstill. The duration of locking varies too from a transitory backward jerk which releases almost instantaneously, to several seconds, or in extreme cases minutes. Temperament seems to govern the reaction to locking; most animals accept it stoically; others seem to panic and make strenuous efforts to release the leg. If it happens at a fast pace it can of course be dangerous for horse and rider. Release is often accompanied by a loud click or clunk and the gait subsequently appears perfectly normal. The intervals between locking episodes vary enormously and it is impossible to predict when the next one will be. Both horses and ponies can be affected and there seems to be no breed or sex predisposition.

Diagnosis

It is uncommon for an animal who exhibits occasional locking to 'perform' for the attending clinician. Turning, backing, and repeated stops and starts are probably the best way to elicit the characteristic signs. Some animals exhibit a partial lock and although there is no obvious fixation in extension the leg will consistently snap into flexion with a jerk, accompanied by an audible click. Occasionally the locking can be provoked by easing the animal into a position where its hind leg is extended and then manually pushing the patella over the top of the femoral trochlea.

Usually, however, it is necessary to rely on the owner's description and on the absence of any other pathology: if there is difficulty in describing the symptoms a little play-acting or mimicry will usually bring delighted recognition! Only two other conditions may be mistaken for upward fixation; they are stringhalt and fibrous myopathy of the semi-membranosus and semi-tendinosus muscles. Neither is common and the similarities are not great!

Treatment

If the animal is noticeably thin, or the symptoms appear during a convalescent phase or at the end of winter, the conservative approach of improving the animal's condition may be effective. Any loss of condition should, of course, be appraised as a separate issue and it may be that the locking patella is the first visible sign of other pathology. Occasionally young and otherwise healthy horses will exhibit this condition but will improve to normality when training begins. This suggests that unfitness and consequent lack of co-ordination may be a factor and that in an unfit and otherwise healthy animal a period of 'fitness training' may solve the problem. Another approach where there is no weight loss is therefore to initiate a programme of controlled exercise to improve fitness and muscle co-ordination.

If conservative measures fail or do not seem to be indicated, surgical relief by section of the medial patellar ligament is a comparatively simple measure.

It is feasible and in fact desirable to carry out the procedure in the standing horse provided its temperament is suitable. In the weight bearing phase of the stride the ligaments of the patella stand out most clearly, are easily identified and, being taut, section easily.

The animal must be *heavily* sedated: an excellent combination is acetyl promazine and pethidine given in *full* therapeutic doses. Xylazine alone is not suitable because it is a clinical observation, not supported by pharmacology or anaesthetists, that its otherwise excellent effects are strangely reluctant to involve the hind legs. Detomidine hydrochloride is a very effective recent addition to the suitable range of drugs.

The area is identified by first finding the tibial crest, surprisingly low down the leg, identifying the three ligaments arranged in a double V proximally and then preparing the area for surgery. With a twitch applied the animal is moved gently backwards and forwards until the ligaments are felt clearly. The foreleg on the same side is lifted and a local anaesthetic skin bleb is inserted with a very fine needle in the distal V between the middle and medial ligaments. After a couple of minutes some 10 ml of 2 or 3% lignocaine are infiltrated behind and in front of the medial ligament using a 4−5 cm medium to fine bore needle inserted through the desensitized skin. It is customary to operate on both hind legs even if only one has seen to be affected so both sides are prepared and anaesthetized before surgery commences.

After a minimum wait of 10 minutes the twitch is reapplied, the ipsilateral foreleg raised and a *small* stab skin incision is made in the distal V between the middle ligaments some 2 cm proximal to the tibial crest. Reidentification of the area is often made more difficult by the swelling caused by the injected local anaesthetic and the incision must not be made until the surgeon is sure of his landmarks. A tenotome, a slim, narrow, solid-bladed scalpel, or, in its absence a pointed No. 11 blade, is inserted through the skin incision, passed deep to the medial ligament and then brought forward with a sawing motion to incise the ligament from back to front. At this stage the surgeon should be ready to withdraw the blade, as sometimes the last few fibres give way with a satisfying crunching sound and the leg collapses into flexion. More often this does not happen and deep palpation is necessary to ensure that the ligament is completely sectioned. Sometimes the ligament tapers medially and the tenotome must be inserted *a little* further and the remaining portion dealt with. Occasionally too the novice surgeon will insert the tenotome through the body of the ligament so that only its medial and superficial portions are sectioned! The skin wound is sutured with a single simple suture or, if very small, left unsutured. Post-operative swelling will depend very much on the speed and deftness of the surgery but there is always some present. The advice given about post-operative rest will vary according to the swelling and discomfort but a month or so should be adequate in most cases.

Under general anaesthesia the surgery is done with the animal on its back and its hind legs stretched out behind it. As an aside, care must be taken not to put any excess downward force on the outstretched legs during preparation or by onlookers, as psoas myopathy can easily occur. The ligaments are not as easily palpated in this position and the legs should be flexed and extended until they are recognized. Once located the leg should be kept in that position otherwise the skin incision or prepared area can shift extensively in relation to the ligaments as the leg flexes or extends. If the ligament cannot be palpated easily then a much more extensive incision and exposure can be made, though in this position of high skin mobility healing of large skin wounds can be a problem. A good indication that the correct ligament has been completely sectioned is provided by the ease with which the leg can be flexed from its extended position. Prior to surgery, if the leg is fully extended, flexion can be difficult because of the locking of the patella on the trochlea. After the tenotomy the leg will glide easily from full extension to full flexion!

Very occasionally the condition recurs following surgery and Hickman and Walker (1964) suggested section of the medial cartilaginous prolongation of the patella as an alternative technique which avoids this subsequent complication. It is a much more extensive piece of surgery and its use as a first line treatment is not really warranted.

Osteochondrosis and osteochondritis dissecans of the trochlear ridge

Aetiology and pathogenesis

The lateral trochlear ridge of the femur is a common site for osteochondrosis (Fig. 6.25). It occurs predominantly in young rapidly growing animals on high feed intakes (see section on osteochondrosis p. 194). Whilst the thickened and weak articular cartilage is undamaged there may be no clinical signs of the disease, but if the joint is badly stressed by for example, a fall, or by the frenetic activity of a foal turned out after a long period of confinement the cartilage can split forming fissures and flaps; thus releasing cartilage fragments and proteins to cause an acute synovitis and joint swelling. Thus owners often link the onset with trauma and the clinician can be misled into thinking that the trauma alone is the cause! In the older animal of 18 months to 2 years the condition often shows first when training

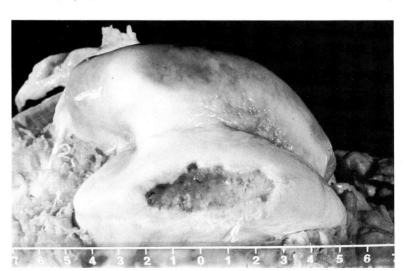

Fig. 6.25 A typical osteochondritis dissecans lesion on the lateral ridge of the femoral trochlea.

begins and the horse is seen to be lame or to be reluctant to work. It would seem that the probable course of events is the development of several abnormal cartilaginous foci within the zones of hypertrophy and provisional calcification of the articular cartilage in the mid-point of the lateral condyle. These eventually become confluent and the large weakened area develops cleavage lines as a result of the 'normal' forces applied via the patella. This downward squeezing force flattens and laterally displaces the soft cartilage. The separation of fragments progresses until they achieve a 'cobblestone' appearance as they lie within the defect bound together by fibrous tissue. Sudden trauma can cause a splitting of the soft cartilage or a complete displacement of fragments resulting in acute signs. In more chronic cases the disruption to the normal contour of the joint causes problems which only become apparent when the animal is brought into work.

Clinical signs

The younger 6 month to 1 year old animal is often presented with the history that it has fallen and damaged its stifle. The older 18 month to 2 year old will usually have been seen to be lame or reluctant to walk. There can be a variable degree of femoropatellar joint capsule distension; this shows best at the level of the three patellar ligaments where it appears as a smooth, soft, domed swelling of variable size. Comparison with the other side may not be of much value as that too may be affected. Similarly, lameness on one side can be masked or reduced by the bilateral involvement.

Diagnosis

Osteochondrosis is an important differential diagnosis in a young or youngish animal presenting with a sudden onset hind limb problem especially if there is a capsular swelling of the femoropatellar joint. There is often a history of some trauma, the owner usually believing the animal to have been kicked or to have 'sprained a ligament'. These suggestions must be taken seriously since they could lead to the same clinical signs; on the other hand trauma may have been the insult responsible for converting the non-clinical osteochondrosis into the clinically significant osteochondritis dissecans. Swelling of the femoropatellar capsule is usually present to some degree, but is worse in the acute cases. Similarly, lameness is variable at both the straight trot and the lunge, if that is feasible; flexion tests too usually have a greater effect in the acute case. Palpation of the lateral ridge of the trochlea will cause only minimal pain response but it is sometimes possible to feel the roughened surface of the articular cartilage. Intra-articular anaesthesia will confirm the location of the lesion although a subchondral bone cyst of the medial femoral condyle, which can present with the same clinical signs, would also be anaesthetized through the communication between the two synovial sacs.

Synovial fluid analysis may be done, though the most rewarding further examination will be radiography.

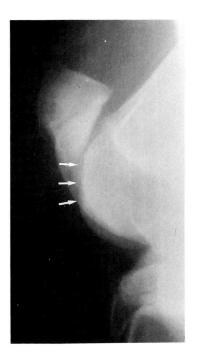

Radiography

Radiographs taken with a beam sufficiently angled in the caudocranial, lateromedial oblique direction will show the lateral ridge clear of the larger medial one. Where lesions are on the lateral aspect or crest of the ridge this view shows them very well. However, lesions on the medial side, within the groove are not so well visualized. These are best seen on well penetrated lateromedial projections, though not so clearly, superimposed on the medial condyle (Fig. 6.26).

The radiographic appearance of the lesions can be grouped into two broad types: Firstly a pronounced irregularity of the subchondral bone at the crest of the lateral ridge usually its middle third (Fig. 6.26), and a second, more well-defined, punched-out lesion looking rather like a bowl full of pebbles (Fig. 6.27). The radiographs should also be evaluated for loose fragments of bone, usually best seen on the straight lateral view lying in the dependent pouch of the femoro-patellar capsule (Fig. 6.28) and for the presence of osteophytes and the articular margins. These are often seen most clearly on the distal patella and indicate osteoarthritis and a poor prognosis.

In very young foals one must be careful about over-interpreting apparent irregularities of the subchondral bone of the trochlear ridges; ossification is often slow at this site and these irregularities can, in

Fig. 6.26 A lateromedial projection of a stifle showing flattening and irregularity of the lateral trochlear ridge: a typical appearance of an osteochondritis dissecans lesion.

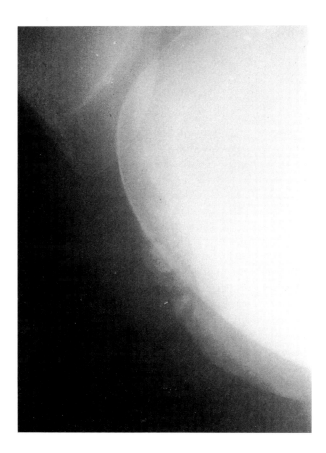

Fig. 6.27 A lateral condyle showing another common radiographic manifestation of osteochondritis dissecans of the lateral femoral trochlear ridge: it has the appearance of a cluster of pebbles in a 'punched out' depression.

Fig. 6.28 A positive contrast arthrogram has outlined the limits of the distal pouch of the femoropatellar joint capsule (arrowed). Heavily mineralized fragments of subchondral bone are seen lying within the pouch. Careful examination will show a radiolucemt halo around the larger fragment indicating a peripheral layer of soft tissue, in this case cartilage. Some of these fragments were firmly adherent to the synovial membrane. The outline of the distal medial ridge is indicated by the thin arrows. It too is bounded by a thin halo of soft tissued opacity cartilage.

the absence of clinical signs to the contrary, be regarded as a normal finding. If doubt exists then a contrast arthrogram can be done to indicate whether there are any cartilage defects. Both stifles should be examined!

Treatment

There are differing views as to the results of conservative and surgical management of OCD of the stifle. One view expressed by Stromberg and Rejno (1978) is that there is little difference in the eventual outcome. However, the other view, that surgery is beneficial, seems to predominate and is typified by Pascoe *et al* (1984). It is the experience of the author too that, without surgery, lameness invariably persists and arthritis rapidly supervenes. However, surgical treatment is not an entirely simple matter and has its drawbacks too. Where feasible the surgery should be carried out under arthroscopic control; where this is not possible or where the lesions are very extensive and there are many loose large fragments an arthrotomy can be done.

With the leg in full extension the lateral condyle can be approached in one of two ways; between the middle and lateral patellar ligament or lateral to the lateral patellar ligament and through the biceps femoris muscle; of the two, the latter tends to provide the better access to the lateral ridge. Unfortunately neither approach gives any advantage when it comes to healing and both are complicated by frequent seroma formation and wound dehiscence. The exposed lesion is curetted to remove all the fragments, leaving a smooth sided depression marginated by normal articular cartilage. The trochlear groove itself and the apposing face of the patella are often affected as well, (Fig. 6.29), though because of the contours these lesions cannot be seen on radiography. These too are curetted smooth and the synovial capsule explored for separated fragments, some of which may be loose or others which may be firmly adherent to the synovial membrane. The joint must be well irrigated, preferably with at least 2 litres

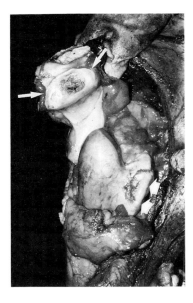

Fig. 6.29 Post mortem disarticulation of the patella revealing lesions on its ventral surface (large arrows) as well as on the lateral ridge of the trochlear (square arrows).

177

of Hartmann's solution, before closing and the wound protected by a stent bandage for recovery. In an effort to avoid the complications mentioned above, the animal, if its temperament allows, should be cross-tied for about 10 days post-operatively. This prevents the stifle from being hyperflexed with consequent stress on the wound as the animal lies down.

In time the defects heal by fibrocartilage though the contour of the lateral ridge never returns to normal but remains flattened. Post-operative management should consist of a scheme of graduated exercise with activity increasing slowly and steadily with the object of a return to training after some 6 months of convalescence.

In essence, the treatment of this condition involves some risk whichever course is chosen; conservative management has only a small chance of a successful outcome, but surgical intervention carries a higher than average risk of wound complications. Although rarely fatal, these do increase convalescent time and often result in a poor cosmetic appearance.

Suggested further reading

Pascoe JR, Pool RR, Wheat JD and O'Brien TR (1984) Osteochondral defects of the lateral trochlear ridge of the distal femur of the horse. Clinical, radiographic and pathological examination and results of surgical treatment. *Vet Surgery* **13**(2), 99–110.

Stromberg B and Rejno S (1978) Osteochondrosis in the horse I. A clinical and radiological investigation of osteochondritis dissecans of the knee and hock joint. *Acta Radiol* **358**(Suppl), 139.

Trotter GW, McIlwraith CW and Norrdin RW (1983) A comparison of two surgical approaches to the equine femoropatellar joint for the treatment of osteochondritis dissecans. *Vet Surgery* **12**, 33.

Medial condylar subchondral bone cysts (stifle cysts)

Aetiology and pathogenesis

The aetiopathogenesis of subchondral bone cysts (SBC) is unclear. Although there is weighty opinion in favour of it being a manifestation of osteochondrosis it is odd that SBCs are not seen in association with the other common manifestation of that condition which affects the lateral trochlear ridge. Theories suggesting that the SBC is a primary avascular necrosis exacerbated by trauma have not been confirmed.

The condition is seen mainly in young, well-grown animals usually of the thoroughbred type. However, the cysts can be present for many years before the overlying cartilage and subchondral bone breaks down releasing cyst material into the joint and causing the appearance of the clinical signs of lameness and joint effusion. In a proportion of cases with simple femoral cysts the symptoms regress spontaneously with rest. Other animals can remain lame for many years with the additional problem of progressive degenerative joint disease. The lesions are often bilateral and 'kissing lesions' in the femur and tibia have been reported.

Clinical signs

Animals suffering from SBC usually present in one of two ways: as a lameness which becomes apparent when the animal is brought into work or training or, as a sudden onset lameness at virtually any period of young adulthood. The onset of lameness is sometimes accompanied by a degree of joint effusion which is visible as a distension of the distal pouch of the femoropatellar capsule just proximal to the tibial crest. The lameness itself is variable in severity though it is usually quite noticeable at the trot and can at times be quite severe. Flexion of the joint will cause only mild exacerbation. Bilaterally affected animals will show a stilted hind limb gait rather than individual leg lameness. Muscle atrophy of the quarter or thigh region is not a feature of these animals with single cysts, though it is often seen in those with multiple cysts or bilateral involvement.

Diagnosis

In young animals a sudden onset lameness with joint effusion should bring to mind both this condition and that of OCD of the lateral trochlear ridge. If the history is vague, then a detailed clinical, nerve block and radiographic examination should eliminate lower limb causes and, along with any capsular distension, focus attention on the stifle.

Intra-articular anaesthesia is quickly and easily carried out, penetration of the distal pouch of the femoropatellar capsule being straightforward, especially if it is distended. Time and a little exercise will be needed to help the local spread into the medial femoropatellar pouch but once it takes effect, there will be a marked improvement.

In both young and older animals the stifle region should be examined carefully for evidence of soft tissue swelling, pain or crepitus as of course trauma must be considered as a differential diagnosis.

Radiography

X-ray examination is essential and should consist of both straight lateromedial and caudocranial views. Surprisingly, the latter is often the easier projection as it does not require a cassette to be placed on the inner thigh. In all but the largest horses the examination can be done standing using fast rare-earth screen/film combinations. Very big horses will usually require a general anaesthetic and the use of a grid on an extended leg. A light beam diaphragm is virtually essential both to allow accurate aiming of the beam, to restrict the beam size and reduce scatter. With a reduced beam area the image is definitely improved but the stifle, buried in muscle masses, may be missed. To avoid this waste of time and films it is a good idea to spend a few minutes palpating and assessing the anatomy of the area and even going to the lengths of drawing the outline of the joint on to the coat with chalk! The cassette is pushed into the flank in front of the patella and the beam directed horizontally and parallel to the sagittal plane of the leg which is often held in an outwardly rotated position.

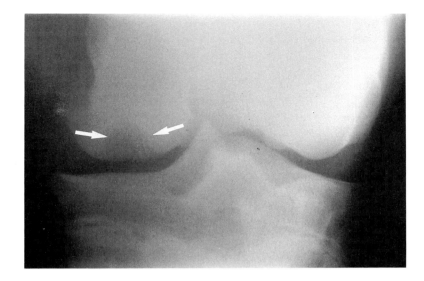

Fig. 6.30 A medial condylar 'cyst' in the distal femur.

The lesions appear in the subchondral area of the medial femoral condyle as a variably shaped circumscribed area of radiolucency with surrounding sclerosis. (Fig. 6.30). The cysts may vary in size from 1–2 cm in diameter to occasionally being so big as to involve virtually the whole condyle. There is often an accompanying distortion or flattening of the subchondral bone contour. Remember that the outline of the cyst will depend, as will its apparent relationship with the articular surface, on the tangent that the X-ray beam makes with the femoral condyle margin. It can therefore change between films! Both stifles should be radiographed.

Treatment

Conservative treatment is not as a rule successful, many animals remaining lame indefinitely. Reports indicate that single cysts affecting only one leg are more likely to respond to rest than multiple or bilateral lesions, about 50% attaining a clinical recovery. Intra-articular steroids are *not* indicated though other non-steroidal anti-inflammatory drugs can be used to give symptomatic relief. The treatment of choice, if the animal is to stand the maximum chance of working again, is surgery, the cyst being curetted through an arthrotomy incision and packed with cancellous bone harvested from the contralateral ilium.

The arthrotomy is performed with the animal lying on the affected side and with the stifle in full flexion. The approach is between the medial patellar ligament and the medial femorotibial ligament, through the fat pad and into the joint. The lesion lies immediately below the incision and appears as a crenellation or indentation in the articular cartilage. The opening is enlarged if necessary to allow a curette into the cyst and the contents removed. Cancellous bone is then packed into the cavity and tapped firmly down. The neck of the cyst is filled to within 2 mm of the articular surface but not flush with it and the arthrotomy closed routinely. A stent bandage is sewn over the wound to protect it.

Because of the mobility of the area, wound dehiscence and seroma formation can be a problem. If the animal's temperament allows, cross tying for a week to 10 days post-operatively would be of great help in reducing this risk.

Up to 9 or 10 months should be allowed for complete graft incorporation before the animal is allowed to recommence work. During that time a programme of graduated exercise should be instituted.

Radiography cannot be used to monitor graft incorporation as there is little correlation between this and radiological appearance. It must be noted here that the cancellous bone is not particularly radio opaque and the cyst will look much the same immediately post-operatively. The first increase in density appears some 3 months later and although some may go on to become completely ossified many will persist with an unhomogenous appearance. At the present time there is no method which allows accurate assessment of graft incorporation and healing though it is clear that full osseous union is not necessary before the animal can resume normal function.

Although there are few reports of long term follow ups it would seem that this technique allows about 80% of affected animals to return to work.

Alternative techniques are curettage without grafting and the use of bone cement. Neither appear to be as satisfactory; the former resulting in greatly delayed healing, and the inelasticity of the cement plug in the latter causing problems as the bone remodels around it and kissing lesions on the apposing tibia are created. To set against this, no healing is involved and recovery is faster and the tibial lesions appear to have little significance if the animal is not to be used for athletic work.

Suggested further reading

Jeffcott LB and Kold SE (1982) Clinical and radiological aspects of stifle bone cysts in the horse. *Eq Vet J* **14**(1), 40−6.

Calcinosis circumscripta (tumoral calcinosis)

Aetiology and pathogenesis

Calcinosis circumscripta is characterized by calcareous aggregations in the subcutaneous tissue usually around the large limb articulations. It also occurs in man and in dogs, usually the larger breeds, in the subcutis of the limbs and foot pads and occasionally in the oral cavity.

Although various suggestions have been put forward regarding its aetiology, principally recurrent trauma, the true cause is not known.

Clinical signs

The development of a hard, pain-free swelling at the margin of one of the large limb joints is the prime clinical sign. By far the most common site is the lateral aspect of the stifle at the level of the proximal tibia. The mass can be very large, commonly up to 12 or 15 cm in diameter, though flattish in cross-section. It has margins which, though indistinct at first, become more obvious with deep palpation and as it is firmly adherent to periarticular fibrous tissue it is relatively immobile. Small masses rarely cause gait problems but larger ones can interfere mechanically with joint mobility.

Diagnosis

The presence of such a mass in the lateral aspect of the stifle should arouse suspicion of calcinosis circumscripta especially as there is little else which can mimic it. At other less characteristic sites this should be a differential of any painless, firm mass.

Radiographic examination will show the characteristic appearance of a loose aggregate of mineralized opacities with fairly well circumscribed boundaries adjacent to the articulation. If it is considered necessary then of course a biopsy can be taken for confirmation of the diagnosis.

Treatment

The course of these tumours is unpredictable; some have been known to regress, others to remain at the same size indefinitely and yet others to expand to clinically significant dimensions.

Surgical removal should not be undertaken lightly: these masses are usually more extensive than they appear and are always well adherent to the periarticular fibrous tissue so that there is always a risk of penetrating the joint capsule. The creation of large undermined skin flaps and much dead space can, in addition, give problems with wound healing, a significant risk anyway in this region adjacent to the joint. At surgery a C-shaped skin flap should be created making sure that as much subcutaneous fascia as possible is left adherent to the skin to preserve its vascular supply. The superficial layer of the mass will dissect away freely but problems are often encountered separating its deep surface from the thick fibrous tissues below it. Every effort should be made to obliterate dead space and tension should be taken off the skin sutures by careful positioning of subcuticular suture layers and the use of a stent bandage. A suction drain system can be used effectively in these cases to prevent fluid accumulation.

If the mass is completely removed then recurrence is not likely. Small masses not interfering with motion and not creating a cosmetic blemish are best left alone.

Patella fractures

Aetiology and pathogenesis

The aetiology of patella fractures is invariably trauma. They occur randomly in the equine population with no known age, sex or breed distribution. Kicks, jumping and trailer accidents are the common causes. There is often a skin wound present. The fracture may be simple or comminuted and sometimes compound. In certain cases the fracture may be small and flake-like, usually lying on the cranial surface of the patella at the point of impact; in others, there may be no overt fracture initially but death of a portion of the rostral patellar bone may occur following an osteitis and ischaemia and result in sequestrum formation. The presence of an infected piece of bone will lead to the formation of a discharging sinus. If left untreated any fracture involving the articular surface will result in the eventual development of degenerative joint disease.

Clinical signs

Major fractures of the patella involving the articular surface will present as a sudden onset, very severe lameness with the animal showing minimal inclination to weight bear even at rest. There will be some soft tissue swelling over the patella and possibly a skin wound. Where the articulation is involved, noticeable joint effusion will be present. These signs are more easily noticeable in the slighter, thinner skinned breeds and may be missed on a superficial examination of heavier or fatter animals with their normally 'podgy' stifles.

If there is only superficial trauma to the patella then the initial lameness can be just as severe, but will last for only a short while, diminishing rapidly after the first few days. However, if a sequestrum forms then it will manifest as a discharging sinus emerging as much as 20 cm distal from the point of the stifle weeks or even months later. During this same period the initial soft, painful, acute swelling will subside to be replaced by a firm, fibrous induration of the parapatellar tissues.

Diagnosis

Where the fracture is recent the diagnosis can be made on obvious local signs and possibly on a history of trauma; though owners will occasionally invent stories to fit the symptoms, later presenting them to the clinician as facts! With less severe fractures and cases of uncertain duration it is sometimes necessary to go through a routine lameness work-up before the cause of lameness is confirmed. Sinus tracts discharging anywhere near the patella should always excite suspicion of a sequestrum.

Confirmation of the diagnosis is by radiography with the emphasis on variously obliqued lateromedial projections taken on a fine-grain screen/film combinations. Sagittal fractures will be difficult to see on these, and a caudocranial projection will be necessary. However, even in this view, visualization of the fracture line can be difficult because superimposition of the femur obscures fine detail as well as necessitating a large increase in exposure. The origin of sinus tracts should be investigated by radiography following the injection of contrast medium into them.

Treatment

Fractures involving the articular surface will result in severe osteo-arthritis if not treated adequately. If possible, fragments should be screwed together using ASIF type screws placed lag fashion. Comminuted fractures can be difficult to repair in this way as individual fragments may be small and the complex shape of the articular surface can make screw placement a major problem. However, it would seem that perfect reduction is not absolutely necessary and even those animals with subsequently severely malformed patellas can lead a reasonable, though not athletic life. Good reduction and compression of fragments is, of course, the ideal! If one or two small fragments are present, the alternative to internal fixation is their removal. The author has removed up to 30% of the patellar articular surface in those cases where reduction and fixation were not feasible with good short and long term results.

The surgical approach in these cases is governed by the nature of the fracture but aspiring surgeons must remember that the patella lies within the tendons of insertion of the mighty quadriceps muscle; and that these cannot be sectioned freely just to gain access to a fracture.

As with all stifle surgery, wound healing can be a problem, and even the effort of rising after anaesthesia can disrupt both the internal fixation and the soft tissue repair.

If sinus tracts originate from a flake fracture or sequestrum then the bone fragment must be removed before the sinus will heal; antibiotics in these cases are of no use whatsoever! Fortunately, the sequestra are usually cranial and are accessible through a C-shaped skin incision followed by resection of the purplish-yellow infected granulation tissue, and curettage of the roughened cranial patellar surface. The subcutaneous tissues and skin are sutured for only two-thirds of the length of the wound, the distal one-third being left open for drainage. An irrigation tube can be sutured in the wound to aid flushing. As the main wound heals, so too will the sinus tract dry up. There is little risk of penetrating the joint capsule with this type of surgery, the main complication being the relatively long time for healing of the open wound. However, the risk of major infection is great if the incision is completely closed so healing must be allowed to take place by second intention.

Suggested further reading

De Bowes RM, Grant BD, Chalman JA and Rantanen NW (1980) Fractured patella in a horse. *Equine Pract* **2**(5), 49.

General stifle trauma and gonitis

Aetiology and pathogenesis

The stifle articulation is large and complex and is subject to many insults ranging from the acute trauma of kicks, falls and collisions to the lesser though repetitive trauma of hard athletic and competitive work. These can result in damage to collateral or cruciate ligaments, the menisci or the joint capsule. The onset may be sudden or, in the chronic conditions, there will most likely be a slow, gradual development of lameness.

Clinical signs

With acute severe trauma the usual local signs of soft tissue swelling, joint effusion, pain on manipulation and even crepitus may be present. The animal will be lame and this will be worsened by flexion. Where damage is irreparable then this state may progress to a chronic stage which will have a reduced local reaction and an improved though permanent lameness. Repetitive trauma can lead to progressive degenerative joint disease with a gradual worsening of lameness over months or even years. In these cases, and those where a single acute episode has resulted in permanent joint pain, atrophy of the quadriceps especially, and other upper thigh muscle masses can occur. Because of the difficulty in comparing sides such an atrophy may not be recognized initially, rather the joint, because of its increased prominence, may be thought to be enlarged or thickened. With degenerative type conditions, both sides may be affected symmetrically, confusing the clinical picture.

Diagnosis

If there is a reliable history of a severe traumatic episode, it is reasonable to infer that a subsequent pain and other local signs are most likely to be a legacy of the initial trauma. With a chronic, slow onset lameness local signs may be minimal and a full lameness work-up will usually be necessary to eliminate other causes before the stifle is implicated. The most satisfactory demonstration is provided by intra-articular local anaesthesia of the compartments of the joint complex (see section on intra-articular anaesthesia, p. 21). Injection of the femoropatellar and the communicating medial femorotibial compartment is relatively simple; slightly less so the lateral femorotibial pouch. Subsequent radiographic examination may show old fractures or the deformity of a healed osteochondritis lesion, but more likely only the subtle change of osteoarthritis will be present. These are usually seen as enthesiophytes on the distal patella, and osteophytes or periarticular new bone at the margins of the two femorotibial articulations.

Treatment

Once established, no treatment will cure osteoarthritis. Only palliation of symptoms and a reduction in the rate of progress of the disease can be expected. If an old lesion of, say osteochondritis dissecans (OCD) is discovered then corrective surgery will not affect the osteoarthritis changes already present and is not really indicated unless it is felt that the lesion is still active and accelerating the degenerative process. Non-steroidal anti-inflammatory drugs may exert some effect and in certain cases where the expense is thought to be warranted, sodium hyaluronate or a similar preparation can be used. However, since the joint capsules are cavernous and the articular surfaces are extensive, the treatment would be expensive and likely to result in only a temporary remission of signs. More realistically, owners should be encouraged to accept a reduced level of performance, or to retire the animal altogether.

The femur

Fractures

Despite its relatively large size and its well protected situation, fractures of the femur are relatively common. In foals fractures often occur during halter breaking or other similar procedures, and their prevalence during this time emphasizes as a side issue the need for early and continuous handling of foals to accustom them to human interference. In adults, any violent trauma or fall can be the cause and there is more likelihood of the fracture being comminuted. In younger animals, simple transverse or, more commonly, oblique breaks are the rule though separation through the proximal and distal physes is also seen.

Clinical signs

Following femoral fracture the animal may well appear permanently recumbent, especially if it is lying on its affected leg. In such a situation when the clinical examination of the accessible portions has not shown any contraindication the animal should be rolled over as gently as is feasible. With its good leg underneath the animal is far more likely to get up and, on rising, will show an immediate and obvious reluctance to bear weight on the affected limb. The leg will appear shorter because of the inevitable tremendous overriding of the fragments, and 'bunching' of the upper limb musculature, which, with the post-fracture haematoma, will usually give the upper thigh a very swollen appearance. Sometimes an upwards fixation of the patella can occur especially with distal fractures and the distal limb then appears extended.

Fractures of the proximal capital epiphysis do not result in such a severe lameness as shaft breaks; the foal will usually bear some weight and there may be some slight swelling over the hip region.

Diagnosis

Shaft fractures can usually be suspected on clinical examination. Manipulation of the limb will elicit abnormal and excessive movement and crepitus. A sound conduction test may provide additional evidence. This is a simple procedure which involves tapping the cannon or another prominent bony area such as the tibial crest with a short piece of wood or metal. Sound is conducted well in the intact leg and can be heard clearly through a stethoscope applied to the point of the ischium; the fracture prevents transmission of sound on the same leg providing an indication of bony discontinuity. In the case of capital epiphyseal, crepitus can be heard best through a stethoscope, or an ear, applied to the area of the trochanter, though occasionally the clinician can be misled by crepitus being referred from the stifle joint.

Radiography

The diagnosis of femoral fracture is usually made beyond reasonable doubt on clinical examination alone. Bearing in mind the impracticality of repair of such fractures in the adult there is little justification in transporting these animals to a place where they can be radiographed. Immediate humane destruction should therefore be advised. Where some doubt exists or where the animal is young and repair may be feasible then radiography may be indicated. General anaesthesia is almost always necessary for the examination so it is wise that, in view of the inhumanity of allowing the animal with an unfixed fracture to recover, both clinician and owner are prepared for either an attempt at repair or euthanasia under anaesthesia.

Although craniocaudal views are desirable they can be difficult to achieve because of the animal's conformation. In practice radiologist and surgeon may have to be content with just lateromedial projections. These are best obtained with the animal lying on its affected side with the uppermost leg being flexed and pulled upwards and forwards out of the way. It may be necessary to angle the beam into the inguinal region and if this is the case grids should not be used, or care taken to ensure the correct alignment of the grid lines. Foals suspected of having a proximal femoral epiphyseal fracture can be radiographed in the conventional ventrodorsal position. If the fracture is not clearly defined in the relaxed 'frog-leg' position then the examination should be repeated with the hind legs gently pulled back into an extended position.

Treatment

With techniques currently available and for the forseeable future, the repair of femoral fracture in animals over about 100 kg is *not* feasible. Consequently when the diagnosis has been made the clinician should not vacillate but rather insist on immediate euthanasia. Even in small and young animals the procedure is extremely difficult and animals should be referred to a centre with the expertise and equipment to deal with major long bone fractures. For travelling the animal should be sedated and ideally fitted with a Thomas extension splint to minimize the mobility of the lower leg. No system of temporary immobilization is ideal but any measures are better than none.

The problems encountered at surgery are many, principally reduction of the inevitable major overriding of the fragment ends and the lack of good exposure of the fracture site. The techniques available are: single pinning with a wide bore clover-leaf nail: 'stack' pinning using multiple conventional Steinman pins, and plating. Though the first two techniques are probably the treatment of choice in calves and pigs, a double plating technique using ASIF plates and screws is infinitely preferable in the foal. The great strength of such a fixation allows a much higher level of mobility which foals need if they are to thrive post-operatively and in which they will try and indulge no matter what.

Fixation with intramedullary pins is generally unsuccessful because overriding of the oblique fracture will generally occur in the immediate post-operative phase whilst the transverse fractures will be subject to rotation. Pins also loosen and migrate in the soft, thin bone of the juvenile.

As with humeral and other neonate fractures, the animal's poor resistance to the stress of fracture repair and subsequent infection, either enteric or at the site of repair, can often be as much of a problem as the fracture fixation itself. Early post-operative progress is often encouraging but all too often signs of infection and later pin loosening or other complications supervene. A wise clinician, therefore, is at pains to discuss with owners every step of the long road to recovery, counselling against too great an optimism in the early stages.

Fractures of the proximal femoral capital epiphysis can be repaired by using a multiple pinning technique (Turner *et al* 1979), the pins being inserted into the epiphysis through the femoral neck following exposure of the fracture site and reduction of the displacement. An initial trochanteric osteotomy is performed to facilitate the approach, the trochanter being replaced later with cancellous ASIF screws.

Following any surgery to a major articulation such as this, degenerative joint disease is a likely sequel and the prognosis for a return to eventual athletic soundness must be very guarded.

In small foals it is tempting to treat this condition with excision arthroplasty much as in dogs. The results are extremely poor, with severely deformed legs and permanent severe lameness and the technique should not be used.

Fracture of the greater trochanter occurs occasionally in foals. It may be treated conservatively with box rest, but internal fixation is entirely feasible if the fragment is large enough using the same technique as when replacing a trochanter following an osteotomy.

Suggested further reading

Turner AS, Milne DW, Hohn RB and Rause GP (1979) Surgical repair of fractured capital femoral epiphysis in three foals. *J Am Vet Med Assoc* **175**, 1198—202.

Coxofemoral dislocation

Dislocation of the coxofemoral articulation is uncommon. In the adult successful permanent reduction is extremely unlikely even in fresh cases. In the extraordinary event of this being successful, severe degenerative joint disease and capsular fibrosis would prevent any hope of complete recovery. In a foal reduction would be easier but its maintenance would be difficult and the subsequent local changes would preclude a return to athletic soundness. The leverage exerted by even the smallest foal limb is enormous and 'toggling' the fracture as in dogs is not a feasible proposition.

Conditions of the pelvis

Pelvic fractures

The cause of pelvic fractures is some form of severe trauma, usually a hard fall. Fractures of the tuber coxae can occur as animals rush through doorways and gates striking the uprights with their protuberant 'pin bones'.

Clinical signs

Clinical signs vary enormously depending on the site and severity of the fracture. Major fractures involving the acetabulum and those with severe displacement of fragments can cause a 10/10th lameness, i.e. no weight bearing; ilial fractures with minimal separation will cause little abnormality at the walk and sometimes even at the trot. Externally the presence of a visible deformity is again dependable on the site and severity though one of the least clinically significant fractures involving the tuber coxae produces a marked asymmetry when viewed from behind as the tip of the pin bone is pulled ventrally by the combined traction of the internal abdominal oblique and tensor fascia lata muscles. Diagnosis of pelvic fracture may therefore be perfectly obvious at first sight, or more usually, one which has to be achieved by a process of elimination of other more common causes of traumatically induced lameness through clinical examination, nerve block and radiography and then by an examination of the pelvic region.

A physical examination should look for swelling or any constant asymmetry of the pelvis. However, care must be taken not to confuse the asymmetry caused by the resting of a painful leg with a true distortion. In long standing cases atrophy will replace swelling as the main feature, though the consequently increased prominence of the trochanter or 'point of the hip' can mimic and be mistaken for a swelling. A rectal examination is essential and a careful comparison made of the two sides. Attempts should be made to elicit crepitus by manipulating the leg in all directions including abduction; this can be heard by auscultating the bony prominences of the hip or by palpation both externally and per rectum. (It is worth noting that rocking a horse's hind quarters when it is standing on concrete or gravel can cause a convincing crepitus to be heard in the upper leg. However it is in fact, only the crunching of the shoes on the ground.)

Radiographic examination

Before advising radiography the clinician should consider whether the induction and recovery from the general anaesthesia necessary for this procedure will cause an exacerbation of the fracture and maybe permanent recumbency. It is obviously impossible to predict accurately but it is a factor to be explained to owners. High powered equipment is needed, and for optimum films a high ratio, preferably cross-hatch, grid should be used. In smaller animals a grid can be dispensed with and rare-earth screen/film combinations used alone. A ventro-dorsal view is used routinely, though in very large animals a reduction in the amount of tissue to be penetrated, and therefore a better picture, can be achieved by rolling the animal slightly over on to its side and exposing one half (the lower half) of the pelvis at a time.

Treatment

Of all the pelvic fractures seen in adults, only those involving the tuber coxae are amenable to surgery; in the other sites the problems of access, reduction of fragments and the magnitude of the stresses placed on implants preclude any attempt at internal fixation. The decision is whether to allow the animal to live and attempt natural healing or to advise euthanasia. This decision must be based on many non-clinical factors as well as on the type of fracture. Fractures involving the acetabulum and/or those fractures where much distortion has taken place have a bad prognosis. There will be perpetual severe lameness due either to misalignments of pelvic and limb structures, disunions and the inevitable degenerative joint disease of the aceta-bulum. If no radiograph is available the decision has to be taken on clinical grounds alone, and severe initial lameness with reluctance to weight bear, marked crepitus on leg manipulation or palpable distortion would all be bad prognostic signs.

Animals with less severe signs, able to walk reasonably well, and with no visible or palpable distortion are candidates for a 'wait and see' programme of conservative therapy with re-evaluation every few weeks. In these cases the initial use of a reasonable level of analgesic therapy is humane.

Fragments resulting from fractures of the tuber coxae can occasion-ally sequestrate, producing a discharging sinus usually in the region of the upper stifle. These fragments must be removed surgically before healing will take place. The author has also seen a few cases where the roughened surface of the remaining ilium has ulcerated through the overlying skin. These cases have responded well to surgical curret-tage and smoothing of the uneven bone surface although the asym-metry is, of course, a permanent feature.

Miscellaneous gait abnormalities

Stringhalt

Stringhalt is a hyperflexion of the hind limb or limbs which occurs at every stride. The flexion may be so exaggerated that the dorsal fetlock strikes the horse's abdomen. The foot is held there momentarily, then brought sharply down. It can develop at any age and its cause in individual animals is not known. In mildly affected cases the animals are usable though with increasing severity their progress is slow and ungainly. The condition does not improve without therapy. Mepha-nesin, a centrally acting voluntary muscle relaxant has been reported to have some effect but the classical treatment is resection of a portion of the lateral digital extensor tendon and parent muscle.

Two incisions are made, preferably under general anaesthesia. The first incision exposes the tendon of the lateral digital extensor just proximal to where it inserts into the common digital extensor. Traction on this causes movement of the muscle belly identifying it to the surgeon. A second incision is made over the distal belly and is continued down through the thick fibrous fascia until it is exposed. After checking that the two structures are joined, the tendon is incised through the distal incision and the proximal portion is pulled up through the tendon sheath by traction on the distal muscle belly and aponeurosis. Sometimes adhesions can make this extremely difficult. A simple apposition of the fascial sheath is used to seal the distal stump of the muscle and help prevent seroma formation. The wounds are then closed routinely. Pressure bandaging of the area is advisable to reduce fluid accumulation, but the dressings are often dislodged by the persistent stringhalt action. This continued exaggerated motion also leads to a high rate of wound breakdown. Resuturing usually results in the same problem and the open wounds are best left to heal by second intention.

Very few animals are returned to complete normality, though most are improved somewhat. Obviously prognosis is difficult and both owner and clinician must wait and see.

Australian stringhalt

The symptoms are similar to those described above, but affected animals can be so severely affected that they may fall or have difficulty rising. It also tends to affect groups of horses. The major difference, however, is that horses affected with Australian stringhalt recover without treatment. As its name suggests, it is seen principally in Australia and also in New Zealand and is believed to be due to the ingestion of a toxic plant or fungus. Although certain plants such as *Hypochaeris radicata*, (catsear or flat weed) have been implicated, its cause remains obscure.

Suggested further reading

Turner AS (1984) *The Practice of Large Animal Surgery* Vol II. Series editor P Jennings. WB Saunders Company, Philadelphia.

Fibrous and ossifying myopathy

Fibrous and ossifying myopathy is relatively rare in the UK but it is more common in the USA in western performance or rodeo horses. This type of work, involving sudden sliding stops and change of direction, puts the hind leg musclature, especially the semitendinosus, semimembranosus and biceps femoris under severe stress. Tearing of muscle fibres occurs and healing results in the replacement of muscle by fibrous tissue. This conversion to scar tissue can be quite rapid after a major rupture or slow and insidious following minor repetitive trauma. Traumatic injuries to the area in the road traffic or jumping accidents can have the same effect. Recently the condition has been described in the newborn foal suggesting the occurrence of congenital fibrous myopathy in horses.

Whatever the cause it produces a characteristic gait which has been likened to the goose-step of marching troops. The leg is advanced normally, but a split second before it is due to be placed on the ground it is snatched back from a height of 10–20 cm. It may be unilateral or bilateral and difficult to spot. The observer is aware that something is wrong but may have difficulty recognizing the exact abnormality. Examination of the muscles involved may show evidence of a thick fibrous scar or, at the other extreme, there may be no discernible change.

In the past, treatment was by myotomy of the affected muscles. A better response is obtained by excising the scar, however, this involves major surgery which must not by undertaken lightly or by the inexperienced surgeon. Problems encountered are: identifying the scarred tissue and its extremities in those cases where percutaneous palpation is not helpful; deciding on how much scar tissue to remove in the very extensively involved cases and post-excision problems with closure of what may be substantial amounts of dead space. Some form of wound drainage, either Penrose or vacuum suction drains, must be employed and the skin wound should be supported by deep-tension, quill-type sutures. Smaller, easily identified lesions carry the best prognosis for surgery with less risk of post-operative wound dehiscence and a better long term outlook. Recent work suggests that functional results equal to myotenectomy can be achieved by simple tenotomy of the tendinous insertion of the affected muscle on to the proximal tibia. This surgery should be easier to perform with better cosmetic results and fewer post-operative complications.

Whatever the surgical technique used, most horses improve, but to an unpredictable extent. Post-operative exercise, in controlled amounts, appears necessary to limit the formation of fresh adhesions.

Suggested further reading

Bramlage LR, Reed SM and Embertson RM (1985) Semitendinosus tenotomy for the treatment of fibrotic myopathy in the horse. *J Am Vet Med Assoc* **186**, 565–7.

Shivering (shivers)

This is a condition of unknown aetiology which, in the majority of sufferers, affects the hind legs. A variety of symptoms occur depending on severity, but the classical signs are the hyperflexion of a hind leg accompanied by violent tremors. The leg can also be partially extended and the animal may lean over on to its contralateral limb to such an extent that it may fall over. The tail is also commonly involved being raised and shaken; in the more extreme cases, the forelegs and the eyes and ears will shiver too. In mild cases it requires some interference with the leg to set it off, or for the animal to be startled but in others, any movement of the horse will trigger this response. Some animals perform a similar manoeuvre when a hind leg, especially the hock, is bandaged. The symptoms are often encountered in previously normal horses after some surgical procedures and may never bother the animal again. Whether this is a very mild manifestation of shivering is not known.

Severely affected animals are dangerous and as there is no effective therapy, euthanasia should be considered. Mildly affected cases can lead a reasonably normal life. Fortunately it is not a common condition.

7: Deformities of the Appendicular Skeleton

Normal growth and osteochondrosis (OC)

The long bones of the skeleton are formed from pre-existing cartilaginous models. The cartilage precursors ossify but, to produce growth in length, certain portions remain cartilaginous. The cells of these regions, the physis or growth plate, and the deeper layers of the articular cartilage, multiply increasing the width of the cartilage band. This is a continuous process during the growth phase and it is matched exactly under normal circumstances by the process of conversion of this cartilage into bone (enchondral ossification). The synchrony of these two processes ensures that bone is formed evenly across the width of the long bone and that no portion of the physis or articular cartilage becomes too thick and unable to bear weight. Cartilage is a remarkable material but, when not intimately supported by solid subchondral bone, it is incapable of withstanding even normal wear and tear.

Osteochondrosis is a disease in which there is a disturbance in the maturation of the chondrocytes in the growth areas and a failure, usually focal, of enchondral ossification. This can lead to such diverse clinical conditions as angular deviations and acute arthritis. Before considering this in more detail it is necessary to have an understanding of the normal process of enchondral ossification!

Enchondral ossification

The growth areas, i.e. the physis and articular cartilage are orientated so that there is proliferation of new hyaline cartilage on the epiphyseal or articular surface side, and through a complex series of events, conversion to bone on the other side.

These zones of proliferation and enchondral ossification are highly organized. They can be divided into four general areas (Fig. 7.1)

1 The zone of resting or germinal cells.
2 The zone of proliferating cells.
3 The zone of hypertrophied cells.
4 The zone of provisional calcification.

In zone 1 the chondrocytes initiate the process of mitotic division. In zone 2 the cells divide to produce small, flattened chondrocytes resulting in an elongation of the columns in which the cells are arranged. These cells are also actively engaged in the production of cartilage intercellular material. Zone 3, occasionally divided into two

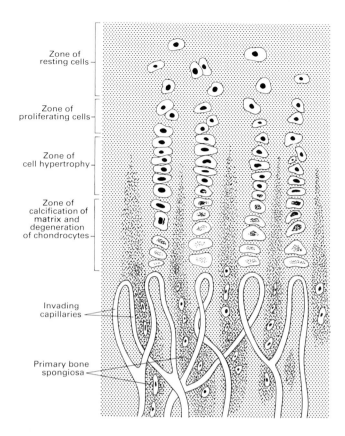

Zone of
resting cells

Zone of
proliferating cells

Zone of
cell hypertrophy

Zone of
calcification of
matrix and
degeneration
of chondrocytes

Invading
capillaries

Primary bone
spongiosa

Fig. 7.1 A diagrammatic illustration of a section through the physis of a growing long bone. The epiphyseal side is at the top of the diagram, the metaphysis at the bottom. The same sequence occurs during enchondral ossification at the articular surface.

separate zones of maturation and hypertrophy, is where these proliferating cells cease to divide and begin to enlarge, becoming vacuolated in the process. The intercellular matrix begins to undergo calcification and the chondrocytes, deprived of nourishment, die. In zone 4 the lacunae of the dead chondrocytes coalesce and are invaded by capillary loops and large multinucleate cells called chondroclasts; these eat away at the calcified matrix leaving only a longitudinally arranged bone scaffolding. On this other cells congregate, this time osteoblasts, which have differentiated from the primitive mesenchymal cells which swarm in from the narrow arteries of the metaphysis. These lay down a thin layer of bone matrix, the 'osteoid seam' which then mineralizes to form primary bone trabeculae.

It is a continuous process during growth, the rate of formation of bone on the metaphyseal side matching the rate of cartilage production on the other side of the physis.

The control of enchondral ossification is poorly understood. However, it is known that a good metaphyseal blood supply is important and that its reduction leads to a reduction in calcification. The converse happens too, if, for example calcification of the matrix does not occur because of experimentally induced rickets. Hormones are also known to play an important part, the pituitary growth hormone somatostatin and its mediator somatomedin being particularly important along with a recently discovered growth inhibiting factor called somatotrophin.

195

Thyroid hormones also affect growth through production of thyroxine and prolactin. Oestrogens suppress growth, by directly inhibiting mitosis of the growth plate chondrocytes and by stimulating maturation and calcification; testosterone on the other hand has the expected opposite effect of accelerating longitudinal growth. The full effects of these hormones are obviously more complex and are interrelated to species, sex and age. Their mode of action is not certain but it may be mediated by their different effects on protein metabolism and not by direct action on the growth area. Cortisone in prolonged dosages has the effect of stunting growth and in hypophysectomized rats even a single dose has a lasting effect. Somewhat surprisingly, the hormones which regulate calcium metabolism seem to have little effect on either the function or morphology of the growth plate.

Neurological factors play a part in growth regulation though their role is not well understood. Cutting peripheral nerves experimentally leads to initial growth acceleration then retardation; clinically this effect can be seen in children suffering from poliomyelitis.

Nutritional factors play a very important role in growth. Absolute deficiency of protein or calorific intake will give rise to stunting, due to their inactivating effect on both the pituitary and thyroid: a diet with a marked Ca/P imbalance, if combined with absolute vitamin D deficiency, will cause a quite severe and complex growth disturbance. However, these circumstances are very rarely encountered in developed countries, undernutrition of horses being a rare phenomenon. Overnutrition, on the other hand, can have equally damaging effects and is as common now in these countries as starvation and undernutrition in the Third World. The most important pathological sequel to overnutrition, apart from obesity, is osteochondrosis.

Osteochondrosis

Several factors have conspired to make this one of the most important contemporary diseases of the horse. The expansion of the equine industry over the last two decades has been exponential. With this development has come increasing economic pressures for rapid attainment of potential and, somewhat paradoxically, an increasing indulgence, especially by the amateur horse owner. Both factors predispose towards rapid growth rates and early attainment of adult size and weight. Increasing affluence and social pressure coupled with a greatly increased agricultural efficiency allow heavy overfeeding of animals to produce the heavily muscled, immature super-athlete or the butterfat yearling ready for showing, or, simply, for 'showing-off'. Osteochondrosis is not restricted to the horse; calves, pigs, turkeys, chickens and even children suffer from it as a consequence of their rapid growth in the contemporary socioeconomic climate.

It is in zone 3 of the growth bands, the zone of hypertrophied cells, that the primary lesion of osteochondrosis occurs. There is focal failure of the enchondral ossification process and, with continued proliferation of cells in zones 1 and 2, the cartilage thickens and the physis, or the articular cartilage, widens. Put simply, the ossification process cannot keep up with the increased production of cartilage!

The nutrition of the articular cartilage is by diffusion from the synovial fluid. As the cartilage thickens there is impairment of metabolism of the deeper layers and subsequent cell death. Large necrotic areas form, and because they are structurally weak, develop fissures which can extend under the influence of stress. Necrotic areas and fissures are less common in the physis probably because the regions are better vascularized. However, it is likely that the cartilage on the metaphyseal side of the growth plate is nutritionally deprived because of its greater distance from the epiphyseal blood supply and it may be more susceptible to axial loading with the eventual development of angular deviations.

As long as the pathological change remains buried below an intact surface of joint cartilage, there are no apparent clinical signs. However, when the fissures extend, usually in the 'tide mark' between the calcified and non-calcified tissue, and reach the surface, synovial fluid penetrates into the clefts and reaches subchondral bone.

This is apparently painful, and in addition, cell debris and inflammatory cells reach the joint cavity and set up a synovitis. A flap of cartilage may develop, its superficial layers receiving nutrition from the synovial fluid, and can persist for some time. Often it breaks off to float around the joint (joint mouse) or become attached to the synovium. When extension of the cleft to the surface has occurred the lesion may then be termed an osteochondr*itis* dissecans.

It is not fully understood why nutrition and rapid growth lead to osteochondrosis, other than the plausible, though slightly glib, theory that cartilage production responds to increased nutritional levels, probably via hormonal mediation, and to genetic selection, the speed of ossification remaining relatively unaffected by either. There seems little doubt that there is an inherited tendency towards developing this condition. Some stallions throw foals, a high percentage of which become affected; the offspring of other sires of the same type, subjected to similar husbandry and conditions can have a very low incidence. There is increasing evidence too that simple overnutrition may not be the complete answer. Excess calcium in the diet is believed to result in retarded cartilage differentiation and copper deficiency, possibly instigated by a high dietary zinc content is also known to lead to a high incidence of osteochondrosis.

The development of the clinically apparent condition of osteochondritis dissecans would seem to be governed by the additional factors of body weight and a vigorous exercise regime. A high body weight will obviously increase the loading on the vulnerable cartilage areas as will strenuous exercise, whether it be intentional training or early breaking, or an uncontrolled half hour's mad-cap tearing around a small paddock. These facts, in addition to a more rapid growth rate, probably account for the increased prevalence in the male too.

In most cases, osteochondritis manifests itself in certain predilection sites. In the horse these are predominantly the stifle and the hock with scapulohumeral and fetlock joints close behind. Osteochondritis is implicated in the aetiology and pathogenesis of cervical spinal malformation (the wobbler syndrome) and new manifestations are being constantly discovered. In addition it is highly likely that undetected osteochondrosis lesions are responsible for the development of many unexplained cases of single joint osteoarthritis and may play some part in the aetiology of the multiple articulation polyarthritis, seen so frequently nowadays in young, often unworked, stock.

Prevention of osteochondrosis is so easy in theory and yet so difficult in practice. As mentioned previously, economic and social pressures encourage the production of bigger, supposedly better, foals earlier and earlier, and it is difficult to fight that trend without being accused of ill treatment or naivety, or facing a reduction in profits. In addition, the practicalities of contemporary agriculture are such that it may be difficult to underfeed. Modern pastures are incomparably lush relative to those on which 'Equus' evolved and this fact, coupled with a carefully selected genetic potential for rapid growth, can negate the best efforts to 'hold back' a foal.

That there is 'little new under the sun' is again illustrated by an old saw common to many countries and communities which says: 'give a foal a good place and you'll ruin him for life'. The reality is that, unless this piece of truth is widely realized, we shall be ruining not just one foal but large percentage of contemporary horseflesh.

Introduction

Two types of deformity occur: those which cause a lateral or medial deviation from the sagittal plane, usually referred to as angular deformities, and those which cause deviations within the sagittal plane with abnormal flexion or occasionally extension of limb joints. These are often called flexural deformities.

In order to describe these conditions it is necessary to subdivide and classify them. However, it must be remembered that their various aspects frequently coexist and overlap and that the divisions are for the author's and reader's convenience and expediency.

Figure 7.2 illustrates the terminology which will be used extensively in discussing these deformities.

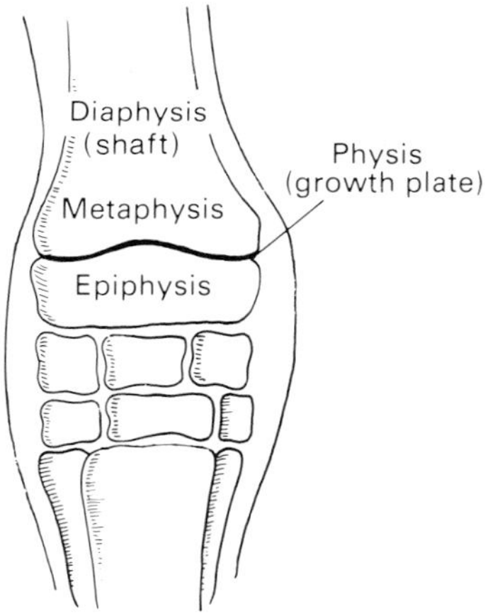

Fig. 7.2 A schematic illustration of a distal radius in an immature animal. The terms which will be used extensively in the section on deformities are illustrated.

Angular deformities of the forelimb

In angular deformities of the forelimb, a distal portion of the limb deviates away from the sagittal plane in either a lateral or medial direction. Often the deviation is referred to as 'lateral' or 'medial' though in some texts the words 'valgus' and 'varus' are used synonymously. Whichever description is used it applies to the deviation of that portion of limb which is distal to the point of angulation and describes the direction of deviation relative to the straight proximal part (Figs. 7.3a and b). The abnormalities are often only slight but, because of the foal's long legs, even minor angulations of a few degrees result in obvious deviations. In addition, the athletic existence of most horses and ponies results in quite profound stresses on their limbs and any deviation from the normal accentuates and concentrates the effects of these stresses within the articulations of the limb, resulting in the inevitable production of degenerative joint disease.

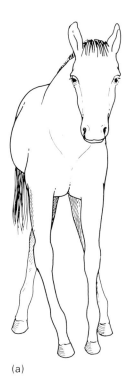

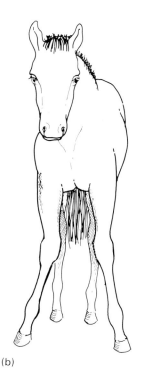

(a)   (b)

Fig. 7.3 (a) A medial (varus) deviation of the right foreleg originating at the carpus or distal radius. (b) A bilateral lateral (valgus) deviation of the distal limbs originating at the carpi or distal radii.

The aetiologies of these deviations fall into two broad categories: those which are caused by abnormalities which develop within joints, principally the carpus and tarsus, and are seen in very young foals; and those which derive from abnormal growth patterns of long bone extremities. Although the latter can compound the angulations of the first category, they *tend* to be seen in slightly older animals.

Deformities present at birth or which develop within the first 2 weeks

Two principal factors contribute to these deformities: congenital laxity of periarticular structures and the plasticity of bone during its cartilaginous and ossification phases.

Most foals are born with some degree of angular deformity in one or more limbs. This is due to a slackness of the supporting structures of joints which have, during gestation, taken no real stress or strain. The laxity is best appreciated in newborn foals; it can be felt by manipulation and seen in the deviation it produces in the carpus and to a lesser extent in other joints such as the tarsus and fetlocks. As the foal goes from strength to strength, muscle tone increases and joint capsules, collateral and intra-articular ligaments tighten up to stabilize the joints and straighten the limbs.

However, in a small proportion of animals the deformities do not correct spontaneously but persist and may even worsen. There are several reasons which can account for this: firstly the deviation may be too great to be corrected by natural means; secondly a weak, sickly or confined foal may not be able to tone-up its periarticular structures sufficiently; thirdly, other factors can counteract the corrective forces. Such counteractive forces include, coexisting deformities of the lower limb, e.g. splayed toes, exerting an outward lever effect on the carpus or tarsus; large, relatively overweight animals putting excessive stress on their joints, and hyperactivity.

The carpal and tarsal bones form by a process of enchondral ossification of cartilaginous precursors. Normal foals are born towards the end of this phase which occupies the last 2—3 months of gestation. However, many are born in a state of absolute or relative immaturity with their bones only partially ossified. Cartilage is not able to withstand even the normal stresses of life if unsupported by subchondral bone and it deforms easily under load; a process called plastic deformation. If the stresses are within reasonable limits and evenly spread across the joint, the deformities are minimal or non-existent and the continuing process of enchondral ossification rapidly produces solid bone capable of withstanding most insults. On the other hand, if stress is localized to one side of the joint, through post-natal joint laxity, then atrophy of cartilage will occur on that side bearing most weight (the concave side of the angulation) and the bones will deform into wedge shapes: if ossification then proceeds, the deformity is permanent! The same effect can result if large foals are allowed to exercise without any check. Certain managemental systems allow only periodic bouts of activity for the dam and these are usually spent racing hell for leather around small paddocks with the foal straining to keep up. Under these circumstances the strains are sufficient to cause an initial deformity which, once present, causes stress concentration and the onset of a cycle of deviation — further stress concentration — further deviation. As the foal gets older, the inexorable process of ossification will make the deformity permanent.

Diagnosis

Joint laxity is easily identified in the newborn foal by the ease with which the deviation is correctable by hand pressure. Radiography will be of little help in its diagnosis, though it is of use in establishing whether carpal and tarsal bones have undergone normal ossification.

In mature, full term foals the underlying osseous portions of the various carpal bones have an almost quadratic shape. The articular cartilage will appear thicker than in the adult, but this is normal. In premature or relatively immature animals the central osseous cores have a more rounded appearance and are smaller, also the surrounding radiolucent cartilaginous precursor appears much wider (Fig. 7.4). This latter factor also makes it difficult to assess the overall shape of the bones and the decision as to whether 'wedging' has occurred usually has to be based on a physical examination.

In summary, any newborn foal which shows reducible deviation is probably suffering from simple laxity of the peri and intra-articular supporting structures of the joint. If this angulation ceases to be reducible after 1 or 2 weeks of life then it is highly likely that plastic

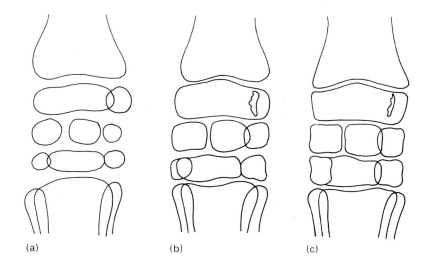

Fig. 7.4 A schematic
representation of the stages of
ossification in the carpi of (a) a
foetus within the last month of
gestation; (b) a very late foetus or
an immature newborn foal and (c) a
mature day-old foal. Note that even
in the normal foal the bone edges
are rounded and the cartilage
lucencies wider than in the adult. In
the immature animal this is much
more noticeable.

deformities of the carpal bone has occurred, and that ossification will, within a further 1–2 weeks, make the deformity permanent.

A foal which begins life with straight legs, or minimal deformity, but which then proceeds to develop significant angulation of its joints, is virtually certain to be deforming the cartilaginous portion of its carpal (or tarsal) bones. Again ossification will, in a few weeks render the deviation a permanent feature.

Treatment

Most angular deformities present at birth are caused by joint laxity; they are manually reducible and most will resolve on their own as the foal exercises and gains tone in its muscles and periarticular structures. The difficulties arise when trying to identify those animals in which spontaneous resolution is not occurring, and especially those in which it appears to occur, but at a rate which is too slow to permit complete correction before deformities of bones occur. The process of correction is usually very gradual and difficult to monitor, and there is also a tendency for foals to minimize the splaying of their legs by adducting their elbows. In doing so they can simulate correction and mislead owners and clinicians alike.

As a rule of thumb it can be said that if there is no significant correction within 1 week then support for the leg is advisable, the temptation to wait another few days 'just in case' must be resisted! During this week, the foal must be allowed to exercise, but sensibly! The mare should be led at a walk and the foal encouraged to follow. At no time should they be turned out suddenly and allowed to tear around until the foal is exhausted. Other categories which benefit from support are those weakly foals who cannot exercise and tone themselves up; also those showing incomplete ossification of carpal or tarsal bones. It has been suggested that all premature foals or those suspected of being immature should be radiographed. Though this may seem a somewhat drastic measure it could well be a worthwhile exercise in the light of the poor outlook for those animals which go on to develop bone deformities.

The most simple and effective support is given by splinting the leg in the straight position. The leg is well padded and bandaged, a suitable length of 10 cm (4") wide plastic guttering is then applied to the outside of the limb from elbow to fetlock. Ideally the foal should be able to bear weight on its foot to prevent the development of tendon laxity. Despite its cumbersome appearance the gutter cast is tolerated remarkably well, even when used on both forelegs. It should be changed every 2–3 days and the obvious pressure points carefully checked. *NB* areas of skin necrosis can hide under an apparently normal hair covering until well advanced. A disadvantage to this method is that careless strapping can exert distorting forces on a limb and with time possibly create an iatrogenic deviation. The use of a full cylinder or tube cast tends to avoid this complication. Tubes or cylinders of plastic are slipped over well padded legs or applied in two halves strapped together; if necessary a sling can be placed over the foal's withers to prevent the cylinders slipping down.

A third method more suited to fetlock or hock deviations is the use of a cast. A conventional cast is applied in the usual way to include the distal two-thirds of the radius or tibia and the whole cannon bone to the level of the proximal sesamoids; or, in cases of fetlock deviation, from just below carpus or tarsus to, and including, the hoof. The leg must be kept straight during the application of the cast, although in doing so it is necessary to take great care not to dent the soft cast by applying local finger pressure. The cast must be light and ideally should consist of an initial layer of easily moulded resin plaster followed by light, ultra-strong fibreglass tape. The cast must be changed every 10–14 days as the animal is growing and the risk of cast rubs is great, especially around the medial epicondyle of the distal radius, the medial malleolus of the tibia and the Achilles tendon.

A technique which causes fewer sleepless nights for the clinician is to wait for the cast to harden and then saw it down both lateral and medial sides. The two halves can be separated and the leg examined daily if necessary. The only proviso is that the same amount of padding must be applied under the cast each day otherwise local pressure points can be set up as the two half shells are refitted and taped together. Care is also necessary to prevent the skin being pinched between the two sides. The cast remains on for a minimum of 3 weeks. Any limb, but especially that of a young foal, when immobilized in a cast for several weeks will develop a degree of disuse osteopenia and tendon and ligament laxity. Therefore owners must be made aware of the potential risk of allowing the patient to exercise unrestrictedly immediately after cast removal.

If the case is caught early and treated promptly as described above then the prognosis for an athletic future is good. If treatment is delayed and there is a permanent deviation, the prognosis must be poor with early onset of degenerative joint disease.

In some instances the clinician is presented with a deformity in a young foal which cannot be corrected manually. If the animal is younger than 2 weeks of age it is likely that the deviation originates in the cuboidal bones of the carpus due to cartilage atrophy. It is often still possible to straighten the leg by the application of pressure. A simple cast will not provide this corrective force, merely holding the leg in its deviated state; however, if a half gutter splint is applied and the strapping so arranged as to provide a straightening effect then over a period of 5–7 days even angulations of the order of 10–15° can be corrected. Cast rubs are a problem and strict attention must be paid to the pressure points; also, if started too late, the inexorable process of ossification slowly reduces, and eventually prevents, further correction. It must therefore be done *early*. It must also be realized that the correction of the deviation does not necessarily mean the restoration of normal relationships within the carpus. The straightening may be due to a combination of factors, including the compensatory atrophy of cartilage on the other side of the carpus and an alteration in the growth of the distal radial epiphysis.

Once the cuboidal bones have ossified the leg cannot be returned to normality. Pressure will have little or no effect and the deviation can only be corrected by altering the growth of the adjacent distal radial epiphysis. Although the leg can be made to look straight its long axis will zig-zag through the induced deviation at the growth plate and the original deviation of the carpal bones. Unequal forces on this joint inevitably result in degenerative disease (osteoarthritis) and the prognosis for athletic use will consequently be poor. A more dramatic form of correction is to remove cartilage and subchondral bone from the surface of the intercarpal joint on the convex side of the deviation, followed by arthrodesis of the proximal and distal rows of carpal bones. This must be regarded as a salvage procedure only.

Epiphyseal and metaphyseal abnormalities causing angular deformities

Deformities arising at the epiphysis (epiphyseal dysplasia)

The distal radial epiphysis (that portion of the bone distal to the growth plate), forms initially by a process of enchondral ossification spreading centrifugally through a cartilage precursor, much as happens in the cuboidal bones of the carpus. Later growth in size occurs by a similar process of ossification in the deep layers of the proliferating articular cartilages and to a lesser extent at the distal margin (or growth plate of the distal radial physis, or growth plate.

Angular deviations of the limb, originating within the epiphysis can therefore be caused in two ways: firstly by plastic deformation or atrophy of the young cartilaginous precursor of the epiphysis; or by later aberrant and unequal growth in size. Like the deviations which originate in the cuboidal bone, deformities originating in the epiphysis are seen in very young, often premature foals. Though occasionally the sole cause of an angulation at the carpus, they usually coexist with and compound the deviation simultaneously present in the two rows of carpal bones. In the distal metacarpus however, epiphyseal wedging may be the only source of deformity.

The aetiology of the deformity will be the same as for the carpal bones, that is, an abnormal distribution of forces across the articular surfaces. This could be a consequence of joint laxity or a distal limb conformational abnormality. It has been suggested that the susceptibility of the lateral aspect of the distal radial epiphysis to compression is due to the presence there of the ulnar styloid process which has its own articular surface and centre of ossification but does not fuse with the radius until about 4 months of age.

Treatment

Prevention is, of course, far easier and more desirable than treatment. It involves early identification of potential sufferers, i.e. premature or immature foals or those with excessive joint laxity, and supporting the limbs as previously described. Animals which are born with, or acquire, a splayed foot conformation are likely to develop this type of deformity and should receive corrective hoof trimming, cutting down the outer wall to exert a straightening leverage on the leg.

If ossification has made the defect permanent the only way of realigning the articular surfaces parallel to the ground is by manipulating the growth of the adjacent growth plate or the physis.

Deformities arising at the growth rate plate and metaphysis (metaphyseal dysplasia)

Most of the growth of long bones takes place at the physis, or growth plates situated at either end of the bone. The remainder, a small contribution, is made by an increase in epiphyseal length. In both radius and metacarpus, the distal growth plate accounts for a much greater proportion of growth than does the proximal one.

The way in which growth rate across the width of the cartilaginous plate is synchronized and kept even is not understood. Somewhat miraculously symmetry is maintained, and growth controlled so that the adjacent joint surfaces are maintained in their correct alignment, parallel to the ground.

Several factors are known to cause asymmetry of growth and hence deformity. The aetiology in each case is likely to be multifactorial and there are also, it is certain, other influences about which we know little. Among the known causes are stress concentration on the growth plate due to a pre-existing malformation; osteochondrosis of the growth plate and (here in the present stage of knowledge we enter the realms of conjecture), forces acting on the growth plate as a result of asynchronous bone and periosteal growth. Salter-Harris type 6 injuries will also prevent synchronous growth and there is increasing evidence that excess or deficiencies of certain trace elements and minerals can also cause defects in the process of enchondral ossification. These factors are now considered in a little more detail.

Trauma. Some degree of carpal deviation at birth is thought to be normal. Most cases, as suggested previously, cure themselves. However, if the abnormality persists for any length of time, possibly masked by the foal adducting its forelimbs, excessive trauma can occur, especially to the outer or lateral aspects of the distal radial, or metacarpal growth plate. The junction of the zone of multiplication and the zone of provisional calcification (see section on osteochondrosis, p. 194) is the weakest, and studies have shown that this area becomes thickened and irregular when subject to excessive trauma. If the compression is maintained or trauma is severe then chondrocytes cease to proliferate and, with the invasion of vessels from epiphysis and metaphysis, the growth plate may be closed by internal bridging. This obviously prevents growth on that side, and, as the other side continues to grow, the leg begins to bend or pivot around the lateral physis. The angulations are accentuated by the long limbs and so quite gross deviations can develop within a week or two.

Trauma will also be the cause of physical injury to the growth plate. A Salter–Harris type 6 injury for example will certainly effect one side and maybe prevent growth there. Other fractures too, if they initiate growth plate bridging, can result in deviations. Salter–Harris types 1 and 2 are probably the least injurious, the split usually involving only the zones of hypertrophy and degeneration. Types 3–6 may involve all layers including the germinal zone (Fig. 7.5).

Osteochondrosis. Angular deformities are reported most often in large, rapidly growing, active individuals, exactly the type in which

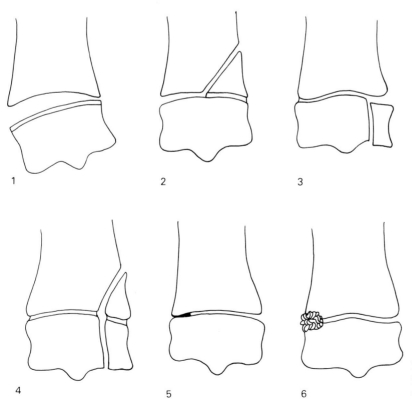

Fig. 7.5 The six types of growth plate injuries according to Salter and Harris.

osteochondrosis is prevalent (see section on osteochondrosis, p. 194). Although osteochondritis dissecans is probably its most well known form, osteochondrosis can affect any zone of enchondral ossification including the growth plates. Its presence, probably in combination with trauma, leads to asynchronous growth and consequent deviation. The causes of osteochondrosis are not fully elucidated as yet. High dietary carbohydrate levels are certainly implicated as is a potential for rapid growth. There is also a strong evidence that the tendency to develop the condition is heritable. In addition mineral imbalances, primarily those of zinc and copper, have also been implicated.

Asynchronous periosteal growth. It was noted some time ago that injuries to the limbs of children which resulted in periosteal damage had the effect of promoting a bone growth spurt on the side of the injury. A development of this was to attempt correction of deviation, not by restricting growth on the convex side, but by promoting it on the concave border by a technique of periosteal section or elevation. One of the theories attempting to explain this phenomenon is that the periosteum acts as a collar around the bone, restraining its growth; when released of this restraint, growth accelerates. Presumably if bone and periosteal growth rate do not coincide then one side of bone may be held back and a deviation occur. On the other hand it is possible that the periosteal/bone relationship may play no part in causing the deviation, but may be merely of use in its correction.

Radiography

Although it is observation of the animal which first reveals the deviation, a simply physical examination of the leg is not sufficient to allow the clinician to decide where the deviation originates and, most importantly, whether there is distortion of cuboidal bones or articular surfaces.

The affected limbs should be radiographed with as large a cassette as possible, so that the maximum amount of bone proximal and distal to the apparent point of deviation is included. Every effort must be made to ensure that it is a true dorsopalmar projection.

On the radiographs, lines are drawn down the exact centres of the radius and the metacarpus in the case of a carpal deviation, and the metacarpus and the 1st and 2nd phalanx in the case of the fetlock angulation. Where these lines intersect will be the exact point at which the limb axis deviates.

If the lines cross at the physis then it will be asymmetric growth in this structure which is causing the problem; if they meet within the body of the epiphysis then it is likely to be epiphyseal 'wedging' either alone, or in combination with a physeal growth disturbance which is to blame. If, however, they meet more distally, within the carpus itself, it is an indication that distortion of carpal cuboidal bones has occurred and the prognosis for eventual complete recovery will be that much worse. A problem with this technique is that perfect dorsopalmar radiographs of the distorted limb are difficult to achieve due, in many cases, to some rotation of the leg distal to the angulation. This rotation is usually outwards and more often encountered in the fetlock. Other positioning problems, e.g. partial flexion of the joint can also lead to discrepancies between radiological and clinical findings.

Other radiographic findings include: flaring of the metaphysis causing its widening and asymmetry: a comparable broadening of the adjacent epiphysis with the increased amount of bone present in the area resulting in an apparent sclerotic band above and below the physis: widening (ectasia) of the cartilaginous growth plate generally but especially at its perimeter with a blurring of its normally fairly clear outline: a sclerosis and broadening of the metaphyseal cortex on the concave, i.e. primary weight bearing side of the leg; and in a proportion of cases a concomitant wedging of the epiphysis. Unusual abnormalities occasionally found are osteochondrosis-like lesions and subchondral bone cysts in the adjacent joints.

Treatment

The treatment of deviations arising from epiphyseal distortion or physeal irregularities, once they are established, is by manipulation of growth at the physis. The main objective is to bring the axis of the distal limb back, either in line with, or within 4° of, the long axis of the limb proximal to the deviation; also to restore the normal parallel relationship of the articular surfaces and the ground.

To date, techniques have involved physical restriction of growth at the adjacent physis on the convex, or more rapidly growing side of the limb. In the foreleg this will be the distal radial, or metacarpal growth plates.

A successful outcome depends, more than any other factor, on early recognition and treatment. For full correction to occur there must be enough growth potential remaining in the other side of the physis to swing the leg back to its normal position. The clinician must remember that, although growth plate closures do not occur until the animal is many months old, it is not they which are important, but rather the periods of maximum growth which, as can be seen from Table 7.1 occur surprisingly early in life.

The earliest technique used was transphyseal stapling. It is a relatively simple procedure in which an incision is made over the area of the physis on the convex side of the deviation. The growth plate is located by walking a needle distally along the bone of the metaphysis until it drops down into the soft cartilage. This normally coincides with the 'peak' of the growth plate distension. Ideally the position of the needle should be checked by intra-operative X-ray as

Table 7.1 Periods of rapid bone growth and ideal age for corrective surgery of angular deviations.

	Rapid growth period (months)	Ideal age for surgery
Distal radius	0–8	2 weeks–4 months
Distal MC and MT III	0–3	Up to 4 weeks
Distal tibia	0–6	2 weeks–4 months

the width of the growth plate and substantial depth of soft tissue distally can sometimes make this an uncertain method if it is done blind. Two or, if there is room, three staples are then hammered home, bridging the growth plate, no pre-drilling being necessary in the soft bone. The fascia and skin are then closed routinely.

Although it is often effective, this technique has several disadvantages. They are: compression is not achieved immediately, some bone growth being necessary before the staples begin to bite; placement of staples across the protrusion of the growth plate means that the points often do not bite deeply into the bone and that they are frequently ejected or spread by the force of the growth; and their exposed position on the tip of the metaphyseal widening results in what is normally a pressure point on a foal's leg becoming even more prominent, hence encouraging wound breakdown as a result of skin devitalization. This complication can arise not only from local trauma but simply from the pressure of protective bandages. If wound dehiscence occurs then the staples must be removed and the wound allowed to heal by second intention before a second attempt is made. By this time, of course it might be too late!

A more elegant technique uses two screws placed each side of the growth plate and joined by wire laid in a figure-of-eight pattern. If ASIF screws are used and the final tightening delayed until the wire is laid, then as the wire loops ride up the flared heads of the screws immediate compression is achieved (Fig. 7.6).

This method avoids many of the complications of staples: the screws bite well, and if necessary the cancellous variety can be used

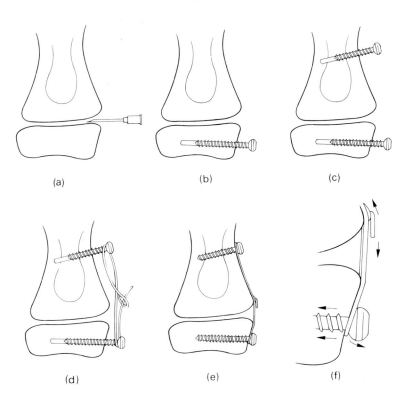

(a) (b) (c)

(d) (e) (f)

Fig. 7.6 A diagrammatic illustration of the steps involved in placement of screws and wire to retard physeal growth. (a) Location of the soft cartilagenous growth plate; (b) and (c) insertion of the epiphyseal and diaphyseal screws; (d) and (e) placement of wire followed by screw tightening; (f) illustration of how, when an ASIF screw is driven home the wire rides up its curved head resulting in an immediate tension and consequent compression of the physis.

in very young and soft bone; the implants are not placed in an exposed position therefore wound complications are infrequent and, as explained above, the effect is immediate.

With both methods, the implants must be removed, either when infection is seen to have become established or, of course, when correction of the angulation has occurred. This latter point must be made strongly to owners as it is not unknown for foals to be returned with the complaint that 'the leg has gone the other way'. If it is unavoidable, the implants can be removed under sedation and local anaesthesia; however general anaesthesia is infinitely preferable. Both staples and screws can become embedded in a mass of fibrous tissue and location of screws especially can be difficult. Here the unique hexagon design of the ASIF screw slot and screwdriver shows its worth as, once engaged, they remain so and removal can be done through stab incisions. It is worth remembering too that, in difficult operating circumstances, only one screw need be removed to stop the compression.

Recently attention has been given to the concept of differential stimulation of growth, rather than its retardation, as a means of correcting these deviations.

The principle is based on the fact that circumferential section of the periosteum at the level of the metaphysis or diaphysis results in a growth spurt in that side of the adjacent growth plate. One of the advantages is that leg length is maintained compared to the previous techniques where there is some mild reduction. In practice this is not important and the major advantage of the technique of periosteal transection is that no implants are used; therefore none have to be removed and the risk of post-operative infection is reduced.

The surgery is carried out on the concave side of the angulation. For distal radial deformities a 6—7 cm skin incision is made on the extreme lateral aspect of the forearm just proximal to the protrusion of the distal radial physis. The fascia is cut to expose the periosteum. Making sure that no tendons or other important structures are cut, the periosteum is incised for 180° around the radius, i.e. the *lateral* hemi-circumference some 4—5 cm proximal to the growth plate and parallel to it. The ulna may sometimes be present but it is a cartilaginous remnant at this level and should be cut with the periosteum.

The only difficult part of the procedure is the incision on the caudal aspect of the radius. Here there are many musculotendinous structures which can limit access. If the carpus is flexed these slacken considerably and the use of a curved No. 12 or stitch-cutting type scalpel blade helps to cut 'around the corner'.

In earlier accounts of this technique flaps of periosteum were elevated off the bone. This has now been found to be unnecessary and simple transection is all that is required.

When the leg has straightened, differential growth ceases and no further action is needed.

Post-operative management for all three techniques involves initial protection of the wound with either a conventional or Stent bandage; severely restricted exercise until soft tissue healing is complete, then an exercise regime graded according to the severity of the deformity and the rate of its correction, returning to normal levels when the leg has straightened and the implants, if any, removed. In addition, it is most important to ensure foot shape on the affected limb is restored to normality by removing any surplus wall.

It frequently happens that owners delay seeking professional attention in the hope that the deviation will self-correct with the result that the time remaining for correction may be limited. This is especially so in cases of deviation arising in the distal metacarpus. Under these circumstances the author has used, with success, a combination of the techniques of growth limitation and stimulation to extract the maximum amount of straightening power remaining in the growth plate.

In certain circumstances, growth plate manipulation will not correct the deviation. If the animal is presented for treatment too late then there will be no potential for corrective growth on either side of the physis. Similarly, in the case of a deviation caused by a major injury to the growth plate, and its permanent closure on one side, no corrective growth will be possible and the deviation must remain permanent unless there is resort to the rather drastic measure of an osteotomy.

Angular deformities of the hind limb

Incomplete ossification of the tarsal bones

Incomplete ossification of the tarsal bones occurs under the same circumstances as described for the carpus; however, the normal angulation of the hock within the sagittal plane introduces a new factor. The transfer of weight between the angled tibia and the vertical cannon results in a concentration of compressive stress at the pivot point, which, surprisingly, is not within the tibiotarsal joint, but, because the joint is a sliding hinge, lies distal to it within the 3rd tarsal bone. If insufficiently ossified, then these stresses will, especially if exacerbated by high body weight and exercise, cause crushing and collapse of the 3rd and the neighbouring central tarsal along with the adjacent joints. Occurring on its own, this will produce a noticeable break in what should be a straight calcaneometatarsal line and a hyperflexed, or so-called 'sickle hock'. This can also occur in conjunction with a lateral or medial deviation at the tarsus caused initially by joint laxity, or with metatarsal or tibial epiphyseal dysplasia, or any of these in combination.

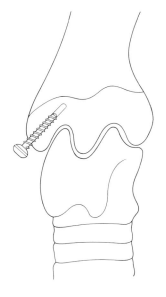

Fig. 7.7 Where a screw and wire technique is used to correct a metaphyseal dysplasia of the distal tibia, the distal screw must be angled as illustrated to avoid the tibiotarsal articulation. In addition it must not transfix the physis.

Diagnosis

Foals affected by this condition show a typical action, well described as a 'bunny hop'. They are sickle hocked and will usually show a noticeable break in the calcaneometatarsal line. Often there will be a coexisting lateral deviation of the limb distal to the tarsus. Radiographic examination is essential to determine whether fragmentation of the 3rd or central tarsal bone has occurred; it is a very important fact in prognosis. In severe cases the dorsal fragment of the bones may be significantly displaced forward. Dorsoplantar views are also useful to assess damage caused by any lateral or medial deviation.

Treatment

If caught early, a cast will provide support until ossification of the bones has progressed sufficiently to withstand the stresses imposed on them. After 2–3 weeks the casts can be removed and the foal allowed to exercise freely.

If fragmentation has occurred then, of course, the prognosis for an athletic future is guarded. However, these animals can be salvaged since the fragmented small bones may well ankylose, if given sufficient support, and produce a natural arthrodesis.

Deviations arising at the distal tibial epiphysis

Deviations arising at the distal tibial epiphysis have essentially the same aetiology and receive the same treatment as in the foreleg.

Deviations originating at the distal tibial growth plate

Deviations originating at the distal tibial growth plate arise and are diagnosed in much the same manner as those in the distal radius. Some caution is needed in interpreting and measuring angulation seen on radiographs, because any deviation from a straight dorsopalmar projection will cause the normal flexed state of the joint to mimic, exacerbate or diminish an angular deviation.

Treatment is by manipulation of growth at the physis with techniques similar to those used in the forelimbs. One difference which must be emphasized is the undulant nature of both the distal tibial physis and articular surface. This means that a screw placed in the epiphysis must be sharply angled proximally to avoid impinging on the joint (Fig. 7.7).

Deviations arising at the distal metatarsal epiphysis

Deviations arising at the distal metatarsal epiphysis tend to be medially directed and secondary to distal tibial angulation. If uncorrected they can produce a 'pigeon-toed' stance as and when the tibial angulation is corrected.

These can often be treated conservatively by hoof trimming and the use of a shoe, fitted so that it protrudes, or is full, on the convex side of the deviation (Fig. 7.8). The process of correction is slow; 4–6 weeks, and it should be accompanied by a concomitant treatment of the distal tibial metaphyseal dysplasia.

Suggested further reading

Auer JA and Martens RJ (1980) Angular limb deformities in young foals. *Proc Am Assoc Eq Prac* **26**, 81–95.

Auer JA, Martens RJ and Williams, EH (1982) Periosteal transection for correction of angular limb deformities in foals. *J Am Vet Med Assoc,* **181**(5), 459–666.

Bertons AL, Park RD and Turner AS (1985) Periosteal transection and stripping for treatment of angular limb deformities in foals: radiographic observations. *J Am Vet Med Assoc* **187**(2), 153–6.

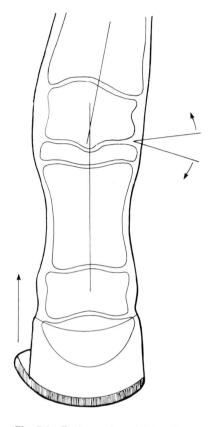

Fig. 7.8 Fitting a shoe 'full' on the convex side of the deviation will produce a straightening effect by reversing the stress concentration which exists on the concave side and by opening up the fetlock joint as illustrated.

Dewes HF (1982) The onset and consequences of tarsal bone fractures in foals. *NJ Vet J* **30**, 129–35.

Fackelman GE and Nunamaker DM (1981) *A Manual of Internal Fixation in the Horse*. Springer Verlag, Heidelberg.

Fretz PB (1980) Angular limb deformities in foals. *Vet Clin North Am* (Large Animal Practice) **2**, 125–50.

Pharr JW and Fretz PB (1981) Radiographic findings in foals with angular limb deformities. *J Am Vet Med Assoc* **179**(8), 812–7.

Flexural deformities

Introduction

Formerly, flexural deformities were called tendon contractions or flexural contractures. These terms were coined before the concept of disparate growth was appreciated and are complete misnomers. Tendons have no innate power of contraction, only of accommodation to increase or decrease in applied tension.

The various types of flexural deformities encountered are divided for descriptive purposes into the congenital, and those which develop later in life.

Congenital deformities

The embryonic limbs develop from ectoderm. Their growth and development up to 6 weeks is entirely under genetic control but subsequently certain extrinsic factors play a part. Until that time limb buds will undergo morphologically normal development even if transplanted. The component parts of the joints also develop initially under intrinsic control, with differentiation of articular cartilage and periarticular support structures. The development of the articular cartilage is interesting in that it derives, not from the central chondrogenic core of the limb but from dense peripheral layers of an interzone, indicating very early on its differences from other cartilage, e.g. epiphyseal cartilage. The joint space develops as a result of cell death within the central portion of the interzone; cystic structures are formed which eventually coalesce to form a synovial cavity.

One of the most important extrinsic factors influencing the normal differentiation of joint components including the joint space, is movement. Without its influence at the right time there is a regression of development, fusion and a fibrous ankylosis. This 'arthrogryposis', as it is known, may involve a single joint or a whole limb. Its cause is probably undue pressure, or confinement, within the uterus. Multiple limb arthrogryposis may be due to any of a large number of known, and, as yet, undiscovered factors, among them viraemias, plant intoxication and mineral deficiency. A number of commonly used drugs, penicillin, streptomycin, caffeine, salicylates and cortisone have also been implicated in other species.

Those foals having multiple limb deformities frequently have axial skeletal asymmetries too, with kyphosis, lordosis and torticollis. Many are aborted early, but some are carried to term with a consequent high risk of dystocia. Some are born alive but the multiplicity of defects makes immediate euthanasia desirable.

Those born with a single limb or joint ankylosis are somewhat more difficult to deal with because the deformities are not so horrific and there can be reluctance on the part of the owners to allow euthanasia. However, if even one major joint is found to be ankylosed, i.e. *completely* immobile, then there is no option but euthanasia. There is no practical or feasible treatment and perseverence will lead to the development of additional unacceptable and distressing sequelae such as severe angular deformities of the contralateral limb.

It is intrauterine positioning which is thought to produce the much more common type of congenital contractures in which the affected joints are formed and mobile. These deformities usually affect the metacarpo/metatarsophalangeal joints (fetlocks), and they fall into two categories: those which are manually correctable and those which are not.

The most frequently seen flexural abnormality in newborn foals is a mild and transient flexion of the fetlocks. The foals are able to stand and can be quite active. As muscle tone builds up and normal agonist/antagonist relationships are established, the defects usually resolve spontaneously. Their resolution can be encouraged by some physiotherapy. The foal is restrained in lateral recumbency and the affected joint manually straightened. Five to 10 minutes, twice a day, is usually sufficient. A device, often used by grooms, is to encourage suckling from that side of the mare which causes the foal to keep its affected leg extended whilst in the suckling position.

Deformities which are refractory to this type of conservative treatment, but which can be manually reduced, can be helped by splinting the articulation into an extended position for about 7–10 days. Great care must be taken with padding as the foal's skin is thin and easily affected by pressure sores. It is worth emphasizing that only those deformities which can be corrected manually should be treated like this. Splinting or pressure devices should not be used to try and straighten gross and irreducible angulation; firstly, they will not be successful and secondly they can cause great discomfort and tissue trauma.

Severe congenital contracture has a poor prognosis. The principal reason is that not only is there likely to be a relative shortening of the main digital flexor tendons and suspensory ligaments, but also the periarticular structures, such as the fibrous joint capsule, will have developed to suit the flexed position. Under these circumstances the joint is physically unable to extend even if it were to be released from all flexor tendon influence. However, if the manipulation only just fails to extend the joint then check ligament desmotomies, as described later in this section, may allow enough extra extension to allow splinting, and the animal's weight, to complete the correction. It has been known for animals with a residual minor degree of metacarpophalangeal deformity to go on to lead a reasonable working life. The development of degenerative joint disease is obviously a major risk in these abnormal joints and must be pointed out to owners contemplating persevering with such a foal.

Congenital hyperextension

Foals are sometimes born with their metacarpophalangeal (MCP) and/ or their interphalangeal joints, especially in the hind legs, in a state of hyperextension. The animal walks on its heels and, in severe cases, on the palmar or plantar surface of its pasterns and fetlocks.

The cause is probably a temporary failure of the agonist/antagonist muscle balance and, as might be expected, most cases resolve spontaneously; occasionally some protection must be given to the pastern and fetlock to prevent 'rubs' but no other treatment is usually needed.

In refractory cases, correct carriage of the foot and improvement of the fetlock angle can be achieved by fitting a heel piece or heel extension to the hooves. It is difficult to put a conventional shoe on the neonate foot and the most effective method is to attach a piece of 1 cm thick plywood, shaped to the hoof but extending into a 5–6 cm tongue out behind (Fig. 7.9). The wood may be wired or stitched on to the hoof but can also be fixed using a resin bonding material, such as Technovit. This material, like all others of its kind, does not bond well to the horn and should be built up like a slipper to provide a physical grip on the foot. The leverage on these shoes is enormous and many become detached; however, perseverance usually pays off in that slowly the foot carriage improves. Exercise should be controlled but not eliminated and the long term prognosis is good.

Casts are not indicated as immobilization of the limb discourages the development of the muscle tone so necessary for permanent resolution.

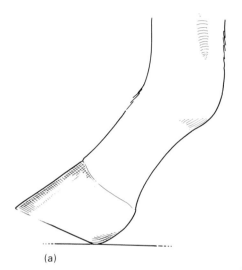

(a)

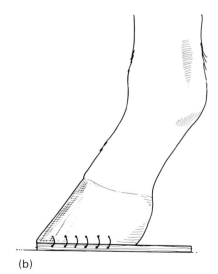

(b)

Fig. 7.9 (a) and (b) Schematic illustration of how a shoe with a 'trailing bar' will correct the hyperextension of the DIP and MCP joints in a newly born foal.

Acquired flexural deformities

Flexural deformity of the carpus associated with rupture of the common digital extensor tendon

The aetiology of the condition is unknown though there is some evidence to suggest an association with inadequate ossification of the cuboidal bones of the carpus: the association may, however, be coincidental. Other theories include straightforward trauma, though with a possible underlying congenital tendon defect.

These foals may be presented for examination during the first week or so of life for either a mild uni or bilateral carpal flexural deformity; or, in the author's experience, just as often because the owner has noticed a swelling on the front of one or both knees. A brief examination will show that, invariably, both signs are present!

The swelling is a distension of the common digital extensor tendon sheath. It is located on the dorsal and lateral surface of the carpus, is slightly elongated, fluid-filled and has an obvious association with the tendon. If palpated firmly the proximal ends of the distal portion of the ruptured tendon can often be felt within. Aspiration of the sheath will reveal the blood contaminated synovial fluid but no evidence of infection.

No attempt should be made to repair the tendon defect, rather attention should be directed towards providing support for the flexed carpi. The deformities are easily corrected with manual pressure and should then be supported by a tube or cylinder cast for a period of about 3 weeks. (Details of the construction of such a cast will be found in the previous section on angular deformities, p. 202.) At the same time exercise should be severely limited. When the cast is removed, fibrosis of the tendon and its sheath will be obvious but the limb should be straight. The long term prognosis is excellent although there is always a minor cosmetic blemish at the site of rupture.

If the legs are not supported the foal continues with its flexural deformity and plastic deformation of the carpal bones ensues. They become wedge-shaped, with the thin end caudally, thus preventing any subsequent correction. When this happens the prognosis for both athletic ability and cosmetic appearance is bad.

Flexural deformity of the distal interphalangeal (DIP) joint
(previously termed deep flexor contracture)

Flexural deformity of the DIP joint develops prior to weaning, from about 6 weeks to 6 months of age. Older animals may sometimes be presented with the condition because of neglect, or due to the owner's belief that it would regress. Affected animals appear as in Fig. 7.10a with the 3rd phalanx in a flexed position relative to the 2nd phalanx. The deformity develops in rapidly growing foals usually those on a high plane of nutrition. It can be created experimentally by firstly retarding and then accelerating growth rate by means of dietary control. This has given strength to the hypothesis that the deformity is due to an asymmetry of growth between the bony structures of the distal limb and that non-muscular portion of the deep flexor tendon (DFT) which runs between the inferior check ligament and the pedal bone. These two structures can be thought of respectively as a bow and its string. If the bow increases in length while the string remains the same, then the bow must bend more if the two ends are to remain attached. The increase in length of the bone (or bow) is brought about by a rapid growth at the distal metacarpal growth plate stimulated by a high protein diet, especially one rich in lysine. The bend in the bow is achieved by flexion at that joint most influenced by the DFT, i.e. the DIP articulation.

The deformity can develop to quite an advanced stage in a relatively short time. As it progresses the hoof is subjected to greater wear at the toe, less in the heels, and assumes a characteristic boxy appearance. With time, the structures on the flexor aspect of the joint, fibrous capsule, navicular suspensory ligaments and paratendinous attachments, all shorten too as they accommodate to the reduced strain imposed on them. In some foals wear at the toe can lead to damage to sensitive structures, with the development of localized inflammatory change; further damage leads to the ingress of infection and sepsis. The pain from the lesions causes the animal to rest the foot thereby compounding the deformity by removing the counteracting force of the foal's own weight. When this happens, the deformity can become severe with the dorsal hoof wall lying at an angle greater than 90° to the ground (Fig. 7.10b).

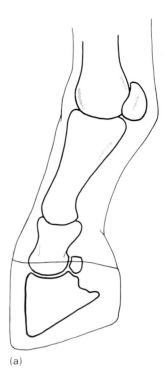
(a)

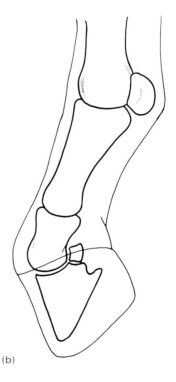
(b)

Fig. 7.10 (a) a mild and (b) severe case of DIP joint flexural deformity.

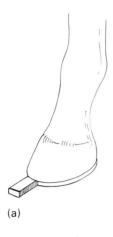

(a)

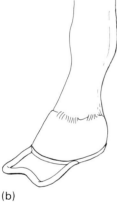

(b)

Fig. 7.11 Two types of toe
extension piece: (b) gives greater
stability to the shoe and hoof than
does (a).

Treatment

If the condition is recognized at an early stage, within the first month
or so, then conservative measures are likely to be effective. These are
simply to reduce the foal's dietary intake substantially, along with
corrective hoof trimming or shoeing. The hoof should be trimmed to
reduce heel length as much as possible whilst sparing the toe. Smiths
are understandably reluctant to be radical and remove the necessary
amount; the initial paring is therefore best done by the clinician. To
hasten the correction, a shoe fitted with an extension piece (Fig. 7.11a)
can be fitted. The extension shown in Fig. 7.11b will give better
stability to the foot though it is, of course, more difficult to construct.
If infection is present at the toe such a shoe is invaluable, provided it
allows access to the infected area. Without it the animal will bear no
weight on the foot and correction will not occur. Under normal
circumstances, with no infection, correction takes about 2 months.

If the deformity is of long standing, or the lesion is refractory to
conservative therapy, then surgical treatment is indicated. In the
latter case the decision to intervene should be made as soon as it is
seen that conservative measures are not working, the longer the delay
the more the periarticular structures will have accomodated to the
new foot shape.

In the milder cases, i.e. when the dorsal hoof wall/ground angle is
less than 90° the treatment of choice is section of the infracarpal check
ligament. This, as it were, detaches one end of the 'bow-string' and
allows the DIP joint to extend.

The inferior check, or accessory ligament is a direct continuation
of the palmar ligament of the carpus, and it may be thought of as the
carpal head of the deep digital flexor. It runs from the proximal 3rd
metacarpus and distal row of carpal bones distally, lying between the
suspensory ligament and the DFT until it joints the latter somewhere
between one-third and half of the way down the cannon bone.

The surgical approach to it is through a 6−8 cm long incision,
placed directly behind, or palmar to, the suspensory ligament and
centred on the junction of the upper and middle thirds of the cannon.
The incision penetrates skin, subcutaneous fascia and then a more
definite fibrous sheath. The approach is the same from both sides of
the leg, except that there is a larger and more intrusive group of
palmar vessels on the medial side. These are not really a problem as
they can be retracted easily out of harm's way and operating on this
side of the leg does have cosmetic advantages.

Section of any structure other than the check ligament can have
dire consequences so it is highly desirable to identify it accurately. It
is a large structure, often thicker than the DFT and at least the same
size. It lies in front of and tightly against the DFT and usually needs
to be separated from the latter by using blunt dissection to find the
cleavage plane between them. It is the author's practice not to cut the
ligament until the four structures — suspensory ligament, check
ligament, DFT and superficial flexor tendon (SFT) — have been identified one by one. The ligament can be elevated before cutting it with
scissors. The deep portion of the ligament will be attached via its

sheath to the SFT; if elevated too vigorously the SFT can be pulled around the DFT and into the gap normally occupied by the check ligament and inadvertently sectioned too! After cutting the ligament almost through, extending the toe will put tension on the few remaining fibres and allow them to be identified easily. Although there is some increase in extensor capability following complete section, the effect is not dramatic until the animal can weight bear and overcome the constraints of the other shortened flexor structures. When making a lateral approach the surgeon must take care not to section the medially placed vessels in the depths of the wound!

The sutured incision is protected by a Stent or conventional bandage and before recovery the foot, if not already pared, should be trimmed as discussed above.

Post-operative weight bearing is essential and this can be ensured by liberal use of analgesics and extensive exercise in hand. Extension of the DIP joint and resolution of the deformity should occur rapidly, the major correction taking place within the first few days. The fitting of shoes with extension toe pieces can be useful if correction seems to be delayed.

Severe flexural deformity of the distal interphalangeal (DIP) joint

Severe flexor deformity of the DIP joint can occur in neglected cases or in an individual where pedal sepsis subsequent to toe wear has resulted in greatly reduced weight bearing and little antagonism to the flexor pull. These DIP joints can be so flexed that the dorsal wall/ground angle is much greater than 90°.

These animals will not, of course, respond to conservative measures, since the geometry of the foot is so altered that even a toe extension piece will not exert any extensor effort. Neither will section of the infra-carpal check ligament produce any significant straightening because of the secondary shortening of the para-articular and tendinous attachments. A more radical approach is needed and is produced by tenotomy of the deep digital flexor tendon itself (Fackelman *et al* 1983). The approach is through a 4–5 cm long straight incision in the midline of the palmar or plantar aspect of the pastern, just proximal to the bulbs of the heels. The flexed position of the foot greatly restricts access to the site, but a more proximal tenotomy seems to be less effective and subsequently more painful for the foal. The skin edges are retracted and the underlying sheath incised to expose the tendon. As much of the sheath as can be exposed is *excised* and then the tendon itself transected. Closure of the wound is routine. Post-operatively the heels of the hoof are trimmed to a more normal shape and analgesics given to encourage weight bearing.

Correction of the deformity is rapid with over-correction, surprisingly, being uncommon. If it occurs then shoes with trailing branches should be fitted. Over a period of several weeks, a scar tissue connection is established between the severed ends of the flexor tendon. This will only occur when the sheath is ablated as described; if it is left intact, proliferating mesothelial cells will heal the transected tendon ends and prevent union. Despite this restoration of apparently normal function, it must be recognized that tendon transection has occurred and it must be a potential weakness. However, many animals do go on to lead normal strenuous lives with no sign of tendon breakdown.

Hind limb flexural deformity

This is an infrequent occurrence and in other than severe cases may manifest itself not by an obvious 'clubbing' of the foot but as a subluxation of the proximal interphalangeal (PIP) joint. The reason for this is thought to be that the shortening of the DFT relative to the bones of the distal limb may be compensated for in ways other than flexing of the distal interphalangeal joint, e.g. by extension of hock and stifle. This could lead to a lengthening of the superficial digital flexor relative to the hind limb skeleton and a reduction in the straightening pull of its tendon on the plantar aspect of the pastern joint.

The clinical signs are of a visible dorsal subluxation of the pastern joint as weight is taken off the limb occasionally accompanied by a popping or clicking sound.

Treatment is probably best carried out by section of the medial head of the DFT in roughly the same area as one would perform an infracarpal check ligament desmotomy. The infratarsal check ligament is small and often not discernible and the medial head tenotomy seems to be a viable alternative.

Flexural deformity of the metacarpophalangeal (MCP) joint (fetlock)
(previously termed superficial digital flexor contracture)

Flexural deformity of the MCP joint is seen in animals of about 1 year of age; older than those showing distal interphalangeal (DIP) joint deformity. Its aetiology would seem to be similar, though in MCP joint deformities the disparity of growth is between that of bone produced by the distal radial physis and the tendon of the superficial flexor which is anchored between the radial metaphysis proximally and the 1st and 2nd phalanx distally. The tendon's attachment to the radius is through the fibrous, inelastic supracarpal check ligament which can be thought of as the radial head of the muscle. The rapid growth of the radius during a period of high nutritional intake outstrips the ability of the check ligament to lengthen and so, to compensate for the lack of effective tendon length, the MCP joint is pulled into a progressive state of flexion. The deformity can be produced experimentally by first restricting and then rapidly increasing the dietary intake; diets high in protein and especially the amino acids lysine and arginine are particularly effective. In the natural state this can happen when poor foals have been sold to new concerned owners, following illness or through heavy feeding in preparation for showing or selling.

The appearance of these animals is very characteristic (Fig. 7.12). The relationship of the hoof to the ground is often normal though in the more severe cases the animal may have to extend its forelegs out in front to keep it so. The condition can be uni, or more usually, bilateral.

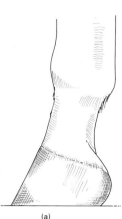
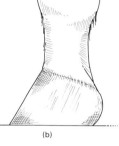
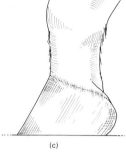
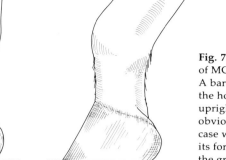

(a)   (b)   (c)

Fig. 7.12 Three stages in severity of MCP joint flexural deformity. (a) A barely perceptible 'breaking' of the hoof pastern angle with slightly upright pasterns; (b) a more obvious manifestation; (c) a severe case where the animal has to extend its forelegs to keep its sole flat on the ground.

Treatment

Once the condition is recognized, treatment must be started as a matter of urgency. If the fetlock stays in the flexed position for any length of time, surrounding tissues will accommodate to the new position. Among the structures affected will be suspensory ligament, infracarpal check ligament, posterior capsule of the MCP joint and the paratendinous attachments of the SFT tendon all of which will shorten or, in some cases, stop growing. The dorsal joint capsule and extensor tendons will also be affected and will slowly lengthen.

It is a common mistake in these cases to attempt correction by elevating the toe of the foot. This will worsen the situation, exerting a flexing effect on the fetlock by increasing the tension in the DFT. In fact it is the opposite effect which is to be desired and it can be achieved by raising the heel, slackening the DFT and removing its support from the palmar fetlock. In mild cases, this method of treatment may sometimes effect an improvement and it is a valuable adjunct to surgery.

The classical surgical treatment of MCP flexural deformity was severance of the superficial flexor tendon in the mid-cannon region. However, this procedure resulted in a great deal of post-operative pain and scarring. It has been completely superseded by the much more elegant though more difficult technique of supracarpal check ligament desmotomy.

Before embarking on this procedure for the first time the surgeon would be wise to perform the technique on several cadaver specimens. The approach is medial through a 10 cm skin incision just anterior and parallel to the accessory cephalic vein (the prominent vein just caudal to the radius) at about the level of the chestnut. Below the skin lies the tough antebrachial fascia; at or about the level of the chestnut this is pierced by a foramen through which passes a branch of the accessory cephalic vein. The foramen can be palpated quite clearly as a soft spot lying below the subcutaneous vessel. It marks the most distal part of the attachment of the check ligament to the caudal radius and the incision length should be adjusted so that some 7 cm lies proximal, and some 3 cm distal to it. Once through the skin and

219

subcutaneous fascia, this branch of the accessory cephalic vein which drains the rete carpi palmaris, should be dissected free and ligated as it dives down through the foramen. It is then sectioned and an incision made through the tough fibrous fascia parallel to the caudal radius and, as in the skin, with two-thirds of its length proximal to the foramen, one-third distal.

The next structure to be identified is the fusiform tendon of flexor carpi radialis in its thin sheath. When this structure and the cut edge of the antebrachial fascia are retracted caudally, the rather amorphous fan-like origin of the supracarpal check ligament can be seen attached to the caudal radius. Identification of the limits of its attachment to the radius can be difficult and it is worth spending some time making sure that they are recognized. Once identified, the rather fleshy ligament can be severed carefully with scissors. Within it lie arteries of the rete carpi palmares and it is unusual not to cut one with spectacular results. Ideally they are identified and ligated before severing but this is often impractical and they must be clamped as they are cut. When the surgeon is satisfied that the whole ligament is sectioned then the antebrachial fascia is sutured followed by subcutis and skin. The wound should then be protected by a Stent bandage or, if the surgery has been prolonged or bleeding severe, a pressure bandage.

Immediately following surgery there is little or no correction of the deformity and it must be realized that this is only the first step, and post-operative management is just as important. This should consist of encouraging the animal to bear weight as much as possible on that leg by a combination of heavy analgesic medication, hand walking, ideally downhill, backing, hopping and corrective shoeing. The latter should raise the heel, provide an extended toe and if necessary a dorsiflexion strap (Figs. 7.13a and b). This device allows normal flexion of the fetlock but puts extensor pressure on the joint when the leg is weight bearing.

In mild cases exercise in hand may be all that is needed; the other measures make sure that full weight is taken on that leg in order to stretch any tissues which may have shortened during the period the joint was in flexion, and may be necessary in more severe cases. The toe pieces ensure maximum extensor leverage on the foot, while the heel elevation, by flexing the DIP joint, relaxes the DFT and removes its support from the palmar fetlock.

Using these measures all but the most severe cases can be returned eventually to a normal or almost normal configuration. However, a careful watch must be kept on them for some time and especially when analgesic therapy stops. At this time any residual soreness can cause the leg to be rested extensively, especially overnight, resulting in regression and a return of a flexural deformity!

Some authors have advocated the treatment of MCP flexural deformity by tenotomy of the infracarpal check ligament. This is based on the belief that the DFT, through its rigid attachment to the cannon via the infracarpal check ligament, is partially or wholly responsible for a proportion of these cases. They report good results with this relatively much simpler surgical procedure but again great emphasis is laid on careful and thorough post-operative management as described above.

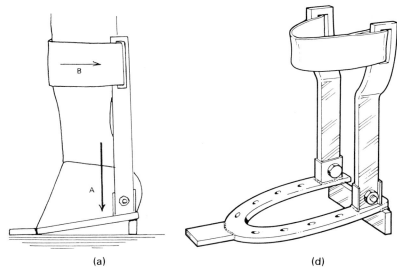

(a)   (d)

Fig. 7.13 A 'dorsiflexion' strap for the treatment of MCP joint flexural deformities. (a) Illustration showing that when the animal puts its weight on the shoe (large arrow) the strap exerts a straightening effect on the fetlock. However, its construction allows the animal to flex its distal limb joints quite freely. (b) The construction of a shoe and dorsiflexion strap. In this version the vertical bars can be removed by unbolting them. For simpler construction they can be welded to the shoe. Each shoe must be tailored to the individual horse for maximum effect. Although cumbersome in appearance the shoe and strap combination can be very effective and is generally well tolerated by the animal. Care must be taken to ensure that the side bars do not rub the sides of the fetlock and that the dorsal fetlock is well padded!

In the author's experience the best results are obtained by a combination of both supra and infracarpal ligament desmotomy. The two procedures can be carried out consecutively. The simple infracarpal procedure adds very little to the total operating time and would seem to hasten resolution by removing from the fetlock the support of a shortened DFT. Again there must be an emphasis on encouraging weight bearing post-operatively but it would seem that cases treated in this way respond well even when long standing and far advanced.

If the condition is bilateral it is better if both legs can be operated on within a very few days of each other. This prevents the favouring of the treated leg and with adequate analgesic therapy does not seem to cause undue distress.

If despite surgical treatment and physiotherapy, an unacceptable degree of MCP deformity persists, then suspensory ligament desmotomy should be considered as a final resort. Although effective it has two major disadvantages. Firstly the integrity of the ligament must be re-established before the animal will be capable of any work, and often the scar tissue bridge which unites the two cut ends is not strong enough to withstand the stresses. Secondly, relaxation of the stabilizing effect of the palmar and dorsal branches of the distal suspensory ligament causes a degree of subluxation of the proximal interphalangeal joint.

The surgery is effective because it places the entire weight bearing load on the remaining periarticular structures and extension does therefore usually take place. The ligament is transected by cutting each branch of its distal bifurcation through two small 2–3 cm incisions, one each side. The branches are best cut from their palmar surface forward so that the palmar pouch of the fetlock joint, which is closely applied to their dorsal surfaces, can be identified and avoided.

Despite its radical nature this procedure is worth doing. In some instances the ligament unites sufficiently well to permit work and the subluxation stabilizes enough not to be too great a problem. Under these circumstances, some athletic work may be possible.

Flexural deformity in the adult

Acquired flexural deformities are occasionally seen in the adult. They can affect fore or hind legs and the author has reported one case in which all four legs were severely affected (Fig. 7.14) (Wyn-Jones *et al* 1985). There is much speculation as to the cause although no evidence has been brought forward to support any particular theory. The condition does bear some resemblance to that of 'palmar fascial contraction' or 'Dupuytren's contracture' in man which is caused by a pathological proliferation and subsequent contracture of the peritendinous palmar fascia.

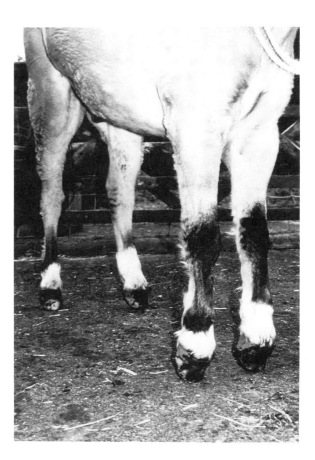

Fig. 7.14 A case of quadrilateral flexural deformity in an adult pony.

The flexural deformity in these cases may be treated by a combination of the surgical techniques mentioned above and consistent and thorough post-operative management. However, there is a strong tendency towards recurrence within a year or so, and even sooner if rigid attention is not paid to hoof care and physiotherapy.

Suggested further reading

Fackelman GE (1980) Equine flexural deformities of developmental origin. *Proc Am Assoc Eq Prac* **26**, 97–105.

Fackelman GE, Auer JA and Orsini J (1983) Surgical treatment of severe flexural deformity of the distal interphalangeal joint in young horses. *J Am Vet Med Assoc* **182**(9), 949–52.

McIlwraith CW and Fessler JF (1978) Evaluation of inferior check ligament desmotomy for treatment of acquired flexor tendon contracture in the horse. *J Am Vet Med Assoc* **172**(3), 293–8.

Wagner PC, Reed SM and Hegreberg GA (1982) Contracted tendons (flexural deformities) in the young horse. *Comp Cont Ed* **4**(3), 101–11.

Wagner PC, Shires GMH, Watrous BJ *et al* (1985) Management of acquired flexural deformity of the metacarpophalangeal joint in equidae. *J Am Vet Med Assoc* **187**(9), 915–18.

Wyn-Jones G, Peremans KY and May SA (1985) Case of quadrilateral flexural contracture in a 10 year old pony. *Vet Rec* **116**, 685–7.

8: Tendon Injuries

Injury to the digital tendons in fast gaited horses
(tendon strain or sprain)

Tendon injury is a common problem in those horses which compete in speed events. In thoroughbreds it occurs primarily in the forelegs, while in trotters there is a higher incidence in the hind limbs. Although all of the tendinous structures on the caudal aspect of the digit can be injured, the superficial digital flexor tendon (SFT) is most commonly affected, followed by the deep digital flexor (DFT).

Aetiology and pathogenesis

The main function of a tendon is to transmit the action of the parent muscle to the bone on which it inserts; accordingly the tendon was thought to act as a simple link between the two. It is now known that these tendons have unique biomechanical properties. Up to a certain level of applied strain the tendon acts as a 'perfect elastomer', returning quickly to complete normality. Beyond a certain point the fibres of the tendon begin to slip past each other and disruption begins.

The elastic qualities of tendon lie in its unique construction. Tropocollagen, the elemental protein building block, is organized into microfibrils; these are then grouped successively into subfibrils, then fibrils, then fascicles which, in bundles, make up the tendon proper. The collagen bundles themselves are not straight, but have a crimped or wavy configuration. The zig-zag crimp has a definite periodicity and crimp angle. During normal physiologic strain, the crimps are straightened out, only to reform when the strain is removed. If the biochemical limits of this elasticity are exceeded, the tendon structure does not return to normal and fibre slippage and disruption occurs.

There has been much discussion in the past about factors which would predispose to this type of tendon injury. Obtaining proof is, of course, extremely difficult, abnormalities of tendon can only be detected on post mortem examination whilst conversely, any predisposing structural aberration will have been destroyed and rendered undetectable by the actual injury.

A great deal of attention has been paid to the blood supply of the flexor tendons and much play has been made of the fact that angiographic, and other studies, have shown a reduced arterial supply to the areas which are most commonly injured — the SFT half way down the cannon, the DFT at the fetlock and the subcarpal check ligament. Since the tenocytes, which control the slow turnover of collagen within a tendon, like any other cells, need nutrition, the suggestion has been made that vascularity leads to a reduction in their functional capacity for this important work of regeneration. It is then further postulated that these areas will not be as fresh, nor as resilient to withstand stress, and therefore more prone to damage. The areas in question have also been shown to be relatively acellular compared with other sections of tendon, and this again is held up as evidence of the existence of a predisposing factor. However, as each argument is raised, others are raised against it and as yet no convincing proof exists of a pre-rupture degeneration.

What is certain is that in certain animals, travelling at speed, the theoretical stress on these tendons may exceed their theoretical capability to withstand it. The forces will obviously be greater in heavier horses and it is likely that this is a major factor in the obvious discrepancy between the high incidence of tendon injuries in thoroughbreds and the rarity of the condition in ponies and light horses. Add to this the length and fine structure of the thoroughbred limb, their speed and the weight they carry and that discrepancy appears less surprising.

Tendon tissue retains its biochemical properties for some time after death so experimental results are quite valid. The tensile strength of equine tendon is in the range $5-10$ kg/mm^2 and the narrowest part of the DFT is only 500 mm^2; the maximum force which can be safely transmitted is therefore $25-50,000$ N (1 N $= 1$ kg/m/sec^2). In a medium thoroughbred at speed, upwards and forwards forces are about 11,000 N. When it is taken into account that the fulcrum action of the fetlock can increase this loading two or three fold it is clear that flexor tendons in this type of animal operate towards the limit of their mechanical strength even with controlled foot movement. Tiredness, inco-ordination, slipping, etc. could take the applied force way above failure level.

When tendon damage occurs it can vary from the most minor to complete separation of tendon ends. Minor lesions involve the separation of a few fibres with some local inflammatory change. More serious disruption results when a large proportion of fibres tear apart with bleeding and inflammatory exudation into the substance of the tendon. If the tearing is within a synovial sheath then synovitis will result with haemorrhage and inflammation of the epitenon and paratenon, the two sheathing structures of tendons.

Given suitable conditions even major lesions will heal, but it will not be by fresh tendon tissue. Repair is by densely cellular and fibrous granulation tissue which contains, not the Type I collagen of tendons, but primarily Type III which is a foetal form and characteristic of repair processes. Type III lacks the crimped structure of tendon collagen and its tensile strength is much lower. Even after long periods of time the composition of the scar remains abnormal with non-alignment of fibres and persistence of excessive amounts of interfibrillar matrix. There is some maturation of the healed tissue with time but the area will always remain weaker than the surrounding normal tendon, and *will always be more prone to further breakdown*!

Clinical signs

In the very mild cases the clinical signs will be detectable only on close examination. Animals coming back from training gallops or races will show slightly lameness. Small amounts of diffuse swelling over the area of damage may accumulate over a matter of an hour or so or, if the injury is within a tendon sheath, a tenosynovitis will develop with an increase in synovial fluid and a sheath distension. These areas may feel warmer to the touch than the normal leg and will be painful on palpation. With more extensive tendon trauma the symptoms will be much more acute, with the animal pulling up severely lame, usually towards the end of a race or gallop, and the rapid development within a few minutes of swelling, heat and, of course, considerable pain. With complete transection there will be peracute signs.

Healing of the torn tendon and paratendinous tissue leaves the animal with a thickened area whose size is roughly proportional to the degree of initial damage. The thickening can be in the mid-metacarpal region, or in the fetlock region with the swelling composed of both tendinous and paratendinous reaction and a synovial sheath distension. Colloquially, these are known as 'bowed tendons' (Fig. 8.1).

Diagnosis

In racing stables, where the possibility of tendon trouble is always present, any suspicion of post-exercise lameness should always provoke a thorough examination of these structures. The clinician must bear in mind that in mild cases swelling may not develop for an hour

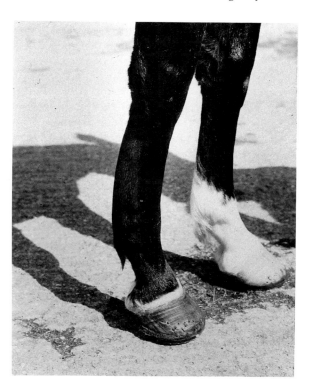

Fig. 8.1 A typical case of 'bowed' tendons, with residual thickening following tendon damage causing the characteristic convexity in the palmar cannon region.

or so after the injury. The tendons should be palpated both during weight bearing, if this is possible, and with the leg bent at the knee to relax the flexor structures. Always compare with the good leg, though bearing in mind that this too might have suffered similar lesions in the past. The edges of the tendons should be clearly palpable and identifiable, especially in the thin-skinned thoroughbred, and should feel like smooth edged steel bars in the weight-bearing position. Any puffiness, lack of clarity of tendon margins, alteration in contour, or a consistently reproducible pain response should give rise to suspicion of tendon injury.

Obvious pain, heat and swelling in the mid-palmar metacarpal region will make the diagnosis self-evident although the reaction will make it well-nigh impossible to distinguish which tendon is involved. Statistically, in this location, it will be the SFT.

DFT damage close to or within the fetlock digital sheath will produce varying degrees of heat, pain and swelling of the palmar fetlock area. Here diagnosis is complicated by the possibility of sesamoid or ligament damage which, in the acute phase, would produce a similar amorphous reaction. In these cases the presence of an obvious fetlock joint distension would arouse suspicion of bone or articular damage.

Complete transection of the DFT would allow hyperextension of the distal interphalangeal joint which would be seen as a 'cocking of the toe of the hoof' (Fig. 8.2). A division of the SFT would not be easy to detect although there might be some hyperextension of the fetlock in the unlikely event of the animal bearing weight on the leg.

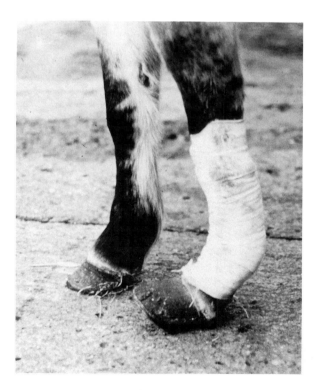

Fig. 8.2 An obvious elevation of the toe indicating that there has been complete division of the DFT in this limb. The fetlock also exhibits a degree of hyperextension, probably as a result of reduced palmar support for this joint.

In the chronic phase, thickening of the region, loss of clarity of tendon margins and their mobility relative to each other and thickening of the tendon outline all indicate tendinous or peritendinous trauma. In cases of rupture at the fetlock region generalized thickening of the structures palmar to the fetlock, distension of the sheath with its possible constriction by the annular ligament, and, in the case of a distal rupture, substantial swelling of the palmar pastern region are all features. As with the acute injuries, generalized reaction prevents the accurate identification of individual structures, only the region involved can give some guide to which tendon is primarily involved.

First aid treatment

The extravasation of blood and inflammatory exudates within tendons and their surroundings has three consequences. Firstly pain because haemorrhage within tendons is known from human experience to be intensely painful: secondly, further disruption of tissues as the blood and exudates separate torn and healthy fibres, strip epitenon and distend tendon sheaths: and thirdly, since all the accumulations of blood and exudate are subject to the same healing process, which, irrespective of the tissue it replaces, lays down fibrous tissue, there is permanent large scale scarring and adhesion formation between the damaged tendon and its surroundings, i.e. the epitenon, paratenon, other tendons and tendon sheaths.

Stopping this accumulation as soon as possible is the aim of first aid. It is best and simply accomplished by the immediate application of pressure in the form of a tight pressure bandage using the minimum of padding and extending from carpus to coronary band. Ideally, the bandage should be applied before the swelling starts so that its application should be considered an *emergency*. The second aim of first aid is to prevent further damage, especially when as so often happens, the animal must be transported soon after injury. A simple bandage will not prevent additional injury as the animal tries to keep its balance in a swaying horse box. The answer is to apply a board cast. A piece of wooden board about 0.5 or 1 cm thick and as wide as the hoof is cut so that, if stood vertically, it would reach from the ground to the top of the cannon bone of the sound leg. With the pressure bandage applied, one end of the board is firmly taped with elastic adhesive bandage to the sole of the hoof. The board is then raised so that it lies behind the cannon bone and firmly taped in that position. The distal limb now acts as a vertical bony strut minimizing the stress on the flexor tendons (Fig. 4.27, p. 87).

The first pressure bandage, if applied correctly, will prevent the accumulation of inflammatory exudates and reduce existing swelling. When this has happened the need is for a more permanent method of immobilization. There is no doubt that the best method is the application of a cast for 6—8 weeks. The cast is applied to just below the knee using the technique (see section on External Coaptation, p. 266). In quiet horses it can be applied with the horse standing. In young or intractable animals, heavy sedation or even a general anaesthetic is necessary. It has been said that casting is contraindicated because it removes the stress necessary to encourage alignment of fibroblasts and collagen. This argument is invalid since casting to the carpus does not stop the parent muscle's traction on the tendon.

In all but the most severe injuries, following cast removal the initial stiffness will wear off over a week or so, revealing a virtually sound animal. Human nature and the economics of racing being what they are, the next problem is to prevent the owner or trainer from working the animal too soon. The concept of maturation of fibrous tissue is a difficult one for a layman to grasp but it must be explained very carefully if the animal is to receive the necessary 12−14 months' rest. The analogy most easily appreciated by many owners is that of newly laid concrete or cement, which, although it sets hard overnight, requires many weeks to become strong enough to withstand stress and up to 50 years to achieve maximum strength!

For the first 6 months of the 12 month rest period, the animal should be stable rested with only exercise in hand being allowed. Small amounts of walking should be started soon after the cast is removed, then increased over the weeks to unlimited amounts by the time 6 months is up. During this period animals must be 'let down' in condition otherwise they will become very unruly. Contrary to most popular opinion, a good hay and water diet is adequate for maintenance, no concentrates, other than a little bran mash, should be fed. After this time they can be turned out; into a small paddock at first, later into larger fields.

The horse should be brought back to work no earlier than 12 months post-injury; earlier than this, and the risk of further damage to the tendons will be unacceptably high. The introduction should be slow and steady, building up over a period of 3 months or so to the fastest gaits. By this time, even though tendon healing and maturation is still taking place, further rest will not significantly decrease the chance of recurrence.

Alternative treatments

Hosing

Hosing of tendons has been a popular water-sport since man first invented the hose-pipe. It has been advocated in all combinations of heat and cold for both acute and chronic pathology. There is no doubt that a strong jet of water will help to disperse accumulated inflammatory fluids; however, its temperature is irrelevant and a pressure bandage does the job much more efficiently. As for any pain relief by hosing, it is likely to be minimal and brief compared with the effect of modern analgesics.

Firing

This technique, often euphemistically called 'therapeutic thermo-cautery' in an attempt to inject an aura of science into it, has had widespread professional and public support in the past, lately, however, much doubt has been cast on its efficacy and its humanity.

The technique of firing consists of burning the skin over and around the area of tendon strain. A more radical method involves the localized burning of the affected tendon itself; this is pin firing. The rationale is that the inflammatory change produced encourages vascularity of the area and thereby promotes healing. Another justification is said to be that the new scar tissue forms a collar around the area, protecting it from further injury; the so-called 'scar tissue bandage'.

The firing is done with specially constructed firing irons, which are heated by gas, electricity or in a furnace. There is strong individual belief in which type of heating method gives the best results, as there is for the various patterns of burns. Some favour firing in straight horizontal lines, other will stagger or interdigitate the burns on each side of the tendon, yet others claim that the only efficacious pattern is the herringbone. The protagonists of ordinary firing say that under no circumstances should the burn penetrate the skin, some practitioners of pin firing also agree; those who support deeper pin firing say that the procedure has no value unless the tendon itself is penetrated. In many cases the other normal leg is done prophylactically! The more radical exponents of these techniques claim that the effects of firing are potentiated by rubbing a strong vesicant or 'blister' into the fresh burns; it is doubtful if any horse treated in this manner would disagree!

Because of professional and public concern over the issue of firing, a research project was established at Bristol (UK) by Professor Silver and his colleagues to evaluate the efficacy and humanitarian aspects of firing.

The general conclusions of the work were that firing techniques which did not penetrate the skin did not produce any quantifiable change in the rate of healing or the nature of the healed tendon but that it did not have any marked deleterious effects either, except on the skin. On the other hand, pin firing into the tendon was shown to be harmful, causing further damage to tendon tissue without affecting the general healing process at all. In addition, neither technique hastened the return of a normal gait.

The work also showed that whilst firing alone was not particularly distressful to animals except in the first 24–48 hours, it concluded that since the procedures were either not helpful, or frankly deleterious, there was no therapeutic justification for their continued use.

Tendon splitting

This is a technique which uses a tenotome (a thin bladed solid scalpel) to create vertical incisions in the injured tendon. The procedure is done through stab incisions in the skin and its rationale is that it stimulates additional blood flow to the tendon and promotes healing. The Bristol group also studied this method of treating damaged tendons and concluded that it was decidedly harmful, creating additional insult to the tendons, delaying healing and the return to normal gait.

Carbon fibre implantation

Collagen in normal tendon aligns with the lines of applied tensile stress, i.e. along the long axis of the tendon. The collagen of healing scar tissue is randomly orientated at first but with about 12 months maturation the longitudinal stresses result in its realignment to a more normal parallel configuration. The idea behind implanting carbon fibres is to give the fibroblasts of the healing granulation tissue a scaffold to which they become attached; collagen fibrils are then formed along the lines of the carbon fibres. If these are implanted along the longitudinal axis of the tendons, the fibroblasts and collagen will do the same from the outset, greatly accelerating the maturation process.

A skin incision is made in the palmar mid-line over the damaged tendon. The paratenon is incised and the tendon exposed. The tendon is divided down its mid-line, almost, but not completely through, with the incision extending above and below the site of injury. A second incision is made at the bottom of the first but at right angles to it. This is directed initially to one side, then the other, creating a T-shaped incision and a pocket within the substance of the tendon. A plaited 'tow' of carbon fibres, some 30,000 in all, is laid within the pocket and the tendon closed over it with simple interrupted sutures. The remaining layers are coapted and the leg is pressure bandaged.

Initial results with this technique were promising, but the new tendons produced still showed, on histological and other examinations, quite abnormal collagen crimp characteristics.

New materials have been evaluated as 'scaffolds'. Nylon and polyester show promising results, both causing more collagen to be synthesized and producing better crimp formation too. In addition the mechanical charateristics of these synthetic fibres approach closer to those of natural collagen than any other.

Work is now directed towards producing a composite tendon prosthesis with characteristics more closely resembling that of normal tendon. Initial evaluation shows that the collagen produced around these new materials is very similar to that of normal tendon.

No long term follow up is available on large numbers of horses treated by these techniques. At the present time they do not seem to confer sufficient advantage to allow them to be recommended as routine treatments for strained tendons.

Summary

Tendon strain is a common condition in athletic horses which compete at speed. It must be taken seriously and initially treated as an emergency. Apart from rest, no other treatment has any scientific rationale or merit, though work with new prostheses shows promise. Where nature is allowed to act without interference, it must be given sufficient time, at least 12 and ideally 14−15 months being the minimum. One of the greatest contributions the clinician can make to long term healing is to explain this concept to the owner and/or trainer and convince him of the wisdom of this rational therapy.

Suggested further reading

Silver IA and Rossdale P (eds) (1983) A clinical and experimental study of tendon injury, healing and treatment in the horse. *Eq Vet J* [Suppl 1]

Webbon PM (1973) Equine tendon stress injuries. *Eq Vet J* **5**, 58–64.

Webbon PM (1977) A post mortem study of equine digital flexor tendons. *Eq Vet J* **9**(2), 61–7.

Tendon laceration

Extensor tendons

Extensor tendons are commonly severed as a result of wounds to the dorsal cannon region. In general, horses manage extremely well without their extensor tendons; although initially there may be 'knuckling' of the fetlock when walking, the animal is able to bear full weight. Attempts at repairing these tendon injuries are not necessary and can in fact hinder the second intention healing of these wounds. The horse learns to flip its foot forward and eventually there will probably be no recognizable abnormality of gait.

Peroneus tertius rupture

Rupture of the peroneus tertius muscle can occur if a hind leg is trapped in a jump and the animal struggles to free itself. The hyperextension which is the cause of the rupture can also be caused by the animal slipping with one leg extended backwards. Wire cuts can also sever the muscle or its tendon. Severance produces a characteristic gait, in that the hock is not flexed as the leg is advanced, ground clearance being obtained by hyperflexion of the stifle. The diagnostic feature of this condition is that while the animal can still bear weight, the reciprocal apparatus does not function, allowing the hock to be extended while the stifle is flexed, a manoeuvre which is normally impossible.

Treatment is conservative with a long period of stable rest. A minimum of 9 months is needed to ensure adequate union between tendon ends. Suturing of the severed ends is not feasible because of the enormous loads imposed on this powerful hock flexor. The outlook is reasonable for a sedentary life but poor for an athletic future.

The flexor tendons

Superficial digital flexor tendon (SFT) lacerations

Lacerations of the SFT are usually caused by kicks, wire or sheet metal cuts. The wounds are often soiled and infected. Partial section of the tendons will produce no change in stance, though complete severance results in a slight drop in the fetlock. Exploration of these wounds by fingers or probes before the animal is anaesthetized is likely to cause more trauma to the area and should not be done. Rather, first aid in the form of a clean dressing, pressure bandaging and, if necessary, a board cast to support the animal during transport is preferable. Contaminated wounds should be allowed to heal by second intention. If the skin wound is lengthy, it can be part sutured after suitable debridement, though a substantial distal portion *must* be left open for drainage. If there is 'pocketing' of the skin distal to the wound then the incision must be lengthened to drain it: to compensate, more of the proximal wound can be sutured. With clean wounds, and complete severance of the tendons, the clinician can contemplate opposing the tendon ends with sutures. A suture pattern which grips the tendon must be used (Fig. 8.3). Nylon is the best suture material as it stimulates more and better collagen production at the gap, and being monofilament tends not to harbour or perpetuate infection. It is likely that the fetlock will have to be flexed to ease the apposition of the severed ends, but if this is the case it must be remembered that later extension of the distal digit will invariably open up a gap between them. This is unavoidable and the technique must be regarded as one for diminishing the gap and not abolishing it. In those cases where there appears to be no infection at the wound site, it is worth seeing if first intention healing of skin can be achieved. Whatever technique is used the foreleg should be cast to the carpus. There is some argument for saying that casts are contraindicated in the hind limb. The reciprocal apparatus is so dominant in hind limb action that, if the upper limb is flexed when the distal limb is held in extension, there will be a tremendous strain exerted on the flexor tendons, resulting in separation of the tendon ends. If a cast is to be applied to the hind limb it should immobilize the hock too for at least 6 weeks or so. Several cast changes may be necessary if the wound is infected. When a cast is not used, a shoe with high heels is often fitted. This is a mistake because raising the heel slackens off the DFT, thus depriving the fetlock of a great deal of flexor support and putting more strain on the SFT and suspensory ligament. A more logical treatment is to raise the toe and increase the tension on the DFT.

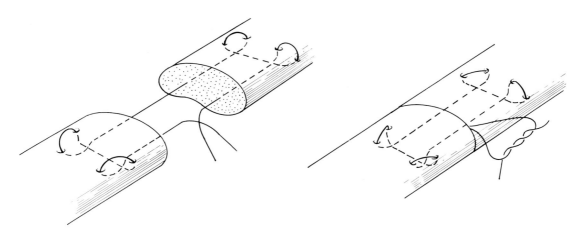

Fig. 8.3 A 'locking loop' suture pattern which, when tightened, grips the substance of the tendon. It is a strong suture, interferes minimally with the blood supply and exposes only a small amount of the suture material to the external surface of the tendon.

The end result is a thickened tendon and paratenon. Healing is by scar tissue which is not, and never will be, as strong as the original. A minimum of 12 months, and ideally 14–16 months, should elapse before the animal is put back to work. The long term prognosis will vary with the severity of the wound, but it is good with partial section though only fair in cases of complete rupture.

Deep digital flexor tendon (DFT) lacerations

Lacerations of the DFT can occur at any level below carpus and hock, but in the author's experience are most commonly seen below the fetlock as a result of wire, sheet metal or overreach cuts. If the wound is above the fetlock, the SFT is usually involved as well (Fig. 8.4). Section of both tendons removes a lot of the flexor support from the fetlock which drops substantially. In addition, there is the characteristic 'cocking' or elevation of the toe produced by the absence of flexor traction on the pedal bone (see Fig. 8.2). Wounds in the mid-cannon should be treated as described for SFT lacerations. Tendon suturing is always indicated in these cases to improve apposition. This must be done even in the face of infection and despite the risk of chronic sinus formation; otherwise, healing will be delayed and the hyper-extension of the lower limb will be permanent. Casting is also essential post-suturing. Frequent cast changes are necessary, especially if the wound is contaminated and healing is by second intention. To obtain and maintain apposition of sutured ends the distal digit often has to be flexed during surgery and maintained in that position during casting. As this and subsequent casts are replaced, the digit should be extended slightly each time. This will help to prevent permanent fixation of the digit in a flexed or semiflexed state. Too much extensor force should be avoided as this can cause breakdown of the bridging scar tissue. In addition, if the leg is cast in this position, then cast rubs can develop on the heels as the limb tries to return to its

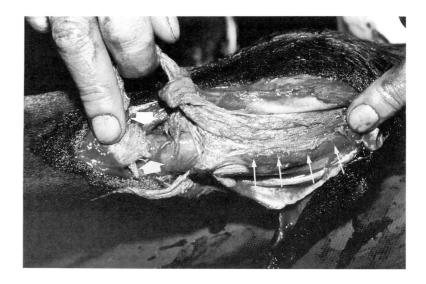

Fig. 8.4 This animal was kicked on the palmar aspect of its distal foreleg creating a small wound some 5 cm proximal to the fetlock. Surgical exploration revealed division of both the SFT and DFT and the animal was euthanased. A post mortem exposure of the DFT (small arrows) reveals extensive damage to the substance of the tendon extending many inches distal to the site of division. The extent of the damage was not apparent during exploration of the original wound when only the clean-cut proximal ends of the DFT (large arrows) was identifiable.

semiflexed state. Some orthopaedic felt padding on the bulbs can help.

Inevitably there will be severe thickening at the site of injury and the animal will never be fit for athletic purposes again. Heel extensions to the shoe can help to relieve the tendency for toe cocking though they themselves can cause problems by traumatizing the elbow and by being trodden on by the hind foot.

When tendons rupture within connective tissue there is a ready and rich source of fibroblasts to initiate the repair. When a tendon ruptures within a tendon sheath, synovial cells, not fibroblasts, grow across the ends creating a barrier and preventing healing. Fortunately, most traumatic tendon lacerations within a sheath will also result in laceration of the sheath itself. This then acts a source of fibroblasts which migrate in to initiate the healing process. It is a slow process but usually it is eventually effective at uniting the severed ends. There will always be severe thickening of the area and, inevitably, adhesion formation.

Wounds of this type in the pastern region are almost always heavily soiled. This is especially true of overreach wounds where grass and earth can be implanted into the sheath itself. Debridement is a necessity but is made difficult by the poor access to this area. Extension of the pastern may help to open the edges of a horizontal wound, but flexion, which slackens the palmar tissues, unfortunately restricts access to the site. If necessary better exposure of the damaged tissues can be achieved by creating an additional incision, usually vertically up the pastern, converting a horizontal wound into an inverted 'T' shape. One of the best ways to debride is to insert a plastic, flexible catheter up and down the remaining sheath and irrigate thoroughly and vigorously, preferably with Hartman's solution. Suturing tendon ends in these wounds is extremely difficult. The proximal end is retracted proximally and is difficult to pull down into the wound; also pulling the two ends together causes hyperflexion of the distal digit, completely blocking access to the site. In general these wounds are best left to heal by second intention. There is always a profuse synovial discharge and wound closure is usually delayed for many weeks. Casting the distal limb helps repair by immobilizing the healing tissues, but cast changes have to be frequent because of the volume of discharge. The leg should stay in a cast for 6−8 weeks in an attitude of slight flexion and then shod with a slightly raised heel and heel extension pieces (Fig. 8.5). The height of the heel is lowered over succeeding weeks but the heel extensions are retained.

Most of the wounds heal eventually but there is always severe thickening of the area, usually a degree of toe elevation and permanent lameness of variable severity. In practice, therefore, the chance of an athletic future for these animals is virtually nil, and the procedure should be regarded primarily as a salvage. Treatment of these cases is also a time consuming, long and extremely expensive business and, as in so many orthopaedic cases, clinicians are well advised to discuss cases thoroughly with owners before embarking on treatment.

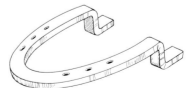

Fig. 8.5 A shoe with a raised heel and heel extension pieces fabricated from a single piece of steel.

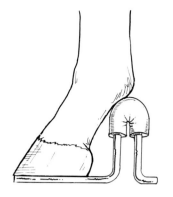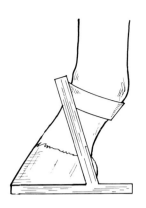

Fig. 8.6 A diagrammatic illustration of two types of shoe which have been used to provide support for the fetlock in cases of traumatic rupture of the suspensory ligament and flexor tendons. Although both shoes are cumbersome they do provide sufficient palmar support during the later stages of healing. Two major problems are pressure rubs at the point of contact and trauma to the elbow as the animal lies down.

Lacerations of the suspensory ligament

Lacerations of the suspensory ligament usually occur in association with laceration of the SFT and DFT. Complete transection of all three has catastrophic effects with complete collapse of the fetlock and elevation of the toe of the hoof. Treatment can be successful in restoring a semblance of normal conformation, though these animals will rarely, if ever, be suitable for even the lightest athletic work. First aid is by the application of a board cast (see section on flexor tendon strain, p. 228). Long term cast support for at least 6 months is essential with numerous cast changes being necessary. Following this, special shoes are fitted to provide support for the fetlock and to prevent hyperextension of the toe (Fig. 8.6). As with other major tendon injuries, full consultation with owners is sensible before starting to treat one of these cases.

Suggested further reading

Nixon AJ *et al* (1984) Comparison of carbon fibre and nylon suture for the repair of transected flexor tendons in the horse. *Eq Vet J* **16**(2), 93–102.

Vaughan LC, Edwards GB and Geering EL (1985) Tendon injuries in horses treated with carbon fibre implants. *Eq Vet J* **17**(1), 45–50.

9: Fracture Fixation Techniques

Fractures of the 3rd phalanx (or pedal bone)

Aetiology and pathogenesis

Fracture of the 3rd phalanx occurs in both horses and ponies and would seem to be a random occurrence with some aberrant trauma or stress being the prime cause. In non-racing horses, fractures are distributed evenly between legs, but in animals which race consistently anticlockwise there is a preponderance of fractures in the lateral aspect of the left pedal bone and the medial aspect of the right. Usually, there is no overt predisposing factor, though bad shoeing, hard surfaces, pedal sepsis and stone bruising have all been implicated from time to time!

Clinical signs

The major presenting sign is a sudden onset of a severe lameness usually when being worked, though occasionally when out at pasture. There is some local heat over the hoof wall and pulsation of the digital artery may be more obvious, though it never quite achieves the 'bounding' quality felt in acute laminitis. As would be expected, the lesion is extremely painful and the animal will react violently to manipulation of the foot and especially to pressure over the site. The lameness remains at a high level for 2–3 weeks and then subsides gradually. However, a low grade 2–3/10th lameness will persist for many months. Full soundness may not be reached for 12 months or more if at all, and subsequently advancing degenerative joint disease will cause a persistence or resurgence of low grade lameness.

Diagnosis

A sudden onset lameness of this severity should immediately raise suspicion of a fracture. Local signs, especially the response to pressure applied with hoof testers or by tapping with a hammer, will show that there is pain in the hoof, and nerve block evidence will confirm this. A palmar digital nerve block (PDNB) will usually improve the lameness somewhat though it requires an abaxial sesamoid block (ASNB) to abolish it completely. If a fracture is suspected, the clinician must resist the temptation to trot the animal as the anaesthesia improves its gait — the difference is easily apparent at the walk!

Conditions which could mimic a fractured pedal bone are a navicular bone fracture, a major solar penetration, laminitis and, if nerve blocks are not done, a host of other minor distal limb fractures.

In a long standing case, the gait abnormality has no characteristic features and the pain source will be localized satisfactorily only with nerve blocks.

The final diagnosis is made with radiography. The foot must be meticulously prepared, the frog clefts carefully and thoroughly cut back to clean horn, not just scraped, and then packed with soft soap or other similar material. Sixty degree dorsopalmar views are ideal for initial screening, with, if necessary, two exposures at different KV values to show the thin dorsal and thick proximal borders clearly. The careful preparation of the foot will eliminate most artefacts but any 'fracture line' should be examined carefully to make sure it begins and ends at the pedal bone borders. If in doubt a horizontal beam projection of the weight bearing foot will give a different view of the fracture line (Fig. 9.1). If wing fractures are suspected then further 60° dorsopalmar oblique projections are necessary to see the fracture line clearly. Whatever the view, the radiograph will sometimes reveal two apparently clear fracture lines (Fig. 9.2). These must not be misinterpreted as two fractures, they are the fissures in the dorsal and solar cortex respectively with an invisible, oblique fracture plane between.

Fresh fractures have sharp, well-defined margins; however, within a few weeks mineral resorption causes the fracture line to broaden and its edges to become indistinct.

Treatment

Conservative therapy consists of shoeing with a bar shoe, followed by a period of rest for up to 12 months. A proportion of animals become sound after this time, but degenerative joint disease can supervene as

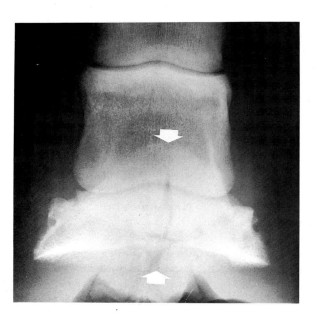

Fig. 9.1 A horizontal beam projection of a fractured pedal bone in a weight bearing leg. The fracture line runs from the top of the extensor process (upper arrows) to the dorsal solar surface (lower arrow).

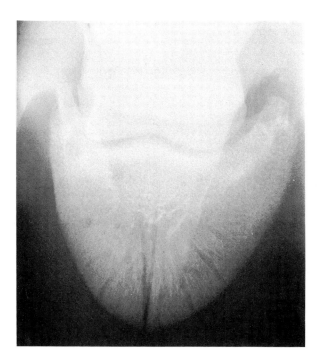

Fig. 9.2 A 60° projection of a fractured pedal bone. The two diverging fracture lines do *not* indicate two fractures, rather the fissures in the dorsal and solar cortices separated by an invisible oblique fracture line.

a result of prolonged synovitis and the eventual formation of intra-articular callus.

The rigidity of the hoof has been said to act as an effective cast for the fractured bone. However, this supposedly rigid structure is surprisingly flexible in response to the forces of weight bearing, and as a result the fracture fragments are not totally immobilized. Internal fixation is therefore of benefit, providing immobilization and compression. With internal fixation, fractures heal quicker, the animal returns to soundness earlier and there is less risk of subsequent arthritis.

Not all fractures are amenable to internal fixation. The simplest to deal with are those in the mid-sagittal plane, or close to it. Fixation is by means of a single ASIF type screw placed lag-fashion across the fracture. The complex curved contours of the bone severely restrict the placement of the screw to a small area which must be located by intra-operative radiographs. Asepsis is vital in any orthopaedic procedure but is more difficult to achieve when the hoof is involved. The patient should be prepared the day before surgery. The hair is clipped up to the fetlock and a layer of superficial horn removed from the entire hoof either by cutting or rasping. When the hoof is clean it is doused in an iodine preparation and bandaged overnight.

At surgery the horse is positioned so that the thinner fragment, if there is one, is uppermost. The iodine is washed off and the point at which the screw is to be inserted (Fig. 9.3) is located using radio-opaque markers on *exact* lateromedial projections of the pedal bone. The thickest, most substantial part of the bone lies directly under the point *x*. There is a tendency to disbelieve the radiograph because the point appears perilously close to the dorsal border. However, if the

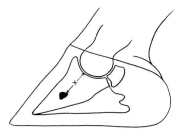

Fig. 9.3 A schematic illustration showing how, on an exact lateromedial radiograph, the point at which drilling takes place is located. A line is drawn between the articular surface and the lucency of the semilunar canal parallel to the dorsal border of the bone. Half way along this line is the site at which the screw should be inserted. Serial radiography using radio-opaque markers enable this point to be found accurately. (In an exact lateromedial projection the two condyles of the 2nd phalanx should be perfectly superimposed on each other and the navicular bone should not appear distorted with multiple outlines.)

projection has been made properly this is the correct point and the temptation of drilling more caudally in the *apparently* solid body of the bone must be resisted. The exact width of the hoof at this point is measured using calipers (tuberculin testing calipers can be modified for this purpose) and the width in mm (A) recorded. The foot is given its final preparation and a slow speed drill (a DIY variable speed drill will suffice if adequately draped) is used to drill a 9.5 cm (3/8th") diameter hole down through horn *and* sensitive laminae to impinge on the pedal bone. An ordinary, preferably new and sharp metal cutting bit can be used, appropriately sterilized, to create this hole which *must* be drilled at *right angles* to the mid-sagittal plane and *parallel* to the bearing surface. This procedure is greatly helped by having a second person watch the angle of the bit relative to the hoof and by laying a 'straight edge' on the sole as a guide. The depth of the hole is measured at its centre (B). If the measurement B is doubled, it gives the total thickness of the horn, which, if subtracted from measurement A (the total width of horn and bone), gives the width of the pedal bone at that site. Total screw length must not exceed this, otherwise the screw will enter the horn on the other side of the bone. A 4.5 mm gliding hole is now drilled in the phalanx, again at right angles to the sagittal plane and parallel to the bearing surface. In the soft bone of this phalanx it is easy to drill too far, so care must be taken until the fracture line is felt with the drill tip. After penetrating another 2−3 mm, the bit is withdrawn. A 3.2 drill sleeve is inserted and the other fragment traversed with a 3.2 mm bit (Fig. 9.4). Bleeding will occur but, if the central artery is not damaged by drilling too distally, it is unlikely to be copious.

The drill holes are now irrigated and the distal portion tapped with a 4.5 mm tap. Following this procedure the hole is well countersunk, irrigated again and a 4.5 mm screw, a few millimetres shorter than the total bone width, is inserted and tightened firmly though not excessively. The soft bone can again cause problems in that it is relatively easy to overtighten the screw and strip the bone threads. If this should happen a 6.5 mm cancellous screw can be inserted in place of the original. It is the author's belief that there is a good case for using cancellous screws as a matter of routine.

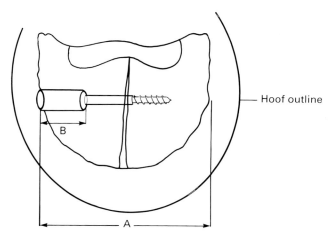

Fig. 9.4 Illustration of the relationship of the drill holes to the 3rd phalanx and its fracture line. Distance A is the total lateral to medial width of the hoof at the exact point where the screw is to be inserted. B is the depth of the hole drilled in the hoof wall and laminae, i.e. the thickness of the horn plus laminae along that same lateral to medial line. A − 2B gives the width of the pedal bone at that site.

Hoof outline

Immediate post-operative radiographs will show little change in the fracture line, and what looks like a very short screw relative to the width of the bone. This is normal and if accurate measurements were taken and adhered to is not a cause for concern.

The hole in the hoof is packed with paraffin gauze and the whole foot bandaged. Care must be taken to seal the top of the bandage to prevent accumulation of straw and shavings, etc. Post-operative anti-bacterial therapy is given for some 5–7 days. The hole should remain dry and odour-free and local pain should diminish rapidly. If there is purulent discharge and persistent or worsening lameness, the implant *must* be removed; antibiotics will not be effective in abolishing infection in the presence of an implant! In uncomplicated cases the animal should be shod with a bar shoe, then box rested for 3 months, followed by a further 3 months of increasing walking exercise in hand. The base of the hole will be covered by horn within 3 weeks or so, although it will never fill completely. Eventually it will grow out with normal wall growth. The screw remains in place for the animal's life. At about 6 months post-operation the animal should be walking normally at which time trotting exercise can begin. When the time comes for the horse to be turned out, it should be into a small paddock to restrict its speed and, ideally, only after a long walk in hand.

Long term radiographic follow-up will show that the fracture line can remain easily visible for up to a year or more. The examination should also include a check for lysis around the screw head and threads, this is an indication of screw loosening or infection. Also, lateral views of the joint are needed to check for the periarticular osteophytes which would be an indication of the development of degenerative joint disease.

The treatment of very oblique fractures and those in the wings is more controversial. Initially there was a high rate of failure after surgery due to infection and loosening of the screws. Because of this the technique fell into disfavour but has recently been revived since it appears that internal fixation, even for a few weeks, is beneficial. Current practice is to insert a screw, leave it *in situ* for about 8 weeks and then deliberately remove it. Fractures at the extreme tip of the wing are not suitable for internal fixation. Treatment in these cases is simply rest. As they do not involve the articular surface the eventual prognosis is good.

Suggested further reading

Fackelman GE and Nunamaker DM (1982) *Manual of Internal Fixation in the Horse.* Springer-Verlag, New York.

Fractures of the navicular bone

Aetiology and pathogenesis

Sagittal fractures of the navicular bone (distal sesamoid) are uncommon, although they occur often enough to warrant consideration in any case of sudden onset lameness. They occur principally in the foreleg, occasionally in the hind leg and are not associated with any particular type of work.

The aetiology is undoubtedly trauma, though, in most cases, there is no unusual event preceding the onset of lameness. Occasionally animals are reported to have stepped on to a kerb stone, or similar structure, only to have the foot slip off when the leg became weight bearing. As with many other features the aetiology is likely to be linked with inco-ordinate movement, possibly with simultaneous torsion and extension of the interphalangeal joint; with external trauma a factor which cannot be eliminated.

It is unlikely that navicular bone osteopenia and synovial fossa enlargement are significant predisposing factors in the aetiology of fractures. They are so commonly seen that, if they were to be important factors, then the fractures too, should be more common. In addition, fractures are seen in 'normal' navicular bones in the hind legs.

The most common manifestation is a simple vertical or slightly oblique fracture running in a sagittal plane abaxial to the central ridge and from 12–20 mm from the bone extremity (Fig. 9.5). Occasionally the fracture will involve the wing of the navicular bone. Because of its multiple attachments the bone itself is comparatively immobile, especially when the distal interphalangeal joint is in extension. For this reason separation or distraction of fragments does not occur. However, mild displacement of the two sides, in the order of 0.5–1 mm can frequently be seen both in proximodistal and dorsopalmar planes.

Clinical signs

There will be a sudden onset, severe lameness typical of a fracture, either during exercise or, possibly, following some traumatic episode.

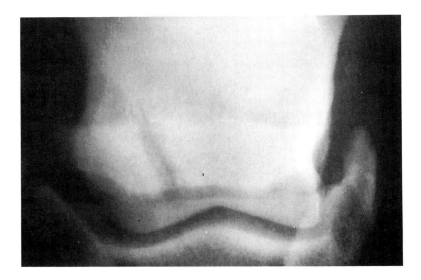

Fig. 9.5 A slightly oblique sagittal fracture of a navicular bone. Demineralization of the fracture line margins indicates that the fracture has been present for some weeks at least.

Occasionally, however, there is a brief period of mild lameness followed by a sudden increase in severity 1 or 2 hours later. Swelling and heat are not features of the fracture, the principle local sign being pain which can be elicited by pressure or manipulation. The pain and hence lameness will remain at a high level for a week or two but then diminish rapidly so that the animal is walking reasonably well. The foot will be rested continuously and with time can become overgrown and narrow at the heels giving it a boxy appearance. The lameness improves slowly for about 3 months or so, by which time the animal is walking normally; however there is an obvious gait abnormality at the trot which usually persists indefinitely. By this time, local pain responses have diminished to a totally non-specific level.

Diagnosis

In the event of an accurate history being available the account of a sudden onset severe lameness should raise immediate suspicion of a fracture. The only likely alternatives are a deeply penetrating foreign body and possibly tendon or ligament rupture.

Many distal limb fractures will produce a similar clinical picture. Observations of gait or stance are of little value since there are no characteristic changes in either. In the initial examination localization of pain is probably the most accurate guide, accompanied by a careful examination of the foot to rule out foreign body penetration. The most reliable route to successful diagnosis is then through a methodical use of nerve blocks. A palmar digital nerve block (PDNB) or, ideally, a navicular bursal block, is virtually diagnostic, resulting in an almost complete return to normality. There may be some residual lameness since fractures of the navicular bone invariably involve the distal interphalangeal joint, and inflammatory change will affect the whole articulation. An abaxial sesamoid block will abolish the pain entirely.

In more long standing cases the severity of lameness can be equalled by advanced navicular disease which will of course respond to blocking in the same way. However, navicular disease is almost invariably bilateral; a response to a PDNB without bilateral lameness should increase suspicion that a fracture exists.

Definitive diagnosis is by radiographic examination. Good preparation of the foot is essential, especially in the frog region. Both abaxial and central sulci must be pared, not scraped, back to clean horn and then packed with soft soap or similar material. Soft soap is ideal for the purpose as it is squeezed into the interstices of the horn as the animal bears weight. Despite this, the deep cleft between the heels of some feet may still produce a very convincing fracture artefact and for this reason the standard 60° dorsopalmar oblique view should always be supplemented by a similar projection at say 50° to the horizontal and, ideally, by flexor projection as well (Fig. 9.6).

Fresh fractures will show a clean, well demarcated fracture line, though in time this broadens and develops indistinct margins due to mineral resorption. As these fractures heal by fibrous union, there will be no evidence of filling of the fracture gap, though new bone can be seen adjacent to fractures on the proximal surface. The fracture

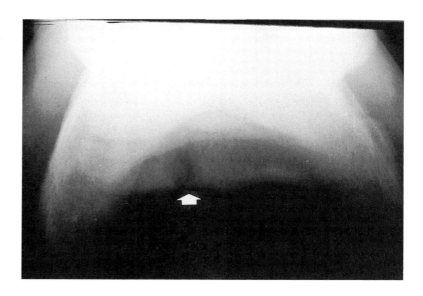

Fig. 9.6 A 'flexor' view of the same fracture as in Fig. 9.5.

line will therefore be visible for many years and maybe for the rest of the animal's life.

Treatment

It is generally agreed that prognosis for untreated cases is grave. Although a small proportion of animals are usable, the vast majority show a persistent low grade lameness which is exacerbated by exercise. Post mortem examination inevitably shows an absence of bony union, the fragments being united by fibrous tissue only and frequently there are strong adhesions between the fracture line and the deep flexor tendon. Because of these factors many authorities have recommended neurectomy of the palmar digital nerves.

Conservative treatment techniques have concentrated on providing immobilization by fitting a bar-shoe over padding and on reducing the compressive load on the navicular bone by raising the heel substantially. The animals are then box rested for many months and following a gradual lowering of the heel some are said to return to normality. The author's experience of this method of treatment has not been encouraging in that the animals, whilst showing considerable improvement, always retain a persistent low grade lameness.

The cause of the inevitable non-union is likely to be interfragmentary movement which, though it may be reduced by rest and surgical shoeing, is unlikely to be eliminated. The only satisfactory way to achieve this would be by internal fixation.

Until recently there was no known way of accurately inserting screws into navicular bone. However, over the last few years techniques have been developed which allow lag-screwing, and therefore interfragmentary compression of navicular bone fractures. The problem of inserting a screw into the long narrow bone buried deep within the hoof has been solved by the construction of a 'jig' or clamp incorporating a series of drill guides. Following careful pre-operative

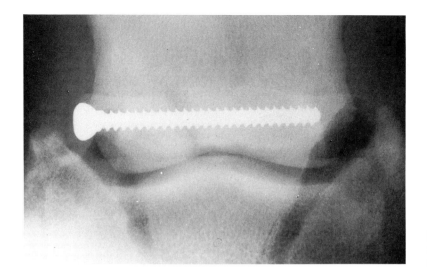

Fig. 9.7 The same navicular bone as in Fig. 9.5 following compression fixation.

preparation of the foot (as described for pedal bone fractures) the jig is placed in position with a fluoroscope/image intensifier system; the drill guides are aligned with the central long axis of the navicular bone and then fixed in position by the clamps. The drill guides are used firstly to drill a 9.5 cm (3/8th″) hole through the horn, soft tissues and lateral cartilage to the edge of the navicular bone.

A second drill guide allows a gliding hole to be drilled under fluoroscopic control to the fracture line. A drill sleeve is inserted into this hole and then a final pilot hole drilled to the far extremity of the bone. After tapping out the thread, an appropriate length screw is inserted and tightened to provide interfragmentary compression (Fig. 9.7).

Initial results using this technique are promising; accurate placement of the screw can be achieved consistently and the few clinical cases treated have shown an encouraging response. As with all fracture fixation, the results depend very much on the age of the fracture. Early diagnosis and treatment are imperative, and suspect fractures must be radiographed early before the fracture has developed into an established non-union with adhesions to the deep flexor tendon and degenerative disease of the distal interphalangeal joint.

Fractures of the extreme tips of the navicular bone are not suitable candidates for internal fixation. In these cases there must be a poor prognosis and neurectomy is probably the only satisfactory course if the animal is to be used again. As all navicular bone fractures involve the distal interphalangeal joint, degenerative joint disease is an inevitable sequel and the relief provided by palmar digital neurectomy is likely to last for only a year or two at most.

Suggested futher reading

Arnbjerg J (1979) Spontaneous fracture of the navicular bone in the horse. *Nord Vet Med* **31**, 429—35.

Wyn-Jones G (1985) Navicular bone fractures. *Vet Annual* **25**, 201.

Fractures of the 2nd phalanx

Aetiology and pathogenesis

In the UK fractures of the 2nd phalanx seem to be less common than those involving the 1st or 3rd phalanx. In the USA however, they are extremely common, especially in Western performance horses whose work involves high speed sharp turns. In American surveys fractures occur more frequently in hind legs, the reason presumably being that they are subject to greater compressions and torque forces in such activities as barrel racing or pole bending. Occasionally however, the fracture seems to occur during light exercise, possibly following fissuring of the bone during earlier hard work. There is a suggestion that heel caulkins, by anchoring the foot to the ground, increase the stress on the bone, and predispose to the fracture.

Clinical signs

There will always be a sudden onset of severe lameness when complete fracture occurs, but it is not unknown for animals to become slightly lame during work, with the onset of severe lameness delayed for anything up to several days. The inference here is that a fissure fracture occurs initially followed by complete breakdown later.

When complete fracture has occurred, the animal bears no weight on the leg, the area is extremely painful to the touch or manipulation and crepitus can often be felt. Because of the location of the bone, half buried within the hoof, swelling is usually minimal.

Diagnosis

Diagnosis is usually on clinical signs alone. Nerve blocks must be used with great caution in any animal suspected of having a distal limb fracture; pain is an invaluable aid in protecting the fracture from further trauma. With pain of this magnitude, location of the general area of the fracture is usually fairly easy. Subsequent examination is by radiography. If the animal is to be transported, the leg must be placed in a cast, no other form of splintage gives adequate immobilization. This can be difficult, since pain causes easing and movement of the leg. However, very rapid setting, resin plaster bandages are now available and they should be part of every equine veterinary surgeon's first aid kit.

A full radiographic examination consists of four views, a dorso-palmar (DP), a lateral and the two 45° obliques. This allows a full evaluation of fracture configuration, and makes decisions as to treatment and prognosis easier.

Treatment

These fractures, because of their location, are rarely compound, thereby removing one source of worry. That location, however, also makes them extremely difficult subjects for internal fixation. In general, only simple fractures and those involving the proximal wings of the bone are suitable. With increasing comminution, the size of fragments diminishes, the fracture lines become more complex and more difficult to avoid, and adequate access becomes a problem. However, where the surgeon thinks fixation is feasible, it provides the best outlook for a return to working soundness. If the fracture involves only the proximal aspect of the 2nd phalanx then a further option is available; that of arthrodesis of the proximal interphalangeal joint. This can be done as the primary treatment in suitable cases or, following healing in a cast, the effects of the secondary degenerative joint disease can be obviated by this technique (see section on pastern arthrodesis p. 68). Where the fracture is comminuted and/or involves the distal interphalangeal joint, then the outlook is very poor for an athletic future.

If the animal is to be salvaged as a pet or for breeding purposes, then the leg should be cast to just below the carpus or hock. Whilst, in emergency, a cast can be applied with the animal standing, one that is to remain on for any length of time should be applied under a general anaesthetic. This is to avoid wrinkles and pressure points which can easily prove as damaging as the fracture. Details of application of casts can be found in the section on external coaptation, p. 266.

Although there is rarely great distraction of the fragments because of the tightly enclosed situation of the bone, the fragments can become separated if the leg is held in certain positions. Radiographs will show in which state of flexion or extension the best apposition is achieved and the leg should be cast in that position. The clinician should bear in mind that if the leg is cast in extreme extension then the natural spring of the tissues may result in pressure rubs on the bulbs of the heels. The first cast remains on for 1—2 weeks, whilst the initial soft tissue swelling reduces. At this time a second cast is applied which, if well tolerated, can be left on for 1—2 months. By then it is likely to have suffered considerable wear and tear and it should be replaced. The cast can finally be removed some 4 months after the initial fracture.

There will usually be marked thickening of the lower pastern, composed of both bony callus and reaction to the extensive soft tissue damage which invariably accompanies this type of fracture. A further period of 3—6 months rest is advisable to consolidate healing before the animal is turned out, although during this time, increasing amounts of exercise in hand should be given.

Although the lameness may subside considerably during this time, the owners should be warned of the inevitable advancement of degenerative disease in the affected joints, and the likelihood of increasing levels of lameness in the future.

Suggested further reading

Calahan PT, Wheat JD and Meagher DM (1981) Treatment of middle phalangeal fractures in the horse. *J Am Vet Med Assoc* **178**, 11882.

Fractures of the 1st phalanx

Aetiology and pathogenesis

In the UK fractures of the 1st phalanx (PI) are much more common than those involving the 2nd phalanx. They probably occur as a result of simultaneous torsion and compression with unfitness, fatigue and momentary inco-ordination being likely predisposing factors. External trauma, hitting fences, etc. is also known to be a cause. The fracture configuration may be anything from a simple incomplete fissure to multiple comminution.

The vast majority of fractures affect the fetlock joint, while some affect both fetlocks and the proximal interphalangeal or pastern joint. A small proportion affect only the pastern and the odd one or two fractures involve neither. There are a certain number of configurations which occur more commonly and some of these are shown in Fig. 9.8.

Any fracture which involves an articulation will eventually cause degenerative joint disease. Its severity will depend on the extent of joint involvement, the presence of any incongruity between the articular surfaces on each side of the fracture line or lines and the method of treatment. This is why, whenever possible, rigid internal fixation should be employed in the treatment of these fractures.

Fig. 9.8 Diagrammatic representations of three of the more common 1st phalanx fractures. (a) The incomplete sagittal fissure which almost invariably commences in or very near the central groove of the articular surface; (b) a curving fracture affecting only the fetlock joint; there is often fragmentation where the fracture line exits the shaft cortex; (c) a typical spiralling fracture affecting both proximal and distal articular surfaces. These fractures must be carefully evaluated radiographically so that the surgeon is fully aware of the direction of spiralling and can place his screws accordingly.

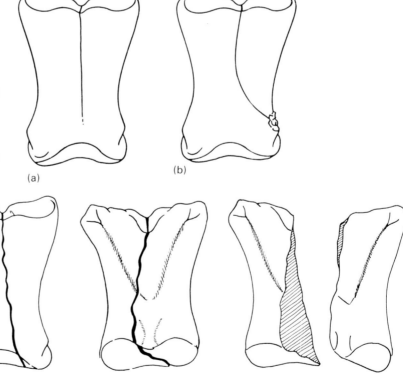

(a)

(b)

(c)

Clinical signs

Clinical signs are very variable. In the case of complete fracture there will be an immediate 10/10th lameness and a complete inability to bear weight. If a horse sustains such a fracture whilst racing, it will often fall or pull up immediately and subsequently refuse to move. In these cases, the jockeys often report that the animal stumbled or 'pecked' earlier in the race. It is possible that a fissure fracture occurs at this time only to be comminuted by the subsequent stress. On the other hand, animals often race well, only to walk off the course with a mild lameness which worsen over the next hour or so. Local signs too will vary. In the case of complete fracture, especially with comminution, crepitus is easily felt. In those with multiple fragments, there is gross mobility and much crepitus, with the pastern area resembling what has been called a 'bag of marbles'. In fissure fractures there will be no mobility or crepitus, but there will be local pain and, if the fetlock is involved, within a few minutes some joint swelling may occur. The leg is carried in the neutral, semiflexed resting position and there is no characteristic gait abnormality. If only fissuring has occurred then the lameness improves rapidly over a few weeks, to a stage where the animal appears normal at the walk.

If no treatment is given, then the fracture can become complete at any time or, if this is avoided, there is a high risk of significant degenerative joint disease preventing a return to complete working soundness.

Diagnosis

The detection of fractures with comminution and multiple fragmentation is easy and needs no further elaboration. Simple fractures, especially the incomplete fissure, can give rise to problems in diagnosis. In those animals which pull up while travelling at speed, the only major orthopaedic differentials are other fractures and tendon or ligament tearing. Simple palpation and manipulation may indicate the area involved, but it may be some time before tissue swelling develops and pin-points an area more clearly. If no tendon or ligament pathology is evident, then *it is essential to assume that a fracture has occurred, until it is proven otherwise*. It is very unwise to dismiss these cases as 'sprained or strained fetlocks'.

Nerve blocks must be used with great caution in suspect fracture cases. Pain is a potent protective agent and its abolition can result in the animal causing further damage to the area. Radiographic examination of the *distal cannon* and *digits* must be thorough. Lesions will only show on well penetrated views, in which the X-ray beam is parallel or nearly parallel to the fracture lines. A dorsopalmar projection is nearly always the most informative initially, but a lateral and two 45° obliques are needed to chart fully the course of the fracture lines. It must be remembered when interpreting these radiographs that fracture gaps usually show up only in the thick cortical bone. A simple sagittal fracture will therefore often have two distinct lines, one in the dorsal and one in the palmar cortex. It is a good idea to use

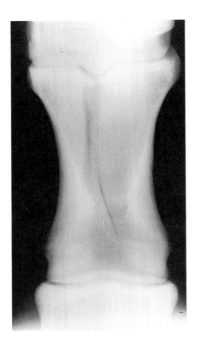

Fig. 9.9 A radiograph of a spiralling, apparently incomplete fracture of a 1st phalanx. However, careful examination shows that there is a 'step' in the relationship of the fragments at the fetlock articular surface indicating that the fracture must be complete. Note the two separate lines of the fracture which indicated the separation of the fragments in the dorsal and palmar cortices. The indistinct wider line represents a fracture plane which is not absolutely parallel to the X-ray beam centre.

Fig. 9.10 (a) and (b) A diagrammatic illustration of the placement of screws in the 1st phalanx to compress a spiralling fracture such as that illustrated in Fig. 9.8c. Note that the gliding hole is continued just beyond the fracture line and the two proximal screws are located one dorsal and one palmar to the extensor branch of the suspensory ligament. The screw heads must be well countersunk into the bone. In the absence of fragment distraction the screws are usually inserted through stab incisions.

a specimen bone on which to map out the fracture line, and essential if internal fixation is contemplated. If the fracture line involves an articular surface, it is most important to decide whether there is a 'step' between the fragments (Fig. 9.9). Any incongruity must be corrected before fixation takes place otherwise the subsequent degenerative joint disease will be severe and disabling.

Treatment

Good first aid is vital. The animal should be moved only the minimum distance, i.e. out of any danger, before a temporary support is applied. Bandages and wooden splints are totally inadequate and the leg should be cast from carpus or hock down. The new very rapid setting resin plasters are ideal and can be applied over a snug cotton bandage which prevents the plaster sticking to the hair. The horse can then be transported safely with the minimum risk of a fissure fracture becoming complete or further damage to fragments and soft tissue. The practice of shooting horses on race tracks is reprehensible in the author's view; a full clinical evaluation is not possible in these circumstances and there are far too many pressures, especially on the young veterinary surgeon. The decision whether or not to euthanase should await radiographic examination and possibly expert advice.

The ideal treatment for any fracture is reduction and compression by internal fixation; however, this is only feasible in a proportion of cases. Incomplete fissure fractures are ideal candidates for internal fixation. Although they will heal in a cast, compression by screwing lag-fashion across the fracture line will speed healing greatly and markedly reduce the risk of subsequent fetlock degenerative joint disease. The technique is relatively simple, the screws being inserted through stab skin incisions at selected sites (Fig. 9.10). Self-tapping Sherman screws can be used, though the ease of insertion and greatly

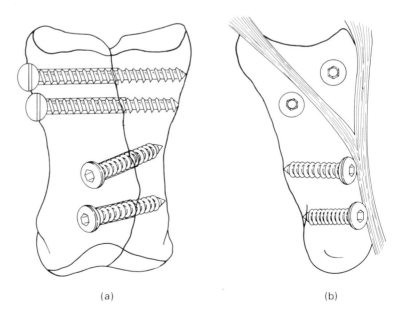

(a)   (b)

increased holding power of the larger ASIF implants makes their use infinitely preferable.

Simple, complete fractures are also best treated by internal fixation. However, accurate reduction of the fracture is essential to prevent massive degenerative change in the affected joint, usually the fetlock. Although desirable, alignment at the proximal interphalangeal or pastern joint is not so critical because of the option of later arthrodesis. Intraoperative radiographic assessment can be difficult and the author prefers to open the joint and check the alignment visually. In the long run, it saves time and is certainly more accurate. Small chip fractures may also be reattached using internal fixation techniques provided they are large enough to accept a screw (Fig. 9.11). Smaller chips are best removed (Fig. 9.12). Before embarking on these techniques the surgeon should be familiar with both the anatomy of the

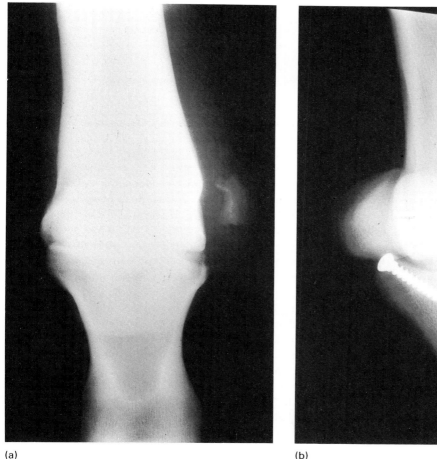
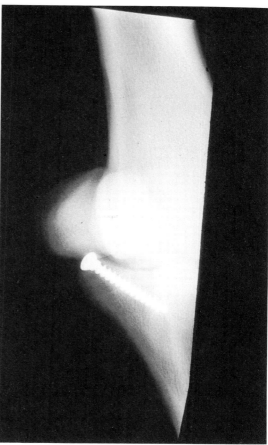

(a)   (b)

Fig. 9.11   (a) This chip of bone was still firmly attached to the joint capsule and following an arthrotomy was relocated and compressed to the parent bone using a suitable length 3.5 mm ASIF screw. (b) The fragment relocated and the screw in place. Despite the fragment having an articular component accurate reduction and compression fixation resulted in the animal returning to working soundness.

251

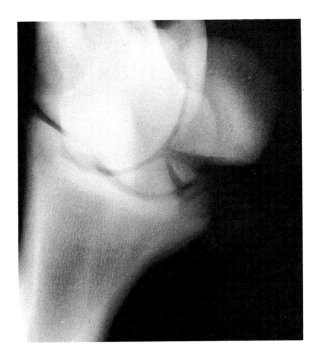

Fig. 9.12 These small chips of bone were too small to be screwed back in place and were removed.

area and of the fracture he is dealing with and, of course the principles of internal fixation.

With increased comminution of the fracture comes increasing difficulty of reduction and internal fixation. It is difficult to make generalizations and each case must be considered on its own merits. However, one useful rule of thumb is that the chances of a successful outcome are substantially increased if there is one fragment which extends intact from the articular surface of the fetlock to that of the pastern. This provides a solid weight bearing strut to which other fragments can be attached. Without this feature the fragments are prone to telescope or compact. When there are numerous fracture lines, the correct placement of screws becomes very difficult and the chance of screwing into a fracture line increases. Also exposure of the fracture sites and accurate reduction becomes a major problem.

With increasing comminution too comes an exponentially worsening prognosis for a return to athletic soundness. Without perfect alignment and compression of intra-articular fragments severe degenerative joint disease is inevitable. Under these circumstances the animal will be fit only for breeding, for keeping as a pet, or, occasionally, for light hacking.

Where the complexity of the fracture would make fixation difficult or even contraindicated, casting the leg is a viable alternative. However, there are limits, and those explosive type fractures which produce myriads of small fragments will not heal even if immobilized. The fragments have no columnar strength, even when confined within a cast, and the forces released on fracture will have severely damaged surrounding soft tissues and compromised the blood supply to this area.

The presence of several large fragments increases the chances of success and many of these cases are worth a try if the economics and the status of the animal warrant it. Remember that casting is an expensive business; two or three casts will need to be applied, and the total cost may be as much, if not more, than internal fixation. Again, full and frank discussion with the owner before embarking on treatment is essential and they must be left in no doubt that this is a salvage procedure only.

Casts which stay on for any length of time must be applied under general anaesthesia. Reduction of these multiple fractures can be a problem and often a combination of extension or flexion, coupled with traction and a compressive force is needed. Ideally radiographs should be taken with the limb in different positions to check which provides the best reduction. The first cast is applied for 1–2 weeks, and then it is changed as reduction in soft tissue swelling will make the cast loose and allow rubs to develop. This second cast should stay on for 3 months or so, and if necessary, be replaced by a third for a further 2 months; a total of some 5 months. Radiography will indicate when the cast can be removed safely.

Following fracture healing the degree of lameness will be variable. In most cases it is tolerable, and the animal will be fit for breeding or as a pet (Fig. 9.13). Some reduction in pain can be achieved by arthrodesis of the pastern joint, and in selected cases by fetlock arthrodesis. The latter is feasible but is technically very difficult surgery and these cases are best referred to an orthopaedic specialist. A recent innovation to try and reduce overriding or telescoping of multiple fragments is the use of external fixation devices. These consist of orthopaedic pins inserted through the bones proximal and distal to the fracture and then stabilized by bolting to vertical bars or encasing in resin pillars. Although successful in some cases, these animals require very intensive and careful management. Infection is a major problem and probably renders the technique one which is best used in referral centres.

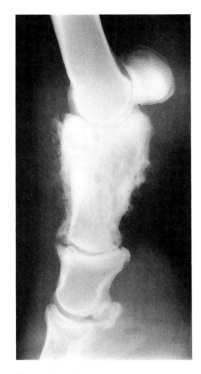

Fig. 9.13 A lateromedial radiograph of a healed comminuted fracture of the 1st phalanx. The fragmentation of the bone was such that internal fixation was not possible and the leg was placed in a cast for 5 months. Note the extensive involvement of both the fetlock and pastern joints.

Suggested further reading

Fackelman GE and Nunamaker DM (1982) *Manual of Internal Fixation in the Horse*. Springer-Verlag, New York.

Markel MD, Martin BB and Richardson DW (1985) Dorsal frontal fractures of the first phalanx in the horse. *Vet Surgery* **14**(1), 36–40.

Markel MD, Richardson DW and Nunamaker DM (1985) Comminuted first phalanx fractures in 30 horses. Surgical versus nonsurgical treatment. *Vet Surgery* **14**(2), 135-40.

Fractures of the 3rd metacarpus cannon bone

Condylar fractures of the metacarpus or metatarsus

Condylar fractures of the metacarpus or metatarsus are uncommon in horses and ponies other than those which compete at high speed.

253

They are therefore seen principally in thoroughbreds in the UK, but also standardbreds and quarter horses in other countries.

Lateral condylar fractures

Aetiology and pathogenesis

Lateral condylar fractures are far more common than medial fractures. The reason is not known, though the fact that the lateral articular facet of the distal cannon is narrower than the medial may be significant. The fracture configuration ranges from incomplete fissures to complete separation with displacement, and, in a proportion of cases, mild comminution can occur. Fragmentation may be found at the thinner proximal portion of the fracture line where it leaves the cortex, but recent reports have drawn attention to the frequent presence of a single, small diamond-shaped fragment within the articulation. It lies at a constant site, where the two different radii of curvature meet (Fig. 9.14). It has obvious implications in the development of degenerative joint disease and may account for the unexpected persistence of lameness in those cases which were thought to have been successfully treated.

Clinical signs

Clinical signs will vary enormously from a mild lameness, detectable only at the trot in cases of incomplete fissures, to a severe, instantaneous 10/10th lameness where complete separation has occurred. Incomplete spiral fractures will also produce a three-legged horse, and this sign, in the absence of separation of fragments should alert the clinician to this possibility. One of the common and misleading scenarios is for an animal to complete and occasionally win a race only to show lameness a few minutes later; the lameness becoming more severe over the next hour or so until the horse is reluctant to bear weight. Local signs too are variable, but with the degree of

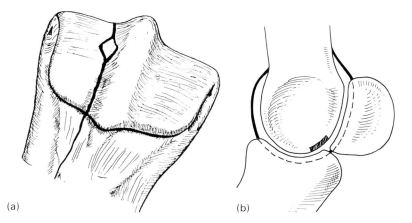

Fig. 9.14 (a) and (b) Diagrammatic illustrations of the position of the palmar fragment in a comminuted lateral condylar fracture.

(a)   (b)

swelling and local pain tending to mirror the level of lameness. However, the clinician must be aware that swelling, both intra and extra-articular, can take a little time to develop and should not be misled into thinking that, for example, a racehorse which pulls up lame cannot have a fracture because there is no swelling at the site or palpable crepitus.

Where fractures remain undetected, the level of lameness will diminish after a week or so. The level to which it eventually drops will again reflect the severity of the fracture and, with undisplaced fissures, the animal may become sound at least while it is not being pressurized. However, degenerative joint disease is an almost certain sequel, becoming evident as a low grade persistent lameness some months or even years after work recommences.

Diagnosis

Many of these cases are not examined properly or radiographed until the lameness from what was thought to be a 'strained fetlock' or 'sprained ankle' has persisted for an unreasonable length of time. By this stage, repair is often impossible, or, at best, pointless because of the onset of degenerative joint disease. The lesson to be learnt from these cases is that it is far better to assume that a fracture has occurred, until is is proved otherwise by X-ray examination. These animals *must* be X-rayed earlier rather than later.

Radiography must be thorough and produce good quality plates; fissure fractures can be extremely difficult to see even on the best films. A DP view is obviously included but since a proportion of fractures spiral, some to the top of the cannon, laterals and obliques must be included, taking in the whole of the bone. If this is not done, then a spiral fracture may be missed and not properly repaired. Even in a simple fracture there will usually be two fracture lines visible. This is not two fractures but the single fracture plane visible separately in the dorsal and palmar cortices. Another factor to bear in mind is that narrow fracture lines are only visible when the beam is nearly parallel to them; even slight obliquity can make them almost invisible, and completely so on poor quality films!

The small distal fragment mentioned earlier will not be detected on conventional views. A 125° dorsopalmar oblique projection (Fig. 9.15) as done for the visualization of osteochondrosis lesions at the

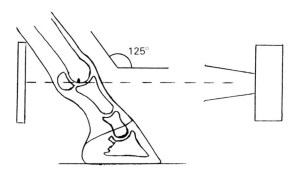

Fig. 9.15 The position of the leg relative to the beam centre in a 125° dorsopalmar oblique projection.

same site is necessary, and, because the presence of the comminution influences the prognosis, should be included in an examination of all condylar fractures.

Treatment

Where a fracture of the distal cannon, or for that matter, any bone in the fetlock region, is suspected good first aid can make the difference between success and failure of treatment. A cast should be applied from distal carpus or hock down to, and including, the foot. The young clinician should not be dissuaded by more 'conservative elements', often found on racecourses, from adopting this eminently sensible and logical measure. This should be done using the rapid setting plaster bandage which is now available and will prevent further trauma to joints and fragments in a complete fracture and in the case of a fissure, prevent it extending. If a casting material is not available, lateral compression can be achieved using multiple layers of sticky elastic dressing which builds up into a fairly rigid structure. Analgesics or NSAIDs should not be given, pain is an excellent protector of fractures!

Fissure fractures can be treated by casting alone; most will heal satisfactorily, but the presence of a fracture line within the joint will always lead to significant degenerative joint disease. Healing will be faster and with less articular damage if the fracture is compressed by lag-screwing across the fracture line. Three or four screws are placed, lag fashion, through stab incisions. The most distal is placed first, usually just distal to the tubercles. The gliding hole must extend to, and preferably slightly beyond, the fracture line otherwise there will be no compressive effect when the screw is tightened. For this first screw there is no need to countersink as the screw head is adequately buried in the origins of the collateral ligament. With small fragments, the most distal screw must be placed in the lateral condylar fossa; this involves separation of the fibres of the ligament so that the screw head seats firmly on bone. Subsequent screws are placed approximately 25 mm apart. These screws must be countersunk to prevent them protruding too much. The most proximal may need to be placed slightly obliquely if the fracture line appears to spiral. Ideally 4.5 mm screws of the ASIF design should be used because of their superior holding power, but ordinary Sherman screws will be adequate if used properly. An ASIF 'C' clamp is available which allows pre-alignment of a guide through which all the holes are drilled. Its use is a matter of preference — it is not essential to use one.

With fissure, or incomplete fractures, alignment of fragments is not a problem. However, it is one of the most important considerations in the treatment of complete fractures. Any discrepancy will result in massive degenerative joint disease within the fetlock in a very short time. If radiographs have shown *clearly* that there is no misalignment then a complete fracture can be treated as if it were a fissure, i.e. by lag-screwing through stab incisions (Figs. 9.16a and b). The most proximal screw should not be too close to the fracture exit otherwise the thin bone of the fragment margin might shatter. Some marginal

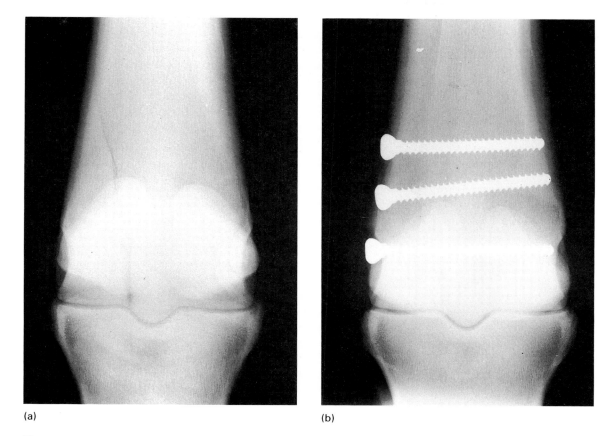

(a)   (b)

Fig. 9.16 (a) A complete non-displacement fracture of the lateral condyle of the metacarpus. (b) The same fracture 3 months after compression fixation. On the original radiograph the fracture line is still faintly discernible.

fragmentation is of no great consequence however, provided the body of the fragment is well secured. Ideally, an intraoperative radiograph should be taken after the first screw is inserted, in case the manipulation has disturbed the alignment. If this shows no discrepancy then the remainder of the screws are inserted and tightened alternately. Screws should be tightened firmly but not over-enthusiastically.

Where there is misalignment it must be corrected. One technique uses a lateral incision to visualize the proximal end of the fracture. The fragment is manipulated so that the fracture margins align at which point the first screw hole is drilled. Fragmentation at the margin of the fracture often makes this difficult and, even when intact, the gently tapering margins of the fragment do not make it an easy task. Far better results are obtained by performing an arthrotomy, when the articular surfaces can be visualized. There is no doubt then that accurate alignment has been achieved and intraoperative radiographs, a time consuming business, are avoided.

If surgery has been delayed for any reason, then it will be advisable to do a complete open reduction with debridement of the fracture faces. Without this, the fragments will not 'mate' accurately.

Anaesthetic recovery should be with the leg in a cast though it can be removed soon afterwards. The animal should be box rested for about 3 months followed by walking exercise in hand for a similar period. After 6 months, and satisfactory check-up radiographs, trotting exercise can begin, progressing *slowly* to full training at 9–10 months post-fixation. With fresh fractures, treated by internal fixation, the prognosis is good. The presence of distal comminution worsens the outlook considerably but improves if the small fragment is removed during an open reduction.

Spiral fissure fractures

Spiral fissure fractures are said to be more common in the hind legs, also in the less frequently affected medial condyles. However, all condylar fractures, irrespective of the leg or side, have the potential to do this and the radiographic examination must take this into account by including lateral and oblique views of the whole of the cannon bone (Figs. 9.17a and b).

The clinical signs and presentation are indistinguishable from complete lateral or medial condylar fractures, adding weight to the desirability of adequate first aid in all such cases. If a spiral fissure fracture dehisces the resulting complete shaft fracture carries a very poor prognosis!

Treatment is identical to the less dramatic simple condylar fissure fracture except that the repair involves compressing the fracture along its whole length with six or seven screws (Fig. 9.18). Although these fractures tend to spiral in the same direction, the fracture line in the dorsal cortex running medially and that in the palmar or plantar cortex coursing laterally, each case *must* be assessed individually. It is a great help to trace out the line of the fracture on a specimen bone prior to surgery.

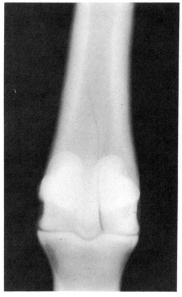 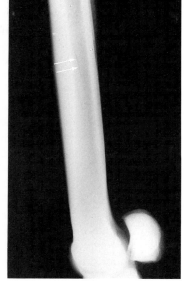

Fig. 9.17 (a) A lateral condylar fracture which appears to 'fade-out' proximally in this dorsopalmar projection. Only a lateromedial view (b) shows the fissure line still running up the cannon bone.

(a)   (b)

Conservative therapy is possible, but casts to above the carpus and hock are not well tolerated and casts to below carpus or hock are not adequate because of the proximal extension of the fracture line. The risk of fracture dehiscence is greatly diminished when the internal fixation is carried out and the prognosis for eventual return to athletic soundness is good.

Suggested further reading

Adams SB, Turner TA, Blevin WE and Shamis LD (1985) Surgical repair of metacarpal condylar fractures with palmar osteochondral comminution in two thoroughbred horses. *Vet Surgery* **14**(1), 32–5.

Fackelman GE and Nunamaker DM (1982) *Manual of Internal Fixation in the Horse.* Springer-Verlag, New York.

Hornof WJ and O'Brien TR (1980) Radiographic evaluation of the palmar aspect of the equine metacarpal condyles: a new projection. *Vet Radiology* **21**(4), 161–7.

Rick MC, O'Brien TR, Pool RR *et al* (1983) Condylar fractures of the 3rd metacarpal and 3rd metatarsal bone in 75 horses: radiographic features, treatment and outcome. *J Am Vet Met Assoc* **183**(3), 287–96.

Shaft fractures

Aetiology and pathogenesis

The aetiology of complete shaft fractures is invariably external trauma, often from kicks, or by foals being trodden on by their dams, etc. In young animals, physeal separations will also occur, usually of the Salter-Harris type II; these are frequently caused by traction during delivery. The cannon bone has little soft tissue covering; vital structures such as nerves and blood vessels run close to the bone and are often irreparably damaged by the explosive forces released as fracture occurs. The skin may also be devitalized as the razor-sharp fragments strip off its underlying fascia. The resulting ischaemia can have effects ranging from the sloughing of a small area of skin to death of the whole distal limb. The former, although not quite as dramatic, can have consequences just as dire, with subsequent massive infection of the fracture site.

Although these factors contribute to the high incidence of compound fractures of the cannon, the prime cause is direct penetration of the skin by bone ends. The risk is greatly increased in oblique fractures which produce lance-like fragments and by the animal's struggles. Inadequate first aid and transport of an animal without rigid immobilization of the leg greatly contribute to the problem. It is a sad fact that more animals are 'lost' during transportation to clinics than ever are by the other numerous complications of fracture. Having said that, not even a cast is a complete guarantee against further damage. Some internal movement is bound to occur, especially overriding in oblique or spiral fractures; this can result in a fracture becoming compound, or at least being further fragmented. Another, less well-known consequence of excess mobility is eburnation, or polishing of the fracture margins. The changes in the bone caused by

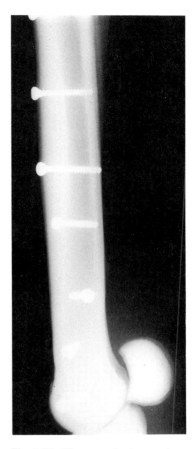

Fig. 9.18 The same fracture as in Fig. 9.17 has been compressed using seven ASIF screws arranged spirally up the cannon bone.

this process retard the primary bone healing which internal fixation and compression is meant to encourage.

Clinical signs and diagnosis

These should not present any problems, however the clinician must be aware of the dangers of enthusiastic manipulation and the potential for causing more damage.

Treatment

The importance of rapid and effective first aid cannot be over-emphasized! Even hopping a short distance with an unsupported distal limb gyrating wildly can be sufficient to cause irreparable soft tissue damage. In emergency situations when animals have to be moved quickly, e.g. on race tracks, good temporary support can be given using two lengths of plastic guttering, 12.5—15 cm (5—6") in diameter, well padded with foam and taped so that they encircle the leg. These should be pre-prepared and kept ready for immediate use.

Before moving the animal any distance, the leg must be immobilized in a cast. Ideally, it should extend to just below the elbow, although a below-the-knee cast is better than none. Very rapid setting resin plaster bandages allow casts to be applied relatively easily in the standing position and should be carried routinely by clinicians attending race meetings, 'point-to-points', etc.

Once a cast is applied the emergency is over and a 'breathing space' is established during which the animal is allowed to quieten down; antibiotic and antitetanus therapy is administered and the animal transported to a place where it can be radiographed. Owners are usually upset or distraught at this time, and the clinician must be aware that much of what he says may not be appreciated or understood. However, discussion of the animal's immediate prospects, the cost of treatment and the long term prognosis must be started as soon as practicable before the costs escalate.

Radiography can be done through a cast using a greatly increased mAs value: although the general configuration of the break can usually be assessed, detail is lost. A quiet or stoical animal can have its cast removed, the leg X-rayed and the cast reapplied without much risk, but in most instances, the case is best served by carrying out the procedure under general anaesthesia. In addition to the better radiographs that can be obtained, the leg can be carefully examined for abrasions, punctures, etc. There is little doubt that, whenever possible, internal fixation of these fractures should be delayed for 2—3 days. During that time, suitably immobilized in a snug cast, the soft tissue damage and swelling will subside, surgery and skin closure especially will be easier, with less risk of wound breakdown; also pre-operative antibiotic therapy will have had time to become effective at sterilizing the operation site.

Some fractures will respond to casting alone. Young foals with closed, relatively stable fracture configurations with no tendency to override, are the most suitable candidates. However, frequent cast changes are necessary as these animals grow rapidly, and the final cost can be greater than if internal fixation techniques had been used. It is also difficult to ensure perfect alignment of the fragments; any angulation is magnified by the length and slenderness of the foal's legs, and the triumph of perfect bone healing is often negated by a residual, small, but unacceptable, deviation of the distal limb.

Casting is highly unlikely to be an effective treatment in adults or youngsters where there is marked distraction of fragments, great obliquity to the fracture line or a degree of comminution. In these animals, internal fixation using plating techniques is indicated; lag-screw fixation alone, as used in incomplete fissure type fractures is not sufficiently strong even with additional cast support.

Double plating is used whenever possible in animals of any size, single plates being suitable only for foals (Fig. 9.19). Two plates are required to provide the requisite strength, but their application can cause problems. They are bulky and there are often problems with skin closure. Large flap incisions are made to provide good cover for the plates which are usually applied to the dorsal and lateral side of the bones. One of the principles of plate application is that they should be fixed wherever possible to the side of the bone under tension. (The metacarpus is axially loaded while the metatarsus has its tension side laterally.)

Overriding of fragments is common and always present in oblique fractures. The surgeon cannot expect to correct this manually but must arrange for some system, usually a block and tackle, to provide the enormous traction force needed. In fact it is often advisable to begin traction before surgery has commenced otherwise the surgeon is kept waiting needlessly. If possible ASIF type implants should be used because of their greater strength. Cannon bone cortex is very dense and hard, and is extremely difficult to penetrate with a hand drill. Therefore, an air drill or other suitable power tool must be available to drill the 20 or so screw holes that could be needed. During recovery the leg must be supported in a cast which extends to just below the elbow.

With increasing comminution, the chances of successful fixation diminish. This is especially so if there is much damage around the area of the nutrient artery with ischaemia leading to greatly delayed bone healing. Multiple small fragments are likely to have lost their soft tissue attachments and will be difficult, if not impossible, to replace. Under these circumstances extensive bone grafting is necessary; this adds to the total operating time and, indeed, may be impossible without a team of surgeons — it may have to be repeated several times! At this point it is appropriate to add that any long bone fixation in the horse is not a task which can be accomplished by the lone surgeon.

Contamination of a fracture site in a compound or open fracture is also a poor prognostic sign. The level of contamination will, of course, vary but even the smallest penetration is a cause for worry. In thick coated animals a small puncture may go unnoticed at first, and may only be found following radiography and the discovery of gas or air

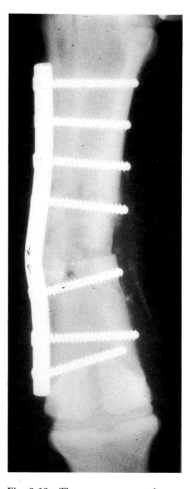

Fig. 9.19 The consequence of inadequate single plating of a comminuted fracture of an adult metacarpus. The lack of stability has resulted in disintegration of the cortex opposite to the plate and bending of the plate itself. On the original radiograph the plate could be seen to be cracked between the two arrows. The fracture became massively infected and the animal was euthanased.

lucencies within the soft tissues of the leg. If soiling of the fragment ends or fracture site is gross or has been present for some considerable time (12−24 hours) without antibiotic therapy, the situation is virtually hopeless. No matter how well the site is debrided, osteomyelitis is certain to develop and these animals should be euthanased. Animals with minor wounds and which have had the benefit of early antibiotic therapy can be treated in one of two ways. In those cases of fractures which are likely to remain stable within a cast, they can be treated conservatively for 7−10 days by casting and heavy antibacterial therapy until the skin abrasion heals, followed by internal fixation. Those fractures which are likely to override or be unstable within a cast should be operated on as soon as possible with thorough debridement and irrigation of the site. The risks of infection are greatly increased even so, but the attempt is worthwhile.

It can be seen that there are many factors to be taken into account when deciding whether to recommend euthanasia or treatment. Cost, future use, the animal's temperament and value are all additional factors. Using strictly technical criteria, smaller, placid animals with simple closed mid-shaft or distal third fractures hold the best chance of success. The prognosis worsens exponentially with increase in patient size, and comminution and/or contamination of the fracture. Lastly, but not least, the outlook is greatly influenced by the orthopaedic expertise of the surgical and anaesthetic team. Surgeons undertaking this type of procedure need to be fully familiar with ASIF techniques and anaesthetists must be capable of monitoring high quality anaesthesia for anything up to 4−5 hours. In addition there must be good recovery facilities and provision for constant supervision in the first few post-operative days!

Suggested further reading

Bramlage LR (1983) Current concepts of emergency first aid treatment and transportation of equine fracture patients. *Comp Cont Education* **5**(3), article 10, S564.

Fackelman GE and Nunamaker DM (1982) *Manual of Internal Fixation in the Horse*. Springer-Verlag, New York.

Turner AS (1981) Long bone fractures in horses. Part I. Initial Management. *Comp Cont Education* **3**(9), article 9, S347.

Turner, AS (1982) Long bone fractures in horses. Part II. Intraoperative Techniques. *Comp Cont Education* **4**(5), article 7, S196.

Turner AS (1982) Long bone fractures in horses. Part III. Post-operative Management. *Comp Cont Education* **4**(6), article 8, S254.

Fractures of the radial shaft

Aetiology and pathogenesis

Fractures of the radial shaft are commonly the result of kicks, road traffic accidents or occasionally collision with fences, etc. It is likely that in some cases, fissuring occurs first, progressing to a full fracture with further stress. Many fractures are 'open' or compound when first seen. The skin break is usually on the medial side because of the paucity of soft tissue covering there.

Clinical signs

A complete fracture of the radial shaft results in a total inability to bear weight on the limb; and usually obvious aberrant mobility at the site of fracture. Soft tissue swelling will develop within a very short time and there may be oedema of the distal limb as well.

Diagnosis

Diagnosis is based entirely on clinical signs initially. There should be little difficulty with this as the evidence is so obvious. The clinician should make sure that the leg is examined minutely for signs of skin penetration; the punctures can be small and concealed by a shaggy coat. The discovery that it is an open or compound fracture will, of course, greatly affect the prognosis.

Treatment

Where a decision as to the animal's future cannot be made immediately, or it is to be transported for radiography or treatment, good first aid is essential. However, in practice this is not so easy. Distal fractures can be immobilized reasonably well in a cast which includes most of the elbow, but in the case of mid-shaft or proximal fractures, a cast may in fact make matters worse. The combined weight of the distal limb and the cast have a pendulum effect which can exacerbate movement at the fracture. The cast can be used in conjunction with a Thomas splint to create a greater rigidity, or by incorporating a wooden or metal proximal extension which, if possible, is bound to the lateral thorax and scapula (Fig. 9.20). This converts the whole leg into a stiff strut and obviates the pendulum effect.

Before embarking on the expensive process of treatment the clinician should be aware of the factors which influence prognosis. Small, good-tempered animals with closed, simple fractures of the distal third of the shaft probably carry the best prognosis. The prognosis worsens rapidly with increasing size of horse, comminution or contamination of the fracture, proximity to the elbow and intractability. Economics too play an important part as fracture fixation and subsequent management is a very expensive business. In cases of doubt the clinician in the field would be well advised to apply first aid as best he can and then seek advice from an experienced orthopaedic surgeon.

In general, the prognosis for shaft fractures is poor, though in individual cases where fixation and recovery are achieved, the outlook is good. Adult horses with severely comminuted fractures should be euthanased since there is no fixation technique currently available which can stand up to the tremendous strains imposed. Other fractures are most likely to be successfully repaired by internal fixation using

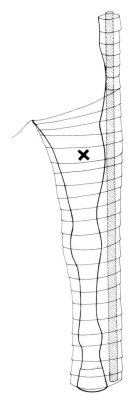

Fig. 9.20 The use of a lateral chest support in conjunction with a Robert Jones bandage or cast to prevent abduction of the limb distal to the fracture at X.

implants and techniques designed by the ASIF group. Aspiring surgeons should be aware that the repair of radial fractures is not easy surgery. It should only be attempted by those with good orthopaedic facilities, proper equipment and by a team of at least two, and preferably three, people experienced in large animal fracture repair. Neither must anaesthesia be forgotten; good facilities must be available as some procedures may require as much as 4 hours or more.

The initial problem at surgery is reduction of the inevitable overriding of fragments. Facilities for applying considerable traction must be set up as soon as the animal is anaesthetized. This is usually done by first stabilizing the body by passing padded rope under the axilla and tying it to the table; then applying a block and tackle or other controlled pulling device to a hobble on the lower limb. Steady traction for up to 45 minutes may be needed. Two plates are used if possible, one of which must be on the tension band side, the cranial cortex. The other can be placed on the medial or lateral side, though the latter is preferable because of better muscle covering for the implants. The plates must span the bone from metaphysis to metaphysis to achieve maximum stability.

With current techniques, most simple fractures can be reduced and stabilized. However, this is only the first step; the most critical period is during recovery from anaesthesia. Distal radius fractures can be successfully protected in a cast during this time, but mid-shaft and proximal fractures are very vulnerable to refracture during the animal's struggles to rise. Very little can be done to help in these cases, since casts can compound the problem as previously explained. Maintaining the animal in recumbency until it is eminently ready to stand minimizes the inco-ordination, but other factors such as pain, myopathies and temperament can lead to struggling or panic.

Even when the animal does rise successfully, the problems are not over. Refracture can occur any time the animal lies down; wound dehiscence, infection, weight bearing laminitis in the contralateral foot and stretched flexor tendons all conspire to produce a relatively low final success rate.

Suggested further reading

As for metacarpal and metatarsal shaft fractures, see p. 262.
Auer JA and Watkins JP (1987) Treatment of radial fractures in adult horses: an analysis of 15 clinical cases. *Eq Vet J* **19**(2), 103–10.
Wyn-Jones G and May SA (1985) Repair of proximal radius fracture in a horse. *Vet Rec* **115**, 516.

Fractures of the tibial shaft

Aetiology

Kicks, jumping accidents and collisions with vehicles have all been known to cause fractures of the tibial shaft. Incomplete, fissure type fractures occur and these can extend with further stress and become complete. Physeal fractures are common in young animals, usually of the Salter—Harris Type II configuration, with a variably sized portion of metaphysis attached. Tibial fractures are usually oblique or spiral and are frequently open, usually on the medial side where there is little muscle covering the bone.

Diagnosis

Detection of the fracture is usually straightforward, with abnormal movement at the site and the animal totally unable to bear weight on the leg. At this stage the decision may be made to euthanase the animal, but if internal fixation is contemplated, then radiography is essential.

Treatment

If an immediate decision about the animal's future cannot be made, or if it is to be transported, an attempt must be made to immobilize the leg. However, this is extremely difficult to achieve and no perfect solution has been found.

Distal fractures can be immobilized in a cast applied from foot to stifle. In proximal breaks, a cast will act as a pendulum and increase the stress of the fracture line. If a cast is used in conjunction with a Thomas splint then some stabilization can be achieved but it is still not good. The expense of applying such a device is, of course, considerable in its own right and can only be justified if there is a reasonable chance of success. As a rough guide, it is not feasible to repair comminuted fractures in adult horses and these should be euthanased immediately on humane grounds. Even in the case of simple fracture, the large adult is not a suitable patient and the chances of eventual success is not good. As with any long bone fracture the best prognosis is given by a simple, closed break, ideally at the distal third of the tibia in a very small, well behaved pony or foal under 150 kg (300 lb). The problems are not so much with the actual reduction and repair of the fracture, which with contemporary techniques are usually feasible, but with initial transport to the clinic and then with anaesthetic recovery and subsequent management. No implants currently available can withstand the enormous forces imparted to the hind legs during the effort of rising, and many beautifully repaired fractures rebreak as the animal rises from anaesthesia. Even if it survives that, the same risk exists for many weeks every time the animal gets up and down. In many types of fracture, casts are no help and may even exacerbate the situation both mechanically and because animals resent full-length hind limb casts and struggle excessively.

In foals or good tempered small adults, distal tibial fractures may sometimes be treated by the application of a cast. This should extend as far up the leg as possible, preferably over the stifle: this is often feasible in these smaller animals because of the smaller bulk of musculature proximal to the stifle. Failing that, if the cast is made to fit snugly up under the patella, it confers an additional amount of rigidity by stabilizing the knee-cap.

If compression plating is used, then at least two plates must be applied. The problem of overriding of the fracture fragments is far greater in the tibia than in the radius. Traction on the distal limb is not always effective and may even have an opposite effect causing distraction because of the geometry and reciprocal system of the hind leg. The plates can be applied to any aspect of the leg apart from the caudal. The medial approach is easier because of the small amount of musculature here but post-operative problems with the wound are greater for the same reason. Lateral and cranial approaches, although technically more difficult, give better long term results.

In the event of a successful repair and anaesthetic recovery, the owner must be warned that this is only a small part of the healing process and that significant risks of infection, wound dehiscence, refracture, etc. still remain; also intra-articular fractures are likely to result in significant degenerative joint disease which may negate the otherwise successful result of surgery.

Finally, aspiring orthopaedic surgeons are cautioned that this type of long bone fixation is difficult surgery, requiring both detailed knowledge and specialist equipment; in most instances these cases are best referred to specialist centres. This topic is discussed at greater length in the section on radial fractures, p. 262.

Suggested further reading

White NA, Blackwell RB and Hoffman PE (1982) Use of a bone plate for repair of proximal physeal fractures of the tibia in two foals. *J Am Vet Med Assoc* **181**(3), 252–4.

External coaptation (splints and casts)

Splints

Splints are not substitute casts; they lack the necessary strength and the conforming qualities. Nevertheless, they have a definite place in emergency fracture treatment, and as a more permanent support in such conditions as angular and flexural deformities.

Splints can be made from a variety of materials. In general, those hastily fabricated from pieces of wood are ineffective: they are difficult to keep in place and tend to slip or rotate around the limb. They are definitely not adequate as a support for fractured long bones during transport.

Good splints can easily be made of plastic (PVC) guttering. Its curved cross-section gives it excellent rigidity and it is extremely light. It can be used as a single length or it can be used 'double' to encase the leg. A 10 cm (4″) diameter is suitable for foals. Larger diameters are available, or suitable sections can be cut from lengths of plastic piping using DIY power tools. These materials, which can be bought from any builders merchants, are usually thermoplastic, and can be moulded to a certain extent after the application of heat. Hot water is usually not adequate and a blow torch is usually required.

The cut ends of the plastic are usually sharp and these and the 'corners' should be rounded off. Because they do not conform to the leg shape, the lengths of guttering must be well padded. This can be done by sticking foam rubber to the concave surface, or by applying them over a heavily bandaged leg. In foals, pressure rubs are a constant source of worry and the splints should be removed every 2 days at least and reapplied after checking the leg. On the other hand, over-padding can have adverse effects, in that too great a thickness will allow movement within the splint, especially when the padding has had time to be compacted.

Single 'channels' are held in place over the padding by sticky dressing or, if applied in two halves, the plastic lengths can be held together by sticky dressing, or by lacing through pedrilled holes. Some means must also be employed to stop the 'tube' from sliding off the limb; this is best done by taping the plastic to the skin proximally and the hoof distally.

The Thomas splint

The Thomas splint has little application in equine orthopaedics. Although of value in ruminants, it is very poorly tolerated by horses. It increases the functional length of the leg, which must then be dragged around rather than advanced, and it also makes getting up and down much more difficult for the more active and less stoical species. It has sometimes been used, incorporated in a cast, for treatment of radial and tibial fractures. In this situation it provides an extension to the cast preventing the rigid distal portion of the immobilized leg acting as a lever at or near the fracture site, whilst also maintaining a degree of distraction on the fragments.

If used it should be stoutly constructed; 12 mm (½") round section mild steel bar is ideal (¼" in foals) as it can be bent by hand, with the aid of a vice. It should be shaped 'on site', to make sure that it fits exactly to the conformation of the animal, and it should, ideally, be welded together, not taped. To keep the leg in extension, holes should be drilled in both the distal tip of the splint and the hoof and the two wired together. Any portion in contact with the animal must be well padded; the ring especially needs careful attention to prevent it chafing the tender skin of the axilla or inguinal region.

The Robert Jones bandage

Originally developed for temporary immobilization of the human limb, the Robert Jones bandage is, in the author's opinion, of limited use in equine orthopaedics. It was meant to stiffen a fractured or traumatized leg or arm so that it could be passively handled, and is in no way adequate to cope with the enormous forces acting on an equine long bone fracture site. Its bulky appearance unfortunately creates a comforting illusion of strength, and animals are often transported for long distances, only to arrive with a bent limb and an 'open' fracture.

Nevertheless, it is better than no support and may be used with some degree of justification as a 'half way stage' between say, the removal of plates and full unrestricted use of the limb.

It consists of multiple layers of cotton wool strapped in place with cotton elastic bandages. Sticky elastic dressing is not essential and merely adds to the already substantial cost of the splint. Successive layers of cotton wool are added, each being held in place with elastic dressing. Each layer is applied tighter than the previous one. At the end of the overall diameter of leg and splint should not be less than some 20−23 cm (8−9″) in an adult or 15−18 cm (6−7″) in a foal. Additional stiffness can be given by incorporating pieces of wood (e.g. brush handles) in the outer layers. A U-shaped metal walking bar can be used to transmit weight bearing to the upper part of the leg. It should be shaped like the distal end of a Thomas splint and have horizontal bars welded at the top of the U to bind in with the bandages.

An unmodified Robert Jones bandage should not be used to give support to fractures above the distal third of the radius or tibia. Its weight only creates a greater lever force on the fracture site without any effective stabilization, thereby exacerbating movement between fragments. It can be made a little more effective in cases of radial fractures by incorporating a lateral chest support (see Fig. 9.20).

Slings

Slings are of limited value, but can in appropriate cases reduce stress on a fracture which has been stabilized by internal fixation, and on the other legs, reducing the risk of weight bearing laminitis and stretched flexor tendons. Only exceptional animals will tolerate slings, most slump in them or thrash wildly at great risk to themselves or their handlers. As an aid to recovery of anaesthetized fracture patients, they can be positively dangerous. Animals should not be supported until they are able to bear their own weight, otherwise they panic and throw themselves about or suffer severe respiratory embarrassment.

Constant supervision is essential, especially in the early days before the animal is accustomed to the strange sensation. In their attempts to get free they can become entangled in the webbing or turn on to their sides. To help prevent this type of behaviour the animal can be surrounded by walls of straw bales which restrict its forward, backwards and sideways movements. Food and water must be given at just below head height, and urine or faecal contamination cleaned daily to reduce the risk of excoriation and pressure sores.

Casts

Casts are used not only in many large animal orthopaedic situations, but also in the treatment of lower limb trauma to immobilize healing tissues and also rapid granulation of wounds. Theoretically the equine distal limb is a very suitable subject for casting in that there is little soft tissue covering to cushion its immobilizing effect. However, casting is less than an ideal solution in that the main stresses of weight bearing act axially, and against these a cast is of little value, impaction and instability occurring as the animal attempts to bear weight.

There are several basic principles which must be heeded when applying a cast to an equine limb:

1 To immobilize a fracture adequately both the joints above and below the fracture must be included in a cast.

2 Casts must not end in the middle of a diaphysis or near a fracture line: the pendulum effect of the heavy distal mass of limb and cast will put a tremendous strain on the area.

3 Casts must be 'snug' fitting. Looseness results in differential movement between cast and leg; differential movement causes rubs.

4 The foot should always be completely included in a cast.

5 Casts are expensive! Broken casts are even more expensive. Without exceeding the obvious weight limits, an extra roll of casting material is well worthwhile!

6 Remember that at some stage the cast must be removed! Full thickness casts on adult horses are well-nigh impossible to remove without a power-driven oscillating saw.

Materials

The traditional casting material, plaster of Paris bandage, is now virtually obsolete in large animal situations. It has low strength for its weight, resulting in impossibly heavy and bulky casts, and the inordinately long time it takes to reach maximum strength (24 hours) means that many casts fracture as animals rise from anaesthesia. However, many alternative casting materials are now available and new ones appear regularly.

The ideal casting material should have three attributes; firstly, it should conform well to the shape of the limb, fitting closely to each contour to prevent rubs; secondly it should be very strong for its weight; and thirdly, it should attain adequate strength in as short a time as possible.

At present, and this may of course change as new materials appear, no one material currently available fulfills all three criteria. Fortunately, an excellent compromise can be made by using a combination of different types of casting agent, using the good qualities of each.

Without doubt, the best conforming qualities are found in the plaster bandage. The new resin-based plasters are very rapid setting, some extremely so, a quality which is extremely useful if a cast has to be applied to a standing horse. If these materials are used to create a first layer, a good snug fitting cast is assured. Strength is then given by applying a second material, one of the lightweight, thermoplastic open-weave bandages (e.g. Hexolite) or a fibreglass resin tape (e.g. Vetcast) on top of the almost dry plaster. It is the author's experience that this latter type of material does not conform well enough to the minor contours of the leg to be used alone. However, in combination with plaster bandage, they produce a lightweight, extremely strong, snug fitting cast.

The practicalities

In an emergency, a cast may have to be applied to the standing horse, and with the rapid setting resin plasters this is quite feasible. However, the inevitable accompanying discomfort is likely to cause some movement, usually at the most inopportune moment when the plaster is just about to harden. This can have two effects; firstly to cause microfracture and disruption of the plaster-to-plaster and layer-to-layer bond; and secondly wrinkling or bunching of the still-soft casting material. The former will result in a weakened cast, and the latter in localized pressure points between the cast and the skin. This means that casts applied in the standing position fracture more easily and are more likely to cause rubs than those put on under the more controlled conditions of general anaesthesia. The clinician must remember that if the two-layer system is used, the inner plaster layer can fracture within an intact outer sheath, resulting in a functionally loose cast and local pressure rubs.

Casts which are destined to remain on for long periods should be put on under general anaesthesia. As well as minimizing the risks outlined above, manipulation of the fracture, including traction, is possible.

The leg must be carefully prepared. If soiled, it should be thoroughly washed and then carefully dried, preferably with a fan heater or hair drier. The hair should then be smoothed or brushed to lie flat. Traction is applied using ropes tied to wire threaded through a hole drilled in the toe of the hoof. The foot can be held in the 'neutral', partly flexed, toe down position, or using other ropes pulling at different angles, in an extended weight bearing position (Fig. 9.21). It must be remembered that if any part of the limb is pulled into an unnatural position before casting, it will, when traction is released, attempt to spring back within the cast, causing localized pressure points. In this situation an earlier cast change may be prudent.

There is no doubt that only the barest minimum of padding should be used under a cast. Padding compresses and allows movement; movement causes rubs, and, as important, may delay or prevent fracture healing. Wounds or incision lines should be dry initially and covered with the minimum size of dressing, preferably the type with a non-adherent plastic film. To prevent the cast from sticking to the hair, the leg should be covered with a tubular stockingette-type bandage. Two layers are adequate to prevent the plaster contaminating the skin and these should initially extend several inches above the proposed proximal limit of the cast. Ordinary bandages should not be used as they will ruck-up and cause local areas of pressure. To prevent chafing at the top of the cast a 5 cm (2″) wide strip of orthopaedic felt should be stuck to the stockingette in a band encircling the leg. At this stage traction is applied and the leg manoeuvred into the position in which it will be cast. If a final check reveals no last-minute adjustment to be made the plaster can be applied.

Until the requisite skill has been acquired it is best to use the rapid setting plaster type and not the very rapid which allows no room for error. Working quickly, but not rushing, apply the first

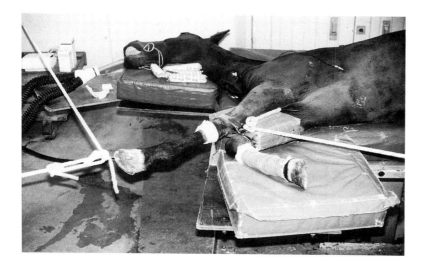

Fig. 9.21 Illustration of how a system of ropes exerting counteracting forces can keep a leg in extension whilst a cast is being applied.

layers, blending them into each other by continuous smoothing movements. The bandages can be rolled on to the leg, provided no tension is put on them and there is no need to construct 'slabs' as in the dog. If the fracture is unstable it is wise to pause after a few layers and, after checking the fragment alignment, wait until the plaster has hardened sufficiently to maintain that alignment before recommencing. Any pressure should be applied through the palm of the hand so as to spread the load. Gripping with the fingers can leave indentations in the plaster which may cause pressure points and cast rubs. The plaster thickness is then built up to the required level, being careful to include the foot and toe extending to the proximal end of the felt 'collar'. In an adult horse the plaster should be about 1 cm thick; in a foal, slightly less.

After some 10−15 minutes the resin plaster cast will be firm and hot, being exothermic in its setting reaction. At this stage the outer sheath of thermoplastic or other fibreglass type bandages can be applied. Again care should be taken to include the foot. Failure to do so will cause the cast to fracture at the coronary band and pressure sores to develop there or on the dorsal pastern region. When this layer has hardened, the stockingette is folded down to cover the sharp proximal rim of the cast and the wire snipped off at the toe.

Three refinements to this basic technique are: firstly to coat the toe and the solar surface of the cast with an acrylic cement or epoxy resin filler. This will serve the double function of preventing wear and waterproofing the sole. Secondly, in casts which extend to below the carpus, a notch should be cut out of the top rim just below the accessory carpal bone (Fig. 9.22). If this is not done the cast will rub on this protruberance causing a pressure sore. Thirdly, the top of the cast should always be sealed with sticky elastic dressing to prevent hay seeds, shavings, etc. from falling into the cast and causing irritation.

Removal of casts

Casts are expensive, especially when added to the cost of a general

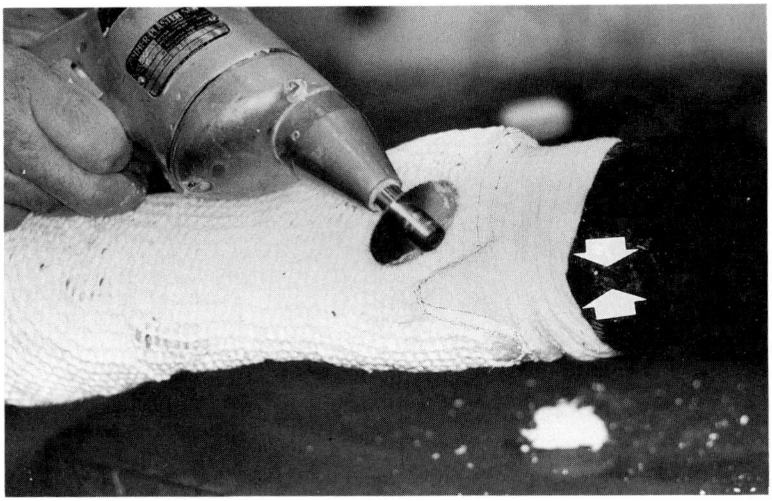

Fig. 9.22 A notch has been cut out of this cast on its proximal palmar surface to prevent pressure rubs on the accessory carpal region (arrowed).

anaesthetic and there is an obvious reluctance to change them unnecessarily 'just to check'. Whilst no absolute rules can be laid down as to when to change a cast (apart from when one breaks), some general guidelines can be given. Early cast change should be considered when

1 The cast has been applied over much soft tissue swelling. This will reduce and allow movement within the cast.

2 The cast has been applied over a wound, either sutured or granulating. In the first instance to check for dehiscence, and in the second, because exudate will soften the cast within a few days.

3 There is a worsening of lameness, which *persists* for more than 48 hours after the application of the cast, or interrupts a gradual improvement. This would, in all likelihood, indicate the development of a significant cast rub. (Sometimes after reapplication of a cast there can be a transient 24—48 hour increase in lameness which then disappears.)

4 When the sole of the cast wears through sufficiently to allow movement of the hoof within. This will rapidly lead to rubs at the coronory band.

Casts can be removed from standing horses of suitable temperament or when they are sedated, though a cast on a partially healed fracture would obviously need to be changed under a general anaesthetic. Casts on horses' legs are well nigh impossible to remove without a special oscillating saw. Whilst these are safe if handled properly, they can cause severe lacerations if they are dragged across skin or applied to skin which has been stiffened by plaster contamination of the hair. They should be used to cut vertically down into the cast, and *not* along it. Unlike dog casts which can be levered open sufficiently to remove the leg, a strong cast on a horse's leg must be cut down both sides, or front and back and removed as two halves. Fighting to remove a partially healed fractured leg from a springy half-sawn cast can lead to problems!

Following cast removal, the clinician must be aware that disuse osteopaenia and joint stiffness will be present, and that exercise should be reintroduced only gradually.

10: Degenerative Joint Disease (Osteoarthritis, Arthritis)

Introduction

Degenerative joint disease (DJD) is a vastly complicated subject which, as yet, is poorly understood in the horse. A detailed discussion on the subject is beyond the scope of this book and those interested should consult the suggested further reading section later.

Much controversy exists over the terminology in this subject and many authorities disagree. A poll of the literature suggests that 'degenerative joint disease' (DJD) is probably the best term for the phenomenon as it occurs in horses, with 'osteoarthritis', or, simply 'arthritis' being the best synonym. In man, some age-related joint changes have no inflammatory component and are given the name 'osteoarthrosis'. This does not seem to be appropriate in the horse, where the clinical syndrome is characterized by inflammatory change.

Rheumatoid arthritis is a systemic, immune system-mediated disease. It results in synovial proliferation and cartilage destruction and affects multiple joints. It is not reported in the horse.

Aetiology

DJD is sub-divided into primary and secondary types. Primary DJD is the state of affairs in which normal ageing changes have caused the degeneration. It is of great concern in man and it is suggested that it might occur in dogs too; however, it can, to all intents, be dismissed as an entity in horses. Advancing age inevitably leads to the accumulation of damage to the body in general, and to joints in particular, and there is no doubt that the incidence of 'secondary DJD', i.e. consequent upon some external insult, increases with age. DJD usually has a multifactoral aetiology though only one or two factors may be important in any one instance. Looked at another way, DJD can be thought of as a collection of pathological joint changes which are the common end-point of many disease processes and physical insults.

Prime amongst the physical insults is direct trauma, from blows, kicks and collisions with fences, cars, etc. A single incident may not result in any detectable change but the worse the trauma, the greater the likelihood of some permanent change. Joint capsule, periarticular ligament and synovial membrane damage can all lead to permanent changes within the joint and especially if there is bleeding into the joint cavity (haemarthrosis). Injuries which involve direct damage to the articular surface and subchondral bone, e.g. articular fractures, usually lead to irreversible changes unless there is very prompt diagnosis and effective treatment.

Repetitive minor trauma may also lead to those irreversible changes though this is extremely difficult to quantify, and associations between cause and effect are often surmised and not proven. The factors which lead to this type of insult are; hard conditions underfoot or excessive road work; poor conformation, possibly the result of poorly corrected juvenile angular deviations and unbanked or badly designed racing surfaces. Activities which call for unnatural gaits or excessive twisting and turning, for example barrel racing can also be a cause; also bad or inadequate training schedules resulting in exhaustion, inco-ordination and hyperextension of limb joints. Infection too, and, of course, the nutritional and managemental practices which, intermingled with certain inherited tendencies, predispose to the ever-increasing incidence of osteochondrosis and its sequelae.

Pathogenesis

The pathogenesis of DJD in the horse has not been fully elucidated. Parts of the story are known, but many are missing and await further research. Two principal factors appear to operate: biomechanical and biochemical. They can probably act both separately and in concert, though their exact interrelationship is not known.

A detailed description of these changes is outside the scope of this book, and those interested should study the relevant current literature. However, a brief summary will be given.

Biochemical changes

The two principal changes to occur involve the proteoglycans, and secondly the intra-articular enzymes.

Proteoglycans are very large, complex molecules synthesized by the chondrocytes. They comprise a linear core protein to which are attached myriads of macromolecular, glycosaminoglycan side chains. The total molecular weight of each molecular complex can be as high as 4×10^{10}. Not only that, but these complexes, once formed, aggregate within the matrix, bound together by hyaluronate, to form truly enormous units with a total molecular weight of up to 100×10^{10}.

The glycosaminoglycan side chains of these huge molecules are strongly negatively charged; they therefore repel each other and those of neigbouring proteoglycan molecules. In addition, the electrostatic forces also attract and hold water molecules, thus hydrating the cartilage matrix and providing compressive resistance. However, the substance of the matrix would have no tensile strength at all if it were merely composed of proteoglycans and water. To give it this quality and its coherence, these gigantic protein molecules are entrapped in a meshwork of collagen fibre arcades, which lie like a series of hoops in the layer of articular cartilage. The combination of collagen fibres, entrapped proteoglycan molecules and bound water gives cartilage its unique properties of compressive stiffness, tensile strength and elasticity.

DJD is characterized by the loss of proteoglycans from the matrix of the articular cartilage causing a decrease in its elasticity and its resistance to compression. The delicate chondrocyte and collagen fibres are therefore exposed to trauma and mechanical damage. The loss of proteoglycans can be quite dramatic in experimentally induced arthritis, and in man has been shown to be directly proportional to the severity of the disease.

Also, a consistent feature of arthritic joints is a reduction in hyaluronic acid concentration. As this substance is responsible for binding the proteoglycan molecules together, it is reasonable to assume that any reduction in its concentration will result in a failure of aggregation, the sequel to which would be the degradation of cartilage mentioned above. The full story is, of course, much more complex and details of the interrelationship of these compounds and the causes of reduced concentrations and interactions are not yet fully understood. It is known however, that some of these changes can occur in immobilized joints or those with a reduced loading, factors which may be significant from both clinical and managemental aspects.

Enzymes also play a major role in the development of DJD. In normal cartilage, synovial membrane and synovial fluid enzyme levels are low, but increases in the concentration of different types occur as the disease progresses. Within the cartilage, the chondrocytes themselves begin to secrete enzymes which degrade the surrounding matrix: why is not certain, but it would appear from this that the early stages of cartilage degeneration are endogenous. With the development of a synovitis for any reason, e.g. external trauma, sepsis or the release of proteoglycans from damaged cartilage, the synovial membrane cells, principally type A, begin to form lysosomes and release exogenous enzymes into synovial fluid. Inflammatory cells also contribute to the total concentration. These enzymes, including hyaluronidase, promote further inflammation and then, once proteases have increased the permeability of the surface cartilage layers, the cartilage matrix too is attacked. The products of enzymic degeneration stimulate further inflammatory change, more enzyme production and the whole cycle repeats itself with increasing vigour.

Biomechanical changes

The biomechanical theory for the aetiology of DJD is sometimes put forward as an alternative to the biochemical one. It is highly likely that it is not so much an alternative but an additional factor, playing sometimes a major role, other times a lesser one: it is probable that no one factor acts in isolation.

It has been well established that cartilage is present in much too thin a layer to have any significant shock-absorbing effect during joint loading. This is the role of the subchondral bone which modifies its structure in accordance with Wolff's law to meet the imposed loads. The biomechanical theory suggests that abnormal stresses cause an increased rigidity of the subchondral bone; the cartilage is then deprived of its proper support, absorbs much more of the loading stresses and begins to degenerate.

The abnormal stresses can occur in a number of ways; for example, as a result of inadequate training schedules, from the absolute overloading of the distal limbs of performance, rodeo type animals or those bred with large bodies and slim legs. Excessive road work could also be the cause; overweight or a heavy rider could contribute too. Whatever the cause the resulting impulse loading is thought to cause microfracture of the subchondral bone. The body's reaction is to remodel the site, lay down new bone and increase the rigidity of the area; cartilage then takes more of the strain and begins to break down. This is probably compounded by lubrication problems caused by the change in cartilage elasticity, and the result is release of matrix compounds into the joint and a resulting synovitis.

Whilst this theory implies that increased stress is the instigator of these changes, the converse may also apply. Reduced activity may lead to deficient nutrition of certain areas of cartilage. If the joint is suddenly stressed these areas may not be able to transmit the loads, and again breakdown of cartilage integrity could occur. This scenario, although sounding implausible at first, is exceedingly common in reality, as children's ponies stand idle all week, working only for a few hectic hours every weekend.

Pathology

Whatever the instigating factors of the degenerative process, once in motion it is a self-perpetuating vicious cycle.

With proteoglycan loss, the normal balance between production and destruction of matrix material is disturbed. One of the first casualties is the water-binding effect of these large molecules. Water is lost from the matrix and the cartilage loses its healthy, wet bloom. The degeneration progresses to the next stage of cartilage fibrillation. Now the collagen fibrils, no longer supported by solid matrix, begin to lift off the cartilage surface; this exposes more matrix and chondrocytes which then die, releasing enzymes and debris into the joint. With time, fibrillation leads to cartilage thinning and fissuring. In turn this results in a reduced ability to resist concussion and loading the process is perpetuated and aggravated.

Unless the initiating factor itself caused some clinical signs, the joint changes which have occurred to this point will have produced no outward signs of pain or swelling; neither will radiographic changes be evident. Debris released by the degenerating cartilage will have been removed by the synovial membrane and the joint cleansing process will be under control. However, if the amount of degradation increases to the point where the synovial membrane cannot cope with the amount of debris such as cartilage and collagen fragments, dead chondrocytes, blood cells, etc. then inflammation, or synovitis results and the first clinical signs begin to show.

The inflammatory change in the synovial membrane consists initially of hyperaemia and oedema. There are changes in the synovial lining cells and accumulation of lymphocytes, leucocytes and plasma cells becomes evident. All these cell types are instrumental in adding more enzymes to the intra-articular pool. With time, changes occur in the synovial fluid so that it becomes a less efficient lubricator and the effect is compounded by increasing disuse of the limb as a result of pain. These factors contribute to the joint's problems, adding yet more impetus to the vicious cycle of events.

At this stage the first characteristic radiographic signs begin to appear. At the junction between cartilage and synovial tissue there is an increasing vascularity which is followed by mineralization of the peripheral cartilage adjacent to the synovial tissue and periosteum. The first discernible changes are a 'squaring off' of the joint margins, followed by distinct lipping and eventually discrete spur formation (Fig. 10.1). It is important to recognize that, by the time even subtle radiographic changes are evident, much pathological change has already occurred.

A second, often radiographically recognizable change occurs in the sub-chondral region with the formation of cysts. These may be formed in the very early stages of DJD as a result of myxoid change in the deep cartilage layers. The cause is increased turnover of proteoglycan without a concomitant shedding of the surplus into the synovial fluid: alternatively, they can be formed around trabecular microfractures in the subchondral bone. A later cause is the forcing of synovial fluid into small fissures in the cartilage face. The resultant cysts would form in accompaniment to the other signs of DJD. These cysts are often clearly seen in some cases of tarsal osteoarthritis or spavin.

In summary, DJD consists of two distinct pathological paths; one leading to loss of articular cartilage with an end-point of exposure of subchondral bone, bone erosion and eburnation; the other resulting in bone remodelling, presumably in an attempt to renew and add to the effective weight bearing surface of the joint. Once at a certain level these processes are all self-perpetuating with each biochemical and physical change wrought by the disease process serving only to fuel the pathological fire.

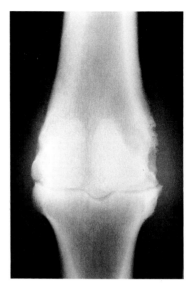

Fig. 10.1 Note the prominent periarticular osteophytes in this advanced case of fetlock degenerative joint disease.

Diagnosis

The diagnosis of DJD is based principally on history, clinical signs and radiology. Other aids such as synovial fluid analysis and synovial biopsy may also be used. The first three criteria are dealt with more specifically under individual joint headings, but a brief account of synovial fluid analysis will be given here.

Synovial fluid analysis

Synovial fluid is a dialysate of blood plasma. Normal samples are clear, pale yellow and contain no flocculent material. It is important to realize that synovial fluid from degenerating joints can be normal, especially in the very early stages. In these circumstances the volume of fluid and the ease with which it was aspirated are good pointers to increased production and joint distension. Red blood cells do not occur in normal fluid although blood streaking may occur as a result of the needle puncture. Recent haemorrhage into the joint will result in a diffuse blood tingeing, older haemorrhage yields a dark yellow specimen. Some blood staining may occur in advanced DJD, as a result of multiple focal damage to the synovial membrane, or through diapedesis of the red blood cells: it can also occur as a result of warfarin therapy. Turbidity of samples can be caused by the presence of large numbers of leucocytes and/or cell and cartilage debris, these would be features of advanced DJD or infection.

Normal synovial fluid will not clot, neither will most samples from joints with uncomplicated DJD. However, fluid from large affected joints and those with marked synovitis may do so. Synovial fluid also exhibits the phenomenon of thixotropy which can mimic clotting as the fluid assumes an almost gelatinous consistency. It is most marked in fluid from small joints and can be distinguished from clotting by the fact that the 'coagulum' can be dispersed by gentle shaking.

Synovial fluid viscosity can be easily assessed by stretching a droplet between thumb and forefinger; or allowing it to drip from a needle. Normal viscosity allows the stretching of a coherent column of fluid to over 2.5 cm (1″) before it breaks. Viscosity is a measure of hyaluronic acid polymerization and should be normal in simple DJD. The viscosity decreases in joints affected by recent trauma or in septic arthritis.

The protein content of synovial fluid is lower than that of plasma with a normal value of some 2.0 g/dl. In early DJD the total value remains relatively unchanged but the albumin/globulin ratio will alter as the larger alpha and gamma globulins enter through more permeable capillaries.

Protein values above 2.5 g/dl indicate an abnormality, usually traumatic arthritis or infection; values above 4.0 g/dl indicate severe inflammatory change.

Only small numbers of leucocytes are present in normal synovial fluid. Fluid from joints with DJD again shows normal values from $0-1000/mm^3$. In the case of acute traumatic arthritis counts can be as high as 30,000, though values of $10-20,000$ are more usual. In cases of infective arthritis the counts will exceed 50,000 with neutrophils being the predominant cell type.

Cytological examination of the leucocytes from a case of DJD will show only normal cells. In severe traumatic arthritis they show varying ageing changes including nuclear hypersegmentation. In infectious arthritis many of the cells will be degenerating.

Histological examination of debris obtained from joint fluid can give a good indication of the pathological process within. Synovial particle analysis can reveal collagen fibrils and flakes of cartilage and chondrocytes. As the erosion penetrates deeper into the cartilage, larger flakes are seen.

Other tests which can be done include measurement of glucose levels, mucin precipitate quality and enzyme levels — aspartate aminotransferase, lactic dehydrogenase and alkaline phosphate levels will all be useful indicators of joint inflammation.

Despite the availability of batteries of tests which can, as outlined above, be used to evaluate synovial fluid, it is necessary to sound a note of caution. Many factors can influence the various parameters discussed, including which joint the sample was taken from, the amount of loading experienced by the joint (i.e. the stage of training or activity of the animal) and the method of handling or storage of the samples. No one sample is likely to be of much value unless the changes are gross; rather serial samples could be used to monitor progressions or response to treatment, or synovial fluid versus plasma values may be used to give more accurate evaluations of joint status.

Treatment

DJD cannot be cured! Once established, the physical change cannot be significantly reversed. Therefore every effort should be directed towards preventing its onset in the first place! Early diagnosis of chip fractures, fissures, etc. and early treatment through surgery, joint lavage and rest is vital and is the geatest contribution a veterinary surgeon can make towards managing this condition. However, it is obvious from the large number of multiple joint problems seen in comparatively young horses that individual joint trauma is not the only cause. Other aetiological factors have been implicated earlier in this section and the author believes strongly that it is also the veterinarian's role to pressurize and influence the horse industry and horse owning public into more sensible and natural ways of husbandry, and to help curb the more outright exploitation of the animal.

Rest

Rest is an invaluable form of treatment. It cuts short the insult to the joint and allows time for the natural reparative processes to get the 'upper hand'. However, in cases where there is mechanical damage to the articulation, rest is no substitute for surgical intervention. It must be realized too that neither rest or any other treatment will allow complete healing.

Too long a period of complete rest can be counterproductive in two ways: firstly it will result in gross unfitness, and secondly prolonged stasis can lead to problems with articular cartilage nutrition and capsular and ligament laxity. After some 3–4 weeks, controlled exercise is indicated and walking in hand, starting with a few minutes a day and building up over some 3 months to unlimited walking, is a reasonable regime in cases of severe joint insult: at this time trotting, again in hand, can begin. One of the dangers which must be stressed is of allowing these animals unrestricted freedom too soon; 2 minutes of kicking their heels up around a paddock can undo the good work of months! A second consequence is to waste a great percentage of the animal's useful life. Twelve months inactivity will result in no better resolution than the regime outlined above, will have cost the owner economically and may have raised false hopes of an eventual 'complete' recovery.

Corticosteroids

Corticosteroids, although much maligned, do have a place in the treatment of DJD. Their bad reputation comes from their overuse in the early days, when there was little appreciation of their adverse effects, and from their association with the racing industry where they have been extensively used to camouflage the effects of injury and keep horses in work.

They are indicated in the treatment of early joint injury to reduce the inflammatory changes which will eventually lead to DJD. A single intra-articular injection will lead to a diminution in the signs of inflammation and a clinical improvement. At the cellular level, synovial membrane inflammation and capillary permeability are reduced, lysosomal membranes are stabilized and enzyme production and action are suppressed. Synovial fluid changes are soon apparent with a decrease in volume and an increase in viscosity. Hyaluronic acid concentration and polymerization are improved.

However, these are short term effects and, provided they are capitalized upon by following up with a period of rest, they can be beneficial. With long term therapy the adverse effects of corticosteroids come to the fore. These consist at the macroscopic level of changes such as thinning, fissuring and fibrillation of cartilage and a decrease in its elasticity. Other effects can be the formation of calcified concentrations on the cartilage surface and, as steroid is deposited in the periarticular tissues, metastatic calcification of fibrous joint capsule, ligaments and tendons. At the cellular level, there is an increased level of nuclear degeneration in chondrocytes and the formation of cysts within the cartilage substances. These and other intracellular changes result in a substantial depression of protein and proteoglycan synthesis which may not recover for many months. These effects seem to be heightened in the presence of cartilage damage, e.g. chip fractures, when steroid injections can result in advanced DJD. Following surgery in treated joints, the incidence of wound problems and intra-articular sepsis is much higher.

In summary, steroids may have a use in some cases of joint trauma. They must be used early on, in the absence of articular surface damage as indicated by synovial fluid analysis, and their use *must*, repeat, *must*, be followed by a rest period of at least 3−4 weeks. Contraindications to their use are: infection in or around the joint; the presence of extensive bony lesions; and where there is evidence that previous intra-articular injections of corticosteroids have been ineffective. In addition it must be remembered that injection of many forms of corticosteroid can itself produce a *transient*, though often marked inflammatory response, the so-called 'post injection flare'. It is likely to be the result of a mechanical irritation of the synovial membrane by the microcystalline structures of the preparation. Although of no clinical significance it can be worrying unless the cause is appreciated.

NB whenever steroids are injected into a joint the strictest possible aseptic precautions must be taken!

Non-steroidal, anti-inflammatory drugs (NSAIDs)

NSAIDs are agents which reduce the synthesis of prostaglandins. Prostaglandins are the cause of many of the symptoms of inflammation — fever, oedema, erythema and pain, the latter by increasing the sensitivity of nerve receptors to stimuli and the effects of pain producing substances. NSAIDs inhibit the essential enzyme cyclo-oxygenase, thereby also inhibiting the synthesis of prostaglandin and blocking the prime inflammatory pathways. They also inhibit kinin formation and can prevent the action of kinin and SRSA (*s*low *r*eleasing *s*ubstance of *a*naphylaxis) on smooth muscle and vascular endothelium. NSAIDs do not appear to be entirely beneficial however, as there is evidence that some actually slow down the synthesis of glycosamino-glycan. However, there is no doubt that overall, their effects are generally beneficial in DJD, possibly by easing the pain of joint movement and thereby improving cartilage nutrition.

In the medical world, aspirin is the most well known and widely used NSAID. It is cheap and very useful in a number of situations. Unfortunately, it, and other similar drugs such as indomethacin, have not found a place in equine therapy, principally because of the high rate of clearance in alkaline urine.

Phenylbutazone ('Bute', PBZ) is the drug most commonly used in horses. Despite its obvious value in the treatment of certain orthopaedic conditions, its use has been the subject of much controversy. Whilst there is no doubt that it is frequently misused, to mask overt lameness at sale or during athletic competition, there is little justification for the often hysterical outcry against its use. The author would have more sympathy with this point of view if those opposing its use appreciated just how many lame horses and ponies are used daily. Their disabilities are not recognized because the animals are affected on two or more limbs and are not showing any easily recognizable gait abnormalities. There is no doubt that these animals would benefit greatly from having their discomfort relieved by daily use of this drug which, in adult horses at standard dose rates, is almost without side effects and which has no stimulant effect other than that produced by alleviating pain.

In cases of DJD the response to phenylbutazone varies with several factors. It is most effective in milder cases, whilst advanced pathology is refractory. The nature of the target joints also seems to have a bearing, with DJD of the relatively immobile articulations, e.g. the small joints of the hock, being most responsive.

It can be administered both systemically and orally. In acute cases of trauma, or post-operatively it may be administered intravenously. Its effect however, will not be immediate as it does not affect the degradation of prostaglandin already circulating. Several hours elapse before an analgesic response is seen and it may be 12 or more hours before physical signs of inflammation begin to regress. An initial dose rate of 8 mg/kg/day can be used, but reducing after about 4 days to 4 mg/kg/day to avoid any possible side effects. These are rare in adult horses but more frequent in foals. Gastric and small intestinal ulceration and colic following oral administration are the most commonly reported signs, with phlebitis at the intravenous injection site and in the portal veins being seen occasionally. These side effects are serious enough in young foals for great care to be necessary when contemplating high level or prolonged therapy after, say, an orthopaedic procedure.

Great care is also needed when treating the equine athletes. In the UK it is an offense to adminster any substance (other than a normal nutrient) which could alter a horse's performance 'at the time of racing'. In addition to artificial stimulation and depression of performance this also means the use of drugs to restore an animal to its normal stage. The veterinary surgeon is, therefore, often placed in an extremely difficult situation, torn between using a perfectly legitimate and effective drug and possibly contravening the rules of racing with disastrous consequences. Many other equine competition rules also ban the use of this type of drug, so clinicians are well advised to ask the owner or the appropriate ruling body before prescribing phenylbutazone or similar drugs.

After oral or intravenous administration, plasma levels return to zero after roughly 24 hours. However, it persists in the urine for at least 36 hours, while the metabolites, especially oxyphenbutazone, can be detected up to 48 hours after elimination of the drug from the systemic circulation.

To summarize; phenylbutazone is a useful drug, within certain limitations. It has no real equal in its role as a cheap, systemically administered drug suitable for long term, low grade pain alleviation, especially that arising from multiple joint DJD. However, it is not curative, it does not significantly reduce pain arising from severe DJD, it only alleviates moderate pain and, in young animals especially, it has some side effects. Its use is also severely restricted by the edicts of the equine beaurocracy!

Hyaluronic acid

The hyaluronic acid in synovial fluid is not to be confused with that produced by chondrocytes within the cartilage matrix. The former is produced by synoviocytes and is associated with a protein to form mucin — this plays an important role in joint lubrication. The degree of polymerization of the hyaluronic acid and its concentration controls the viscosity of synovial fluid. In DJD polymerization and hence viscosity are reduced.

Interestingly, it would seem from experimental work that it is the protein-containing fraction of the complex which is responsible for the lubricating effect and not hyaluronic acid, though this may have a function in reducing wear. Rather its purpose is probably to lubricate the soft tissues which, it has been calculated, may account for up to 10% of normal joint stiffness.

Hyaluronic acid, as the sodium salt, is used in the treatment of DJD. Its mode of action is not fully understood though any explanation must account both for its immediate action and its sustained effect long after the surplus drug has been cleared from the joints.

There is no doubt that the injection of high molecular weight hyaluronic acid effectively improves soft tissue lubrication, increasing joint movement and reducing pain and this would explain its immediate effects. Explanations for its long term effects include a binding of the preparation to proteoglycans at the cartilage surface, restoring it to some extent and preventing further leakage of cartilage components;

a binding and inactivation of those irritant proteoglycans which have leaked into the joint; a stimulation of further hyaluronic acid synthesis by synoviocytes and many others. The effects of intra-articular sodium hyaluronate on the healing of cartilage defects would appear from the findings of several workers to be minimal; indeed one report suggests a deleterious effect.

Sodium hyaluronate is marketed under several brand names. No standardized dosage regime is available at present and recommendations vary greatly. Such experimental work as has been done suggests a minimum dose of 20 mg for a carpal or fetlock joint, increasing for larger joint compartments such as the stifle. One intra-articular injection is usually sufficient, though some workers advocate two, several weeks apart. A rest period of 1 week or so following injection is probably indicated, followed by a slow return to work via walking and trotting exercise. The immediate effects of hyaluronate injection are not dramatic and indeed there are reports of an occasional transient increase in lameness. However, in 4–5 days, in those cases which are responsive, an improvement will occur and will persist for a variable period. The duration of improvement probably depends on the severity of inflammation, the degree of permanent change which has taken place and whether there is intra-articular damage such as a chip fracture.

Despite the uncertainties as to mode of action and the long term benefits, there is no doubt that in cases of single joint DJD, without major changes or untreated fractures, the use of intra-articular hyaluronate is beneficial. It constitutes a thoroughly physiological approach to the treatment of DJD and, provided too much is not expected of it, is an extremely useful addition to the clinican's armamentarium.

Synovial fluid transfer

Sterile transfer of normal synovial fluid from a large articulation such as the stifle to a diseased joint will confer many of the benefits listed above. The technique is comparatively simple and above all is inexpensive! It should be considered following any routine arthrotomy and as a possible alternative to the more expensive intra-articular preparations.

Glycosaminoglycan polysulphate

Glycosaminoglycan polysulphate has been used for the treatment of DJD with apparently good results. Most of the available literature concerns its use in man, and as yet little information is available on its action in equine DJD. However, it is now available in the UK as Adequan (Luitpold Werk) for use in the horse.

The compound is a polysulphated glycosaminoglycan, said to resemble closely the naturally occurring chondroitin sulphate. It is believed to act in several beneficial ways.

Following injection, catabolic lysosomal enzymes which sustain the degenerative process are inhibited, so the cartilage is protected

283

from further damage. Other inflammatory mediators are also suppressed, so synovial inflammation, pain and swelling are reduced too. It also is said to stimulate the production of highly polymerized, good quality hyaluronic acid, thus improving joint lubrication.

Its main advantage however, is that its ionic structure allows it to bind with the cartilaginous matrix in areas of cartilage destruction. It also seems to stimulate chondrocyte metabolism thus improving the strength, elasticity and other properties of cartilage. In short it would seem to stimulate cartilage healing!

Despite the drug's ability to cross synovial membranes (in man it is available as an intramuscular preparation) the drug is offered for use in horses as an intra-articular preparation. Five weekly injections of 250 mg of the active agent are recommended. In man this is the minimum dose level with 10−15 injections being the apparent optimum course. Somewhat surprisingly, the use of the drug is contraindicated in active inflammatory conditions, when appropriate initial anti-inflammatory therapy is advised. Although this drug has not been properly evaluated in the horse, its mode of action would seem to be highly promising. It is the only therapy which appears to promote cartilage regeneration and therefore offer a more physiological means of treating degenerative joint disease. The repeated intra-articular injections will certainly pose some problems to the clinician and it is desirable that further attention should be given to the other modes of administration. If this were possible and the claims for the drugs' action are substantiated, then treatment of multiple joint DJD might come a step closer.

Joint lavage

The rationale behind joint lavage is that it removes cartilaginous and other debris from the joint cavity along with synovial enzymes, etc. Ideally the lavage should be through two needles or catheters placed at opposite extremities of the joint. In a distended joint, placing the first needle is usually staightforward; the second can be difficult unless joint distension is maintained or actually increased by injection of irrigating solution. Sterile technique is mandatory and the procedure is best done under general anaesthesia.

The ideal irrigating fluid is a balanced electrolyte solution with a compatible pH (Hartmann's is ideal). Three to 6 litres are suggested in the literature, though practically 2 litres can take a long enough time to run through and will usually show a good result. Irrigation is effective at reducing inflammation and is well worthwhile in acute joint trauma and early DJD as well as in cases of septic arthritis where its use is probably better known. Its effect in individual cases may be monitored by serial examination of synovial fluid samples.

Arthrodesis

A few articulations in the equine limb lend themselves to the ultimate cure for DJD — that of arthrodesis.

The proximal interphalangeal (pastern), the proximal and distal intertarsal and the tarsometatarsal joints are the most frequently treated in this way. Occasionally metacarpophalangeal (fetlock) and pancarpal arthrodesis can be carried out, but usually for other reasons such as sesamoid dehiscence or multiple fracture of the carpal bones. The latter two are essentially salvage procedures while the pastern and hock surgery have a high success rate in restoring the animal to athletic soundness.

Suggested further reading

Fessler JF (1982) Functional anatomy and physiology of dierthrodial joints and degenerative joint diseases (osteoarthritis). In *The Practice of Large Animal Surgery*. Ed. PB Jennings. WB Saunders Co, Philadelphia.

Hackett RP (1982) Intra-articular use of corticosteroids in the horse. *J Am Vet Med Assoc* **181**(3), 292–4.

Hamm D, Goldman L and Jones EW (1984) Polysulphated glycosaminoglycan: a new intra-articular treatment for equine lameness. *Vet Med* **811**, 811–16.

Lees P and Higgins AJ (1985) Clinical pharmacology and therapeutic uses of non-steroidal anti-inflammatory drugs in the horse. *Eq Vet J* **17**(2), 83–96.

McIlwraith CW (1982) Current concepts in equine degenerative joint disease. *J Am Vet Med Assoc* **180**(3), 239–50.

Nizolek DJH and White KK (1981) Corticosteroid and hyaluronic acid treatment in equine degenerative joint disease: a review. *Cornell Vet* **71**, 355–75.

Septic arthritis and osteomyelitis in foals
(Joint ill, navel-ill, septic polyarthritis and septic epiphysitis)

Septic arthritis and osteomyelitis are inextricably intermingled in the foal and will be dealt with together.

Aetiology and pathogenesis

Foals can be infected *in utero* if the mare has a systemic infection or through the endometritis–placentitis complex. Following birth, the infection can gain entry, not just through the umbilicus but through the respiratory and digestive tracts too; the term 'navel-ill', therefore, is not always appropriate. Some factors predisposing to the development of infection are poor sanitary conditions, poor ventilation and maybe overcrowding. Stress will also increase the chances of infection as will the indiscriminate use of drugs, especially steroids. The most important factors, however, are those which result in failure to achieve adequate passive transfer of immunoglobulins from the dam's colostrum. This could be due to maternal illness, failure of the foal to suck, management problems and many others. Whatever the cause, it results in a hypogammaglobulinaemia. The establishment of infection, once introduced, is helped in the young animal by some inherent inadequacies in its defence mechanisms; the reduced phagocytic and bactericidal capacities of its leucocytes, an immature reticuloendothelial system and an increased glucocorticoid synthesis all increasing the foal's susceptibility.

The first signs will be those of a septicaemia. This can obviously vary from the peracute which leads to death within a few hours to a more chronic type with depression, listlessness, pyrexia, etc. In some the septicaemic phase can pass unnoticed, or at best the owner may notice that the foal is not quite so lively, or progressing as well as it was. The onset of lameness is often very sudden, so rapid in fact that the foal is often thought to have been 'stepped on' or otherwise damaged by the mare. This is especially so if the foal is not systemically ill or perhaps shows a degree of 'puffiness', i.e. para-articular oedema. Unfortunately this often results in the owner not seeking veterinary attention until much later!

Once in the blood stream, bacteria enter the bone via the nutrient and synovial membranes via their capillary networks, though also by direct extension from bone.

Within the metaphysis, the nurient artery forms loops which open out into venous sinusoids. The sudden slowing down of the blood as the vessel diameter increases allows bacteria to settle on the walls and begin to multiply, forming a focus of infection. There is an initial period of acute inflammation which progresses in a few days to bone ischaemia and necrosis. An abscess may form which can expand and possibly penetrate the periosteum to infect adjacent soft tissues. In the very young, bacteria can enter the physis and epiphysis via transphyseal vessels or enter the epiphysis through its own nutrient arteries.

It is in the metaphyses of long bones that osteomyelitis is most frequently seen, but other bones such as scapula, pelvis, carpal and tarsal bones, rib or vertebrae can become infected in much the same way. This is because these bones, although they do not form in the same way as long bones, have a similar vascular arrangement of articular loops and venous sinusoids adjacent to their cartilaginous regions, which trap blood-borne bacteria. These have been given the name of 'metaphyseal equivalent locations'.

Joints become infected by direct extension from surrounding tissues, or by the direct vascular route with bacteria passing through the capillary networks of the synovial membrane to colonize the synovial tissue. The infection causes inflammation which subsequently results in thrombosis of the vascular network and changes within the synovial cells. This prevents normal dialysis of plasma producing abnormal synovial fluid which is more acidic. Leucocytes invade the joint and harmful proteolytic enzymes are activated and superoxide radicals are generated. Subsequent changes include: a dilution and enzymic degradation of hyaluronic acid which is not replaced by the damaged synovial tissue; a change in the predominant white cell type from mononuclear to polymorphonuclear; an increase in protein constituents, and the formation of fibrin clots through the action of pro-thrombin, fibrinogen and activating factors.

At this stage the articular cartilage begins to suffer. Normally it receives most of its nutrition by diffusion but, with the change in the nature of the synovial fluid, this process diminishes drastically and may be stopped entirely by pannus or granulation tissue. Cartilage degradation begins and is further promoted by the effects of the proteolytic enzymes. Products of this degeneration are released into

the joint cavity, initiating further inflammatory change and instigating
a vicious cycle of inflammation, degradation, inflammation, etc.

CHAPTER 10
Degenerative Joint Disease

Diagnosis

Of those foals presenting with a sudden onset lameness, a high
proportion will be developing osteomyelitis or septic arthritis. Weakly
individuals, or those with any problem which prevents normal suckling,
must be considered prime candidates. It is simple and very tempting
to ascribe all the signs to trauma and especially so if the owner is
convinced, though usually with little factual evidence, that the dam
has trodden on the foal.

The foal's physical condition can vary enormously from apparent
normality, to a sick, listless, pyrexic animal. A clinical examination
should try to find evidence of capsular distension or puffiness around
the joints and the metaphyseal regions. Pressure over long bone ends
and manipulation of articulation should also be used in an attempt to
elicit pain.

It can be difficult to distinguish early cases from the effects of
genuine trauma. Where the facilities are available, radiography and
synovial fluid analysis from suspect joints will help clarify the picture.

For the first 48 hours or so after infection has become established
there will be no detectable radiographic changes; the main purpose of
the examination at this stage is to eliminate fractures! However, the
changes in synovial fluid following the onset of septic arthritis occur
more rapidly and will present to some extent within a few hours.
When these examinations are not immediately practicable then the
clinician should assume that he or she is dealing with infection and
start antibiotic therapy sooner rather than later.

The first radiographic signs of osteomyelitis are patchy areas of
lucency in the metaphysis, epiphysis or in metaphyseal equivalent
locations. They can develop within about 72 hours, so if nothing was
evident on the first examination, a second is advisable 3 days later.
Good quality plates are essential! The characteristic signs of septic
arthritis, para-articular periosteal proliferation and narrowing of the
joint space do not occur until much later, up to 2–3 weeks after the
onset of infection. However, radiographs are valuable in prognosis
and in monitoring the progress of infection and healing.

Analysis of synovial fluid is one of the best indicators of joint
involvement. Even a naked-eye examination can give valuable information with a reduction in viscosity (thumb and finger test), presence
of turbidity and blood staining all pointing to infection (see section
on synovial fluid analysis, p. 278). When a full analysis is done the
most telling sign is a vast increase in the number of segmented
neutrophils, with counts of over $50,000/mm^3$ being common. A practical point for those doing their own counts is that normal saline
should be used instead of the routine blood diluents; their acidity can
cause coagulation of hyaluronic acid, clumping of cells and inaccurate
counts.

Identification of the causal organism and determining its antibiotic sensitivity is of great help in choosing the correct therapy. Unfortunately this is difficult if only synovial fluid is taken. Despite severe changes in the nature of the fluid, bacteria are few and far between, preferring to colonize the synovium. For best results a synovial membrane biopsy should be done, or, on a more practical level, aspiration of fluid directly into blood culture medium. Failing this, fluid can be centrifuged and the sediment used to innoculate the media. Aerobic and anaerobic bacteria can be found causing septic arthritis in the horse, and both types should be looked for. A more direct method is to Gram stain the synovial debris and look for characteristic bacterial forms; it gives rapid result and is useful too if previous antibiotic therapy inhibits growth in culture. On a more esoteric note, the use of chromatography techniques now allow the identification of bacteria through analysis of their short chain and total fatty acid composition, without the need for culture.

Organisms commonly isolated from joints are *Salmonella* sp., *Actinobacillus equuli, Streptococcus* sp. and *Escherichia coli. Staphylococcus aureus, Klebsiella* sp. *Bacteroides* sp. and *Corynbacterium equi* are also frequently found.

Treatment

Prompt and vigorous treatment is essential in both osteomyelitis and septic arthritis. In infected joints, delay means an increased likelihood of cartilage damage, and this, despite the young animal's ability to regenerate articular cartilage to some extent, means a considerably worse prognosis due to the inevitable subsequent osteoarthritis.

In early cases there is rarely any indication of which organism is involved or its antibiotic sensitivity. The antibiotics chosen must therefore have a broad spectrum of activity and be used at full therapeutic doses. (Remember that joint aspiration must be done before therapy commences.) In the light of subsequent bacteriology results, the antibiotic may need to be changed, but whichever drug is finally chosen it must be maintained for at least 2 weeks after clinical signs have subsided. If repeated injections cause problems, an antibiotic preparation which can be given orally, e.g. the potentiated sulphonamides, can be used, provided it has an appropriate spectrum.

The inflamed synovial membrane is very permeable to antibiotics and so intra-articular therapy is not necessary in these early cases. In fact, multiple needle puncture of joints under field conditions is as likely to introduce fresh infection as to cure it. Also, most antibiotics are irritant to the synovial membrane and are likely to cause an additional synovitis. In these early stages, steroid therapy, by any route, is completely contraindicated as it suppresses what may already be a deficient immune response.

Almost as important is the ancillary supportive treatment given to the foal. If possible its immune status should be assessed using the zinc sulphate turbidity test, or Single Radical Immunodiffusion Assay. If there is a deficiency a transfusion of 20 ml/kg plasma from a suitable donor should be given. If these tests cannot be done then the animal should be assumed to be immunodeficient and the transfusion carried out regardless. Warmth, a dry environment, and, if necessary, fluid therapy will help tip the balance in favour of the foal.

Chronic infection

The keys to successful treatment of any chronic enclosed infections are drainage and debridement: this applies equally well to osteomyelitis and septic arthritis. In established pathology antibiotics alone are very rarely effective and should be used in conjunction with surgery.

Where osteomyelitis persists, fistulous tracts often form. These invariably originate from necrotic infected bone and the treatment of choice is surgical exposure of the affected area, curettage of the dead bone followed by provision of good drainage. This is obtained by leaving the wound open or only part sutured and allowing healing by second intention to occur. Full closure of these wounds invites disaster and should not be considered unless an effective drain system can be implanted. Drains can be difficult to maintain unless the foal is under constant, competent supervision. Part sutured wounds generally heal well with only the minimum of attention. One of the major problems occurs when tracts do not form and the infection becomes 'damped-down' by the antibiotic regime but not eradicated. Under these circumstances symptoms may flare up when therapy is stopped. Several changes in antibiotic type will help prevent the development of antibiotic resistance and treatment may have to be carried on for several months. As the metaphysis, physis and epiphyses are usually involved, premature closure of affected growth plates is a distinct possibility. The consequent angular deformities are difficult to treat because there can be no subsequent compensatory bone elongation on that area and treatment by growth manipulation will not work.

Septic arthritis can be considered to be in a chronic phase when there is no regression of symptoms or only partial improvement with antibiotic therapy, or where the condition has been present for more than about 48 hours. This is an arbitrary figure and rapidly progressing infection may instigate irreversible changes earlier than this. At this stage it becomes obvious that antibiotics alone will not affect a cure and physical cleansing of the joint is required.

Several methods are available but all rely on irrigation of the joint cavity to remove bacterial contamination, toxins and the ensuant debris. The irrigating fluids must be innocuous to synovial tissue and virtually all the common transfusion fluids, normal saline, lactated Ringer's and Hartmann's solutions can be used. The latter two are especially suitable because of their pH compatibility.

Distension irrigation is the simplest. A wide bore needle is inserted into the joint and a three-way tap is attached to it. A large syringe is used to alternately inject and withdraw irrigating fluid, the contaminated mixture being discarded each time. Unfortunately, as well as being the simplest, it is the least effective technique. There is no overall movement of fluid within the joint cavity and therefore little flushing effect, also parts of the joint distant from the needle will barely be affected.

A more effective technique is through-and-through irrigation with irrigation fluid entering through one needle and exiting through a second placed as far away on the other side of the joint as possible. Whilst it is possible to carry out distension irrigation under sedation alone, this technique really requires general anaesthesia. Wide bore needles, or preferably catheter needles to minimize trauma, should be used to allow a good flow rate and a minimum of 4 litres of irrigating solution should be run through. This may seem excessive, especially when the fluid runs clear after a few minutes but there is no doubt of the increased beneficial effect of large quantities. Insertion of the needles can present problems; the first is usually easy because of the distended joint capsule; the second can be difficult, unless the distension is maintained or increased by pumping in fluid through the first needle.

White cell counts done before and several days after irrigation will provide a good indicator of its efficacy and the need for further irrigation. If in doubt, irrigate again!

These techniques, though beneficial in the early case are rarely effective once joint changes have become well established and fibrin clots have formed. Being leucotactic themselves the clots enlarge, rapidly becoming too bulky or viscous to be removed through even a large bore needle. As a rough guide this will have happened some 5 days or so after the onset of infection. At this stage, simple irrigation will not be wholly effective, and it becomes necessary to perform an arthrotomy. The joint can then be thoroughly debrided and flushed and the arthrotomy left open to ensure maximum drainage.

Surprisingly, the biggest problem is keeping these arthrotomy wounds open; they close rapidly, sometimes before drainage is completed. To keep them open, a Penrose drain of soft rubber can be inserted. An irrigation catheter can also be placed into the joint and used to flush the cavity several times a day. The drains should enter and leave the joint at points as far distant from each other as possible, and with the exit point at the most dependant part of the capsule. In joints which can be kept clean by bandaging, both drain and flushing catheter can be led directly into the joint. In joints such as stifle or elbow the contamination of the joint can be minimized by leading both drain and catheter subcutaneously for 10–12 cm before entering and after leaving the articulation.

Wherever possible heavy bandaging is used to protect the area and to impart a degree of rigidity to the joint. Ideally flushing should be carried out 2–3 times a day for at least 1 week. When the clinician is happy that the joint is 'clean' then the tubes can be withdrawn and the arthrotomy incisions then heal, usually without any problem.

Ancillary therapy which can be useful, and certainly humane, is the use of non-steroidal anti-inflammatory drugs. The ones which are prostaglandin synthetase inhibitors are especially useful since they reduce the pain and swelling caused by prostaglandin release from the inflamed tissue.

Intra-articular corticosteroids can also be used in the later stages of this disease. Cartilage degredation, etc. can continue even when the joint is sterile and physically cleaned, so the marked anti-inflammatory properties of the steroid can be used to halt this process. They act by suppressing prostaglandin synthesis, preventing enzyme release, inhibiting capillary and fibroblastic proliferation and in many other ways. However, they are also immunosuppressive and *must be used cautiously and under conditions of careful monitoring.* Effective antibiotic therapy must be continued whilst they are in use and frequent synovial fluid analysis done. If there is any sign of resurgence of infection their use must be stopped immediately and joint lavage begun anew to remove infection and residual steroid.

Although no positive evidence exists to support the case, it is likely that, following the sterilizing and cleansing of an affected joint, drugs such as sodium hyaluronate, and more especially the poly-sulphonated mucopolysaccharide drugs which are reported to stimulate cartilage regeneration, would be beneficial. They are expensive and must be given into the articulation, but in a potential athlete with single joint involvement, they could be worthwhile.

Finally, whenever a joint has been affected by a septic process, some degradation will have taken place. Degenerative joint disease is therefore a certain sequel. Its severity will probably parallel the severity of the septic arthritis and in mild cases, treated early and vigorously, the subsequent effects are minimal. However, it must be a fact to take into account when embarking on what might well be a prolonged and expensive course of treatment for an established case of septic arthritis in a potential athlete.

References

Adams OR (1974) *Lameness in Horses*. Lea and Febiger, Philadelphia.

Auer JA (1980) Equine Lameness: diseases of the carpus. *Vet Clin North Am* (Large Animal Practice) **2**, 81–90.

Colles CM (1979) Ischaemic necrosis of the navicular bone and its treatment. *Vet Rec* **104**, 133.

Colles CM (1982) Navicular disease and its treatment. *In Practice*, **March**, 29–36.

Colles CM and Hickman J (1977) The arterial supply of the navicular bone and its variations in navicular disease. *Eq Vet J* **9**(3), 150–4.

Comben N, Clark RJ and Sutherland DJB (1984) Clinical observations on the response of equine hoof defects to biotin supplementation. *Vet Rec* **115**, 642–5.

Dyson S (1985) Sixteen fractures of the shoulder region in the horse. *Eq Vet J* **17**(2), 104–10.

Edwards GB (1982) Surgical arthodesis for the treatment of bone spavin in 20 horses. *Eq Vet J* **14**, 117–21.

Ellis D (1979) Fracture of the proximal sesamoid bones in thoroughbred horses. *Eq Vet J* **11**(11), 48–52.

Eyre P, Elmes PJ and Strickland S (1979) Corticosteroid-potentiated vascular responses of the equine digit: a possible pharmacologic basis for laminitis. *Am J Vet Res* **40**(1), 135–8.

Fackelman GE, Auer JA and Orsisni J (1983) Surgical treatment of severe flexural deformity of the distal interphalangeal joint in young horses. *J Am Vet Med Assoc* **182**(9), 949–52.

Gabel AA (1979) Prevention, diagnosis and treatment of inflammation of the distal hock. *Proc Am Ass Eq Prac* **28**, 287–98.

Hickman J and Walker RG (1964) *An Atlas of Veterinary Surgery*, 1e. John Wright and Sons, Bristol.

Hoppe F (1984) Radiological investigations of osteochondrosis dissecans of standardbred trotters and Swedish Warmblood horses. *Eq Vet J* **16**(5), 425–9.

Hornof WJ and O'Brien TR (1980) Radiographic evaluation of the palmar aspect of the equine metacarpal condyles: a new projection. *Vet Radiol* **21**(4), 161–7.

Leitch M (1977) A review of treatment of tuberscapulae fractures in the horse. *J Equine Med Surg* **1**, 234.

Mason TA and MacLean AA (1977) Osteochondrosis of the head of the humerus in two foals. *Eq Vet J* **9**, 189–91.

Nickels FA, Grant BD and Lincoln SD (1976) Villonodular synovitis of the equine metacarpophalangeal joint. *J Am Vet Med Ass* **168**(11), 1043–6.

Nyack B, Morgan JP, Pool R and Meagher D (1981) Osteochondrosis of the shoulder joint of the horse. *Cornell Vet* **71**, 149–63.

Obel N (1948) *Studies of the Histopathologies of Acute Laminitis*. Almqvist and Wiksells, Bokprickeri, ab upsala.

Ostblom L, Lund C and Melsen F (1982) Histological study of navicular disease *Eq Vet J* **14**(93), 199–202.

Pascoe JR, Pool RR, Wheat JD and O'Brien TR (1984) Osteochondral defects of the lateral trochlear ridge of the distal femur of the horse. Clinical, radiographic and pathological examination and results of surgical treatment. *Vet Surgery* **13**(2), 99–110.

Palmer SE (1982) Radiography of the abaxial surface of the proximal sesamoid bones of the horse. *J Am Vet Med Ass* **181**(3), 264–5.

Pettersson H and Ryden G (1982) Avulsion fractures of the caudoproximal extremity of the 1st phalanx. *Eq Vet J* **14**(4), 333–5.

Poulos PW (1983) Correlation of radiographic signs and histological changes in navicular disease. *Proc 29th Ann Conv Amer Ass Eq Prac* **29**, 244–55.

Renando VT and Grant B (1978) The equine third phalanx: its radiographic appearance. *J Am Vet Rad Soc* **19**, 125–35.

Rooney JR (1977) *Biomechanics of Lameness.* R.E. Krieger Publishing Co. Inc., Florida.

Rose RJ, Allen JR, Hodgson DR and Kohnke JR (1983) Studies on isoxsuprine hydrochloride for the treatment of navicular disease. *Eq Vet J* **15**(3), 238–43.

Sack WO and Orsini BS (1981) Distal intertarsal and tarsometatarsal joints in horse: communication and injection sites. *JAVMA* **179**(4), 355–9.

Saxe JG (1936) *The Blind Man and the Elephant: the Best Loved Poems of the American People.* Selected by Hazel Fellemen. Gandern City Books, New York.

Schmitt GR, Dueland R and Vaughan JT (1975) Osteochondrosis dissecans of the equine shoulder joint. *Vet Med Small Animal Clin* **70**, 542–7.

Sisson S and Grossman JD (1975) *The Anatomy of the Domestic Animals,* Vol 1, 5th Edn. W.B. Saunders Co., Philadelphia.

Stromberg B and Rejno S (1978) Osteochondrosis in the horse. I. A clinical and radiological investigation of osteochondritis dissecans of the knee and hock joint. *Acta Radiol* **358**(Suppl), 139.

Svalastoga E (1983) Navicular disease in the horse — a microangiographic investigation. *Nord Vet Med* **35**, 131–9.

Svalastoga E and Nielsen K (1983) Navicular disease in the horse — the synovial membrane of the bursa podotrochlearis. *Nord Vet Med* **35**, 28–30.

Svalastoga E and Smith M (1983) Navicular disease in the horse — the subchondral bone pressure. *Nord Vet Med* **35**, 31–7.

Turner AS, Milne DW, Hohn RB and Rause GP (1979) Surgical repair of fractured capital femoral epiphysis in three foals. *J Am Vet Med Assoc* **175**, 1198-202.

Wright IM (1986) Navicular suspensory desmotomy in the treatment of navicular disease: technique and preliminary results. *Eq Vet J* **18**(6), 443–6.

Wyn-Jones G and May SA (1985) Repair of proximal radius fracture in a horse. *Vet Rec* **115**, 516.

Wyn-Jones G and May SA (1986) Surgical arthrodesis for the treatment of osteoarthrosis of the proximal intertarsal, distal and tarsometatarsal joints in 30 horses: a comparison of four different techniques. *Eq Vet J* **18**(1), 59–64.

Wyn-Jones G, Peremans KY and May SA (1985) Case of quadrilateral flexural contracture in a 10 year old pony. *Vet Rec* **116**, 685–7.

Yovich JV, McIllwraith CW and Stashak TS (1985) Osteochondritis dissecans of the sagittal ridge of the third metacarpal and metatarsal bones in horses. *J Am Vet Med Ass* **186**(11) 1186–91.

Index

abaxial sesamoid nerve block 12
   hind limb 14
abscessation of the heel 37
accessory carpal bone
   fractures 112—14
   avulsion 114
Adequan *see* glycosaminoglycan
     polysulphate
adrenaline 10—11
alcohol block in navicular syndrome
     60
anaesthesia
   diagnostic regional 9—15
   intra-articular 9, 15—22
   intrabursal 15—22
   local 10—11
analgesics 59, 280—2
anamnesis 2
angular deformities
   forelimb 198—210
   hind limb 210—11
ankylosis, congenital 213
annular ligaments of the fetlock
   constriction 90—1
   resection 91
appendicular skeleton deformities
     198—223
arc of flight, alteration in 5
arthritis *see* degenerative joint
     disease, septic arthritis
arthrodesis, surgical
   DIP joint 68
   in DJD 284—5
   in spavin 148—9
   PIP joint 68—9
arthrogryposis 212
articular ring-bone 66
'articular thoroughpin' 150, 162
articular wind-gall 74
ASNB *see* abaxial sesamoid nerve
     block
aspirin 281
Australian stringhalt 191

'back in the knees' 106
'back lameness' 1
'bench knee' 95, 106
bicipital bursitis 130—1

bilateral branch desmitis 93—4
biotin, role in horn formation 30
'blood spavin' 143
board cast 86—7, 228
'bog spavin' 150—1
bone
   formation 194—6
   grafts in SBCs 180—1
   reaction to abnormal stress 275—6
'bone spavin' 142
bones, long, normal growth 194, *207*
'bowed knees' 106
'bowed tendons' 226
'boxy' hoof 132
bucked shin complex 101—2
'bunny hop' gait 210
'Bute' *see* phenylbutazone
'button' 95
'buttress foot' 50—1

calcaneometatarsal ligament strain
     167—8
calcinosis circumscripta 181—2
calcium, role in osteochondrosis 197
cannon bones
   bucked shin complex 101—2
   fractures
      condylar 253—8
      cortical fissure 102—3
      shaft 259—62
      slab 101
      spiral fissure 258—9
capped elbow 120—1
capped hock 166—7
Carbocaine 11, 15
carbohydrate intake, relationship
     with laminitis 44
carbon fibre implantation in tendons
     230—1
carpal blocks 18—19
carpal canal (tunnel) syndrome
     114—15
carpometacarpal joint 18, 104
   see also carpus
carpus
   acute trauma 116—18
   anatomy 104, *108*
   arthrotomy 110

Note: Page numbers in italic refer to figures

biomechanics 105−6
chronic swelling 118−19
clinical examination 106−7
degenerative joint disease 107−8
flexural deformity 214−15
fluid swellings 115−16
fractures
    chip 108−10
    multiple 112
    slab 110−12
ossification 200−1
radiography 104−5
carpus valgus 106
carpus varus 106
cartilage 194
fibrillation 276
plastic deformation 200
reaction to abnormal stress 275−6
reaction to trauma 37
case history 2
case record 1
cassettes, radiographic 24−5
casts 268−9
application 270−1
board 86−7, 228
gutter 202, 266
materials 269
removal 271−2
catsear, implicated in Australian
    stringhalt 191
cellulitis 150
cervical spinal malformation 197
chestnut 29
clinical examination 1−22
'clover-leaf' nails 127
coffin bone see pedal bone
coffin joint see distal interphalangeal
    (DIP) joint
'cold splint' 96
copper deficiency, role in
    osteochondrosis 197, 206
corium 28
'corns' 39−40
coronary band 28
coronary cushion 28
cortical fissure fractures 102−3
corticosteroids 279−80
intra-articular in DJD 81
    relationship with slab fractures
    111
in laminitis 47
see also cortisone
cortisone
effect on growth 196
intrabursal injection 59
see also corticosteroids
cow hock 141, 167
coxofemoral joint
block 22
dislocation 188−9

cryoneurectomy in navicular
    syndrome 60
cunean tendon
anaesthesia 21
bursitis 145
tenotomy 148
curb 167−8
cysts see sub-chondral bone cysts
    (SBC)

debridement 235
deep digital flexor tendon (DFT) 53
'contracture' 215
division 227
lacerations 234−6
mineralization 58
sheath distensions 161−5
strain/sprain 224−31
tenotomy 218
degenerative joint disease (DJD)
aetiology 273−4
carpus 107−8
diagnosis 277−9
DIP joint 64−6
MCP joint 78−81
in navicular syndrome 62, 63
pathogenesis 274−6
pathology 276−7
PIP joint 71−2
stifle joint 185−6
treatment 279−85
see also tarsal osteoarthritis
desmitis 92
bilateral branch 93−4
main ligament body 93−4
single branch 92−3, 93−4
detection of lameness 3−8
DFT see deep digital flexor tendon
    (DFT)
diagnosis of causes of lameness 1−22
digital extensor tendon
resection 191
rupture 214−15
DIP joint see distal interphalangeal
    (DIP) joint
directional nomenclature 11
distal interphalangeal (DIP) joint
block 16, 17
congenital hyperextension 214
degenerative disease 64−6
extension 7
flexural deformity 215−18
phalangeal exostoses affecting
    66, 68
distal intertarsal (DIT) joint
block 20−1, 144
see also tarsal osteoarthritis
distal sesamoid see navicular bone
disuse osteopenia 85, 86

DIT joint *see* distal intertarsal (DIT) joint
DJD *see* degenerative joint disease
'dorsiflexion strap' *221*
'dropped elbow' stance 122

eburnation 259−60
eggbar shoe 47, 62
elbow joint 121
  block 19
  luxation 121−2
  septic arthritis 125−6
  swelling at point of 120−1
enchondral ossification 194−6
  in newborn foals 200−1
endotoxins, role in laminitis 44
enthesiophytes
  navicular bone 58
  pedal bone 50
  in spavin 142, 145, *146*
  see also osteophytes
enzymes, intra-articular, role in DJD 274, 275
epinephrine 10−11
epiphyseal dysplasia 203−4
  distal metatarsal 211
ergot 29
extension tests 6−7
extensor process of the pedal bone, fracture of 51−2
extensor tendons, laceration 232
external coaptation 266−72

femoral capital epiphysis fracture 188
femoropatellar joint 21, 168
  see also stifle joint
femorotibial joint 21, 168
  see also stifle joint
femur fractures 186−8
fetlock joint *see* metacarpophalangeal joint
fibreglass resin tape 269
fibrous and ossifying myopathy 191−2
  gait alterations in 5
fillers for horn 32
films, radiographic 25
firing 147, 229−30
1st phalanx fractures 248−50
  fixation 250−3
flat weed, implicated in Australian stringhalt 191
flexion tests 6−8
  carpal 106
flexor tendons *see* deep digital flexor tendon (DFT); superficial digital flexor tendon (SFT)
flexural contractures *see* flexural deformities

flexural deformities 212
  acquired 214−23
  congenital 212−14
'footy' gait 5
forelimb
  angular deformities 198−210
  distal nerve distribution *12*
  regional nerve blocks 11−14
  see also individual bones and joints
four-point block 13
  hind limb 14
4th metacarpal *see* splint bones
fracture fixation
  femur 187−8
  pelvis 190
  post-operative complications in neonates 127, 188
  techniques 237−72
frog 28−9
  penetrating injury 33−7
  preparation for radiography 42, 238
  trimming 29−30

gastrocnemius bursa, distension 162
generator 23
'ghost sesamoids' 85, *86*
glycosaminoglycan polysulphate 81, 108, 283−4
grass cracks 31−2
greater trochanter, fracture of 188
grids, radiographic 23−4
growth
  asymmetrical 204−6
  normal 194
  periods of maximum *207*
  retardation 207−9
  stimulation 209−10
growth plate 194−5
  asymmetric growth at 204
    treatment 207−10
  distal tibial 211
  osteochondrosis 205−6
  radiography 206−7
  Salter−Harris injury classification 205
  trauma 204−5
gutter casts 202, 266

head carriage in forelimb lameness 3−4
heel
  abscessation 37
  traumatic wounds 39
high ring-bone 66
hind limb
  angular deformities 210−11
  deformity 218

full flexion 8
regional blocks 14—15
see also individual bones and joints
hip joint *see* coxofemoral joint
history taking 2
hock
    capped 166—7
    regional local anaesthesia,
        diagnostic 21
    swellings in the plantar region
        161—8
    swollen 139
    see also hock joint
hock joint
    anatomy 138, *139*
    block 14—15, 19
    flexion 7
    physical examination 138—9
    radiographic examination 139—40
    see also tarsal osteoarthritis;
        tibiotarsal joint
'hock lameness' 138
hoof
    cracks 31—2
    infection 33
    overgrowth 29—30
    overwear 30
    paring 29
    penetrating injury 33—7
    structure 28—9
    trimming
        in DIP joint flexural deformity
            216
        in laminitis 47—8
        in navicular syndrome 61—2
hoof oil 30—1
hoof testers 9
hormones, role in growth 195—6
horn
    growth rate 29
    quality 30
    ridges in laminitis 45, 46
    structure 28—9
    see also hoof
hot splint 96
humeroradial joint *see* elbow joint
humerus, fracture of 126—7
hyaluronic acid
    level in DJD 275
    therapy 81, 108, 282—3
hygromas 115—16
Hypochaeris radicata, implicated in
        Australian stringhalt 191

immobilization of fractures during
        transportation 187, 259, 265
indomethacin 281
infectious arthritis of the tibiotarsal
        joint 156—9
infracarpal check ligament 104
    section of 216—17, 220—1

infrapatellar joint, capsule distension
        169
injection technique 10
intercarpal joint 18, 104
    see also carpus
interference boots 97
'interfering' 95—7
intra-articular anaesthesia, diagnostic
        9, 15—22
intrabursal anaesthesia, diagnostic
        15—22
isoxsuprine hydrochloride
    in laminitis 47
    in navicular syndrome 61

'Jack-spavin' 143
joint
    aspiration of fluid from cavity 157
    lavage 158—9, 284, 289—90
    laxity in newborn foals 199—200
        diagnosis 200—1
        treatment 201—3
joint-ill *see* osteomyelitis in foals
joint mouse 197

keratoma 40—1
knee *see* carpus
kneecap *see* patella
'knock knees' 106
kyphosis, congenital 212

lamellar horn 28
lameness
    definition 1
    detection 3—4, 5—8
    score systems 5
laminitis
    aetiology and pathogenesis 44—5
    clinical signs 45
    diagnosis 45
    epidemiology 46
    prevention 48
    treatment 46—8
lateral cartilages 42
LBD 23
lidocaine hydrochloride 10—11, 15
light beam diaphragm 23
lignocaine hydrochloride 10—11, 15
local anaesthetic agents 10—11
lordosis, congenital 212
low ring-bone 66
lunging as an aid to the detection of
        lameness 5—6

magnetic field therapy 102
MCP joint *see* metacarpophalangeal
        (MCP) joint
meclafenamic acid 59

medial patellar ligament section 172–4
median block 13–14
mephanesin 191
mepivacaine 11, 15
metacarpi *see* cannon bones; splint bones
metacarpophalangeal (MCP) joint
  anatomy 73
  block 17, 18
  chip fractures 82–3
  congenital hyperextension 214
  degenerative disease 78–81
  disease in young animals 76
  flexion 7, 143
    congenital 213
  flexural deformity 218–22
  local anaesthesia 74
  osteochondritis dissecans 76–7
  pathology 74
  physical examination 74
  radiography 74–5
  susceptibility to injury 73
  villonodular synovitis 77–8
metaphyseal dysplasia 204–10
matatarsal bones *see* cannon bones
methionine
  role in horn formation 30
  therapy in laminitis 47
metranidazole 33
Monteggia fracture 121
myopathy, fibrous and ossifying 191–2

navel-ill *see* osteomyelitis in foals
navicular bone
  anatomy 53
  arterial distribution 43, 53
  chip fractures 58–9
  focal osteopenia 57, 58
  medullary sclerosis 58
  osteophytes 58
  radiography 56, 243–4
  sagittal fractures 241–4
    fixation 244–5
  synovial fossae 57
  see also navicular syndrome
navicular bursal block 16
navicular suspensory ligaments, section of 62
navicular syndrome 54, 62–3
  aetiology and pathogenesis 54
  association with polyarthritis syndrome 63
  clinical signs 55
  diagnosis 55–6
    radiographic 56–9
  treatment 59–62
nerve blocks, diagnostic 9–22
nerve distribution in distal forelimb 12

nerves, peripheral, role in growth regulation 196
neurectomy
  dorsal digital 52, 68
  in navicular syndrome 60
non-steroidal anti-inflammatory drugs (NSAIDs) 59, 63, 81, 280–2
nutrient foraminae in navicular bone 57
nutrition, role in growth 196

OCD *see* osteochondritis dissecans
oestrogens, role in growth 196
olecranon
  bursitis 120–1
  fractures 122–5
omarthritis of the shoulder joint 135–6
osteoarthritis *see* degenerative joint disease, tarsal osteoarthritis
osteochondritis dissecans (OCD) 197–8
  fetlock 76–7
  growth plates 205–6
  shoulder joint 131
  tibiotarsal joint 151–6
  trochlear ridge 174–8
osteochondrosis 194, 196–8
  growth plates 205–6
  shoulder joint 131–3
  trochlear ridge 174–8
osteomyelitis in foals
  aetiology and pathogenesis 285–7
  chronic infection 289–91
  diagnosis 287–8
  treatment 288–9
osteopenia 35
  disuse 85, 86
  focal, in navicular bone 57, 58
osteophytes 65, 71, 72, 79, 107, 277
  in spavin 142, 145, 146
  navicular bone 58
  see also enthesiophytes
overnutrition, effects on growth 196

pain relief in navicular syndrome 59–60
palmar block 12, 13
palmar digital nerve block 11–12
palpation 8
pastern joint *see* proximal interphalangeal joint
patella 168
  fractures 182–4
  luxation 170
  upward fixation 170–4
PBZ *see* phenylbutazone
PDNB 11–12
pedal bone 28, 42

arterial distribution *43*
conditions in 44−52
fractures 237−8
   extensor process 51−2
   fixation 238−41
   marginal 49, *50*
   osteitis 35, 49, *50*
   quittor 37−8
   radiography 42−4, 238
'pedal osteitis' 49, *50*
pelvic movements in hindlimb
      lameness 4
pelvis, fractures of 189−90
penetration, solar 33−7
periarticular ring-bone 66
perioplic horn 28
periosteal exostoses 49, 67
periosteal growth
   asynchronous 206
   new 95−7
periosteal transection 209
peroneal block 14−15, 145
peroneus tertius rupture 232
phalangeal exostosis 66−9
phalangeal fractures 246−53
phenoxybenzamine therapy in
      laminitis 47
phenylbutazone (PBZ)
   in DJD therapy 81, 281−2
   in navicular syndrome 59
   prohibition 63, 282
   reaction with warfarin 61
physical examination 8−9
physis *see* growth plate
pin-firing 147, 230
pincers 9
PIP joint *see* proximal interphalangeal
      (PIP) joint
PIT joint *see* tarsal osteoarthritis
plantar digital nerve block 14
plaster bandage 269
podotrochleosis chronica aseptica *see*
      navicular syndrome
polyarthritis syndrome 63, 64, 81
polysulphated glycosaminoglycan 81,
      108, 283−4
post injection flare 280
post-operative complications in
      neonates 127, 188
'pottery' gait 5, 55
prolactin, role in growth 196
'proppy' gait 5, 55
prostaglandins, role in DJD 280−1
proteoglycans, role in DJD 274−5
proximal interphalangeal (PIP) joint
   block 16, *17*, 18
   congenital hyperextension 214
   degenerative disease 71−2
   phalangeal exostoses 66
   subluxation 218
   surgical arthrodesis 68−9

proximal intertarsal (PIT) joint
   block 19, 144
   see also tarsal osteoarthritis
proximal sesamoids 84
   dehiscence 89
   fractures
      in adults 87−9
      axial 89
      T 89
      in young foals 90
   'ghost' 85, *86*
   inflammation 84−7
   vascular channels in 85−6
purges 46
'pyramidal disease' 50−1

quadriceps, wasting 169
quittor 37−8

radiocarpal joint 18, 104
   see also carpus
radiography
   equipment 23−5
   processing 25−6
   techniques 26
   through a cast 260
   viewing 26
   see also specific joints and bones
radius, fractures of
   fissure 119−20
   shaft 262−4
rest as treatment in DJD 81, 279
restraint 10
rheumatoid arthritis 273
ring block 14
ring-bone 66−9
Robert Jones bandage *263*, 267−8

sagittal ridge, demineralization 79,
      80
Salter−Harris classification of growth
      plate injuries 205
sand cracks 31−2
sausage boot 121
Saxe, John Godfrey, quoted 54
SBC *see* sub-chondral bone cysts
      (SBC)
scapula, fractures of 133−5
scapulohumeral joint *see* shoulder
      joint
'scar tissue bandage' 230
score systems for lameness 5
screens, radiographic 25
'Seat of spavin' 147
2nd metacarpal *see* splint bones
2nd phalanx, fractures of 246−7
sedation 173
'seedy toe' 45

septic arthritis
  elbow joint 125−6
  in foals
    aetiology and pathogenesis
      285−7
    chronic infection 289−91
    diagnosis 287−8
    treatment 288−9
  tibiotarsal joint 156−9
septic epiphysitis *see* septic arthritis
septic polyarthritis *see* septic arthritis
sesamoiditis 84−7
seton 37
SFT *see* superficial digital flexor
      tendon (SFT)
shivering (shivers) 192−3
'shoe boil' 120−1
shoeing, corrective
  congenital hyperextension 214
  DFT laceration 235−6
  DIP joint flexural deformity 216
  distal metatarsal epiphyseal
    dysplasia 211
  MCP joint flexural deformity 220,
    221
  navicular syndrome 61−2
  suspensory ligament laceration 236
shoes
  badly fitting 39−40
  plaster 47
shoulder blade *see* scapula
shoulder joint
  bicipital bursitis 130−1
  block 19
  omarthritis 135−6
  osteochondrosis 131−3
'shoulder lameness' 1, 128
shoulder region
  clinical examination 128−9
  radiology 129
'shoulder slip' *128*, 136−7
sickle hock 141, 167, 210
single branch desmitis 92−3, 93−4
slings 268
sodium hyaluronate *see* hyaluronic
    acid
sole 28
  flat 49
  penetrating injury 33−7
somatomedin, role in growth 195
somatostatin, role in growth 195
somatotropin, role in growth 195
sound conduction test in fractures
    126, 186−7
spavin *see* tarsal osteoarthritis
splint bones 95
  fractures 97−100
  periosteal new bone growth 95−7
'splints' 95−7
splints, use of in fracture fixation
    266−7

'spurs' on navicular bone 58
stifle joint 168
  block 21−2
  degenerative disease 185−6
  gonitis 184−6
  physical examination 168−9
  radiography 169−70
  sub-chondral bone cysts 178−81
  trauma 184−6
  tumoral calcinosis 181−2
  see also patella
'straw cramp' 171
stringhalt 190−1
  gait alterations in 5
sub-carpal block 13, *14*
sub-chondral bone cysts (SBC) 70−1,
    277
  medial condylar 178−81
superficial digital flexor tendon (SFT)
    166
  'contracture' 218
  lacerations 232−4
  section 219
  strain/sprain 224−31
supracarpal check ligament
    desmotomy 219−20
suprascapular nerve paralysis *128*,
    136−7
suspensory ligament 92
  desmitis 92−4
  desmotomy 221−2
  lacerations 236
  sesamoiditis 84−7
sustentaculum, marginal fracture 165
Sweeney *128*, 136−7
synovial fistulae 117−18
synovial fluid
  analysis 277−9
  transfer 283
synovial fossae in navicular bone 57
synovial membrane
  biopsy 75
  inflammatory changes in DJD
    276−7

talus, fractures of 161
tarsal bones, incomplete ossification
    210−11
tarsal osteoarthritis
  aetiology and pathogenesis 140−2
  clinical signs 142−3
  diagnosis 143−5
  radiographic examination 145−7
  treatment 147−9
tarsocrural joint *see* tibiotarsal joint
tarsometatarsal (TMT) joint
  block 20−1, 144
  see also tarsal osteoarthritis
Technovit 32
'tendinous thoroughpin' 150, 162

tendinous wind-gall 74
tendon
  carbon-fibre implantation 230−1
  contractions *see* flexural
      deformities
  laceration 232−6
  splitting 230
  strain/sprain 224
    aetiology and pathogenesis
        224−5
    clinical signs 226
    diagnosis 226−8
    first aid 228
    treatment 228−31
  sutures 233
tenocytes 224−5
testosterone, role in growth 196
'thermocautery, therapeutic' 147,
      229−30
thermoplastic open-weave bandage
      269
3rd metacarpal *see* cannon bones
3rd phalanx *see* pedal bone
Thomas splint 126−7, 263, 267
thrush 33
thyroxine, role in growth 196
tibia
  block 14−15, 145
  fractures 161
    shaft 264−6
tibiotarsal joint 138
  block 19
  distension of the capsule 150−1
  infectious arthritis 156−9
  intra-articular fractures 159−61
  osteochondritis dissecans 151−6
  septic arthritis 156−9
  see also hock joint
TMT joint *see* tarsometatarsal (TMT)
      joint

toe dragging 4
  in spavin 143
torticollis, congenital 212
traction
  in cast application *271*
  in fracture fixation 264
'trailing' 4
  in spavin 143
transphyseal stapling 207−8
trochlear ridge, osteochondrosis in
      174−8
tropocollagen 224
trotting as an aid to detection of
      lameness 3−4
tumoral calcinosis 181−2

ulna
  block 13−14
  fractures 122−5

vascular channels
  in navicular bone 57
  in sesamoids 85−6
villonodular synovitis 77−8

wall horn 28
  removal 31
Wamberg's operation 147−8
warfarin therapy
  in navicular syndrome 60−1
  prohibition 63
'white line' 28
wobbler syndrome 197

zinc, role in osteochondrosis 197, 206
zones of penetration 34